Theory
and Research in
Behavioral Pediatrics
Volume 4

Theory and Research in Behavioral Pediatrics
Volume 4

Edited by

Hiram E. Fitzgerald, Ph.D.

Professor of Psychology
Michigan State University
East Lansing, Michigan

Barry M. Lester, Ph.D.

Associate Professor of Child Psychiatry/
Human Behavior and Pediatrics
Bradley Hospital
and Women and Infant's Hospital
Brown University
Providence, Rhode Island

and

Michael W. Yogman, M.D.

Director, Infant Health and Development Program
The Children's Hospital Medical Center
Assistant Professor of Pediatrics
Harvard Medical School
Boston, Massachusetts

PLENUM PRESS • NEW YORK AND LONDON

The Library of Congress has cataloged this title as follows:

Theory and research in behavioral pediatrics — Vol. 1- — New York, N.Y.: Plenum
Press, c1982-
　　v.; 24 cm.
　Biennial.
　Editors: Hiram E. Fitzgerald, Barry M. Lester, and Michael W. Yogman.
　ISSN 0735-6897 = Theory and research in behavioral pediatrics.

　　1. Pediatrics — Psychological aspects — Periodicals. 2. Child Development — period-
icals. I. Fitzgerald, Hiram E. II. Lester, Barry M. III. Yogman, Michael W.
[DNLM: 1. Child Behavior — periodicals. 2. Child Development — periodicals. 3.
Pediatrics — periodicals.　W1 TH123Y (P)]
RJ131.T54　　　　　　　　　618.92′02′9 — dc19　　　　　　　　　　82-646646
　　　　　　　　　　　　　　　　　　　　　　　　　　　　　AACR 2　MARC-S
Library of Congress　　　　　　　　　[8607]

ISBN 0-306-42882-2

© 1988 Plenum Press, New York
A Division of Plenum Publishing Corporation
233 Spring Street, New York, N.Y. 10013

Printed in the United States of America

Contributors

Thomas F. Anders, M.D. • Department of Psychiatry and Human Behavior, Division of Child Psychiatry, Bradley Hospital, Brown University Program in Medicine, Providence, Rhode Island

Marc H. Bornstein, Ph.D. • Child and Family Research, National Institute of Child Health and Human Development, Bethesda, Maryland, and Department of Psychology, New York University, New York, New York

Mary A. Carskadon, Ph.D. • Department of Psychiatry and Human Behavior, Division of Child Psychiatry, Bradley Hospital, Brown University Program in Medicine, Providence, Rhode Island

Susan Crockenberg, Ph.D. • Department of Applied Behavioral Sciences, University of California, Davis, California

Cynthia T. Garcia-Coll, Ph.D. • Section of Pediatrics, Brown University and Women and Infant's Hospital, Providence, Rhode Island

William Hole, M.D. • Department of Psychiatry and Human Behavior, Division of Child Psychiatry, Bradley Hospital, Brown University Program in Medicine, Providence, Rhode Island

Wade F. Horn, Ph.D. • Department of Psychiatry, Children's Hospital National Medical Center, Washington, D.C., and George Washington University Medical School, Washington, D.C.

Nicholas Ialongo, Ph.D. • Department of Psychology, University of Virginia, Charlottesville, Virginia

E. Shea, Ph.D. • Department of Psychology, University of Massachusetts, Amherst, Massachusetts

Edward Z. Tronick, Ph.D. • Department of Psychology, University of Massachusetts, Amherst, Massachusetts

Betty R. Vohr, M.D. • Brown University Program in Medicine, Women and Infant's Hospital of Rhode Island, Providence, Rhode Island

Preface

Formation of the Society for Behavioral Pediatrics in 1982 together with adoption of the *Journal of Developmental and Behavioral Pediatrics* as its official journal and the publication of volumes such as Russo and Varni's (1982) *Behavioral Pediatrics: Research and Practice*, Krasnegor, Arasteh, and Cataldo's (1986) *Child Health Behavior: A Behavioral Pediatrics Perspective*, Levine, Carey, Crocker, and Gross's (1983) *Developmental—Behavioral Pediatrics*, and Magrab's (1978a,b) *Psychological Management of Pediatric Problems* (Volumes I and II) provide clear evidence that the field that Richmond (1967) helped to define over 20 years ago has come of age. In a previous volume we suggested that one objective for behavioral pediatrics is to encourage integration of biological and behavioral science in order to promote a clinical, relevant perspective on child health (Fitzgerald, Lester, & Yogman, 1982). Each chapter in the current volume is consistent with this objective and captures the other distinguishing features of behavioral pediatrics: multicausality of etiology; interdisciplinary approaches to child health and development; prevention, health promotion, and well-care; behavioral modification; biobehavioral aspects of pediatrics; and developmental perspectives.

In Chapter 1, Betty R. Vohr and Cynthia T. Garcia-Coll review the extant literature on developmental outcome of low-birth-weight infants. Although biomedical technology can be credited with significant reductions in mortality and morbidity of 1500- to 2500-g infants and has reduced mortality in 500- to 1500-g infants, morbidity among ≤1500-g infants remains high. Respiratory, metabolic, and central nervous system disorders often require prolonged hospitalization and stress the caregiver—infant relationship. Thus, not only is the extremely low-birth-weight infant at risk but the parent—infant relationship also is at risk. According to Vohr and Garcia-Coll, individual differences among low-birth-weight infants combine with developmental changes in their presenting state characteristics to weaken our ability to predict long-term developmental outcome. However, one fact seems clear. A major variable contributing to the low-birth-weight infant's developmental outcome is the quality of the caregiving environment.

What defines the quality of the caregiving environment? In Chapter 2 Marc H. Bornstein provides a scheme for investigating three aspects of caregiver–infant interaction, aspects he terms nurturant, social, and didactic. Although Bornstein focuses on mother–infant interactions, he carefully points out that the three aspects of caregiver–infant interaction apply equally well to father–infant relationships. Bornstein reviews the results of his systematic research program, focusing on the development of cognitive competence framed in the context of nurturant, social, and didactic interactions. His research suggests that caregiver consistency is an important aspect of developmental outcome.

Surprisingly, there is relatively little systematic developmental research investigating aspects of maternal personality as possible mediators of quality caregiving. Self-esteem, for example, may have an indirect effect on the mother–infant relationship via its influence on maternal adaptation to motherhood. In Chapter 3 E. Shea and Edward Z. Tronick survey the literature on general and specific components of maternal self-esteem and conclude (1) that infant health and family support are two key variables affecting the woman's adaptation to motherhood and (2) that lack of objective measures interferes with our ability to understand how maternal self-esteem changes developmentally. Shea and Tronick attempt to fill this void with the Maternal Self-Esteem Inventory. They describe steps taken to establish face, concurrent, internal, and external validity of the instrument. Their research suggests that a variety of variables influence maternal adaptation for motherhood indirectly through maternal self-esteem. Moreover, in some instances, direct strengthening of maternal self-esteem may be a more effective way to influence the quality of mother–infant interactions than efforts to enhance interactions themselves.

In Chapter 4, Susan Crockenberg reviews a broader literature assessing the extent to which social support benefits infants, parents, and families at risk. One important aspect of Crockenberg's research is that it indicates that social support bolsters parenting both for high-risk families and for ("low-risk") families that only have to deal with the routine problems of everyday life. Thus, social support effectively strengthens child development in families with handicapped infants and in single-parent, low-income, and abusing families. It also can strengthen the coping abilities of parents who have just had their first child. What types of social support are valued? Those that provide emotional support to caregivers and those that provide assistance with child care. According to Crockenberg, family members, professionals, friends, and parent groups are all good sources for social support.

In Chapter 1, Vohr and Garcia-Coll noted that learning disabilities are a characteristic of low-birth-weight infants. One factor that contributes to learning disability is the child's inability to pay attention in the classroom. In some instances, inattention can be a sign of a disorder that accounts for nearly half of all child referrals to outpatient mental health clinics, namely, attention deficit disorder. Currently over one-half million children are treated with psychostimulant drugs in an effort to control their hyperactivity, inappropriate inattention, impulsiveness, or aggressiveness. In Chapter 5 Wade F. Horn and Nicholas Ialongo report the results of a research program designed to determine whether psychostimulant therapy is more effective in suppressing the symptoms of attention deficit disorder when used alone or when used in combination with other therapeutic approaches. One important outcome of their research suggests that therapeutic treatments are most effective when they are matched to the symptom characteristcis presented by individual children.

In Chapter 6, Mary A. Carskadon, Thomas F. Anders, and William Hole summarize scientific and clinical studies of sleep disturbances, one of the more common problems of infancy, childhood, and adolescence. During the early years of development common sleep disturbances include night waking, difficulty falling asleep, and night terrors. During childhood, sleep disturbances often involve sleepwalking and bedwetting, whereas during adolescence insomnia, narcolepsy, and insufficient sleep are the more common disturbances. At any period of development, but especially during infancy, sleep disturbances can be especially disruptive to the caregiver–infant relationship. Fatigued and frustrated parents are not well prepared to deal effectively with their infant's erratic sleep cycles and incessant crying. Often in such situations, relatively simple behavioral management strategies can be introduced to regulate the caregiving environment, or support systems can be identified in an effort to reduce caregiver stress and increase caregiving quality.

We believe that at least three general themes bind the contributions to Volume 4 of *Theory and Research in Behavioral Pediatrics*. First, evidence that progressively stronger environmental influences on the organization of behavior occur developmentally with the net effect being that our ability to predict developmental outcome must be based on dynamic, change-based models rather than linear causal models. Second, the aspects of the environment collectively referred to as social support systems can be extremely influential in minimizing the effects of caregiver stress and promoting more optimal caregiver–child relationships. Third, knowledge about prevention of or intervention in various developmental disorders can be enhanced considerably by systematic study of the comparative effectiveness of biologically and behaviorally based treatment approaches, when used alone or in combination. Results of such research will assist practitioners in their efforts to match treatment strategies with symptom characteristics.

HIRAM E. FITZGERALD
BARRY M. LESTER
MICHAEL W. YOGMAN

REFERENCES

Fitzgerald, H. E., Lester, B. M., & Yogman, M. H. (Eds.). (1982). *Theory and research in behavioral pediatrics.* (Vol. 1). New York: Plenum Press.

Krasnegor, N. A., Arasteh, J. D., & Cataldo, M. F. (Eds.). (1986). *Child health behavior: A behavioral pediatrics perspective.* New York: Wiley.

Levine, M. D., Carey, W. B., Crocker, A. C., & Gross, R. E. T. (1983). *Developmental–behavioral pediatrics.* Philadelphia: W. B. Saunders.

Magrab, P. R. (Ed.). (1978a). *Psychological management of pediatric problems.* (Vol. 1). *Early life conditions and chronic diseases.* Baltimore: University Park Press.

Magrab, P. R. (Ed.). (1978b). *Psychological management of pediatric problems.* (Vol. 2). *Sensorineural conditions and social concerns.* Baltimore: University Park Press.

Richmond, J. B. (1967). Child development: A basic science for pediatrics. *Pediatrics, 50,* 649.

Russo, D. C., & Varni, J. W. (1982). *Behavioral pediatrics.* New York: Plenum Press.

Contents

CHAPTER 2.   MOTHERS, INFANTS, AND THE DEVELOPMENT
             OF COGNITIVE COMPETENCE   67
             Marc H. Bornstein

CHAPTER 3.   THE MATERNAL SELF-REPORT INVENTORY: A
             RESEARCH AND CLINICAL INSTRUMENT FOR
             ASSESSING MATERNAL SELF-ESTEEM   101
             E. Shea and Edward Z. Tronick

CHAPTER 4. SOCIAL SUPPORT AND PARENTING   141
Susan Crockenberg

Follow-up Studies of High-Risk Low-Birth-Weight Infants
Changing Trends

BETTY R. VOHR AND CYNTHIA T. GARCIA-COLL

1. THE LOW-BIRTH-WEIGHT INFANT

1.1. A Historical Perspective

The tiny, premature infant, with that initial unique and somewhat pathetic appearance, an uncanny ability to survive, and a steadfast potential for normal growth and a "normal life," has long been a source of interest not only to physicians but also to the lay public. This was demonstrated in the first half of the twentieth century with public exhibits of premature infants, first in the Hess Incubator at Coney Island Amusement Park in New York and subsequently in the Century of Progress Display at the 1933 World's Fair in Chicago (Smith & Vidyasagar, 1983).

Although Dr. Julius Hess (1876–1955) made great inroads in the care of premature infants and developed the Hess Incubator, it was not until the 1960s, as a direct result of the progressive sophistication of neonatal intensive care units (Rawlings, Stewart, & Reynolds, 1971; Williams & Chen, 1982; Paneth et al., 1982; Kitchen, Lissenden, Yu, &

Betty R. Vohr and Cynthia T. Garcia-Coll • Brown University Program in Medicine, Women and Infants Hospital of Rhode Island, Providence, Rhode Island 02908.

Bajuk, 1982; Hack, Caron, Rivers, & Fanaroff, 1983) and the development of regionalization programs (Walker, Vohr, & Oh, 1985; McCormick, Shapiro, & Starfield, 1985) that survival of very-low-birth-weight infants (≤1500 g) began to improve significantly. Survival of ≤1500-g infants now approaches 90% in most neonatal centers. With regionalization of defined geographic areas high-risk mothers and/or their infants are being brought to perinatal tertiary care centers where the level of care is geared to addressing their "at-risk" situation.

The first neonatal intensive care unit was developed at Vanderbilt University by Dr. Mildred Stahlman in 1964 (Smith et al. 1983). Since that time, many modern perinatal centers have emerged in which maternal–fetal medicine, neonatology, and follow-up programs have successfully collaborated to provide optimal acute and longitudinal care for the at-risk mother and her infant. The high-risk pregnancy (the high-risk mother and/or her high-risk infant) now had the advantage of sophisticated technology for identification, surveillance, and treatment. For example, the obstetrician or perinatologist can with the use of fetal ultrasound assist the neonatologist by providing early diagnoses of fetal age, multiple gestation, congenital anomalies, fetal head growth, and rate of fetal growth, thereby facilitating immediate appropriate neonatal care.

1.2. Improving Survival

There has been a steady improvement in the survival of very-low-birth-weight infants (≤1500 g). In the state of Rhode Island, for example, survival improved significantly after the establishment of a regionalized tertiary care center at the Women and Infants Hospital in 1974. Data for infants born in the state of Rhode Island with a birth weight less than 1500 g between two time periods, 1974–1975 (first two years of the Neonatal Intensive Care Unit Regionalized Program) and 1979–1980 (well-established regionalized program), are shown in Figure 1. Perhaps the most dramatic ongoing improvement in neonatal survival has been seen in the weight category of 500 to 1000 g (Hack et al., 1983; Buchwald, Zorn, & Egan, 1982; Bennett, Robinson, & Sells, 1983; Walker, Feldman, Vohr, & Oh, 1984). Data from Rhode Island demonstrating this trend between 1981 and 1986 are shown in Table 1. In 1986, survival of infants ≤1000 g was 58%.

1.3. Early Follow-up Studies

As neonatal centers have documented increasing numbers of these tiny survivors, the issue of the quality of survival has continued to be

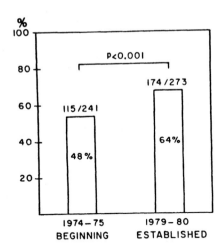

FIGURE 1. Survival rates for infants with a birth weight less than 1500 g born in Rhode Island for 1974–1975 (beginning of regionalization period) and 1979–1980 (well-established regionalization period).

debated. Iatrogenic disorders have occurred as part of the evolution of treatment procedures and have, therefore, strengthened the importance and value of the follow-up component of neonatal care. It was actually in 1953 (pre-intensive-care era) that Dr. Julius Hess, whose primary interest was the care of the premature infant, published the first follow-up study of premature infants born at the Sarah Morris Hospital in Chicago between 1922 and 1950 (Hess, 1953). The purpose of his 30-year longitudinal study of infants with birth weights ranging from 605 to 1250 g was, according to Dr. Hess, "the question of whether these very small, premature infants are worth saving."

The manuscript includes a number of photographs of prematures in the first weeks of life and at subsequent ages, a blueprint of the nursery, a description of the nursery organization, and details of a component of its financial backing. The organization of the neonatal and follow-up data is meticulously reported. The mortality data are present-

TABLE 1. Inborn Survival Statistics—The 1980s
(Women and Infants Hospital of Rhode Island)

Birth weight	1981	1982	1983	1984	1985	1986
500– 999 g	20/63	16/52	33/69	43/79	34/62	39/67
	32%	31%	48%	54%	55%	58%
1000–1499 g	48/54	69/77	52/59	76/86	72/87	84/91
	89%	89%	88%	88%	83%	92%

ed in 250-g increments between 1000 and 2500 g, and the timing of death is specifically subdivided into time segments of ≤ 24 hours, 24 to 28 hours, 48 to 72 hours, and ≥ 72 hours, leading to the conclusion that the most critical period determining premature survival is the first 24 hours.

The study sample is substantial for the 30-year period and includes 445 premature NICU graduates, 45 of which were postdischarge deaths, with only 30 survivors not available for follow-up study. A total of 335 survivors were evaluated for medical, sensory, neurological, cognitive, and physical parameters. The overall outcome was good with 85% of the survivors having average or better cognitive physical development and 90% having average or better development. Risk factors such as intramuscular blood transfusions, low social and environmental status, and treatment, specifically breast milk, are discussed anecdotally. Although the long-term 30-year neurodevelopmental outcome of ≤ 1250-g premature infants reported by Hess was relatively favorable, infant survival remained poor at that time.

With changes in care patterns and the introduction of unproven therapeutic techniques, subsequent long-term follow-up studies of the 1960s published both abroad and in the United States were less promising (Drillien, 1964; Lubchenco et al., 1963). Drillien followed a cohort of 50 survivors weighing ≤ 1360 g born between 1948 and 1956 to 5 years of age. Fifty-three percent of these children had one or more physical defects; 50% were considered uneducable; and 78% were reported to have behavior problems. Drillien categorized the mothers of her population into three cohorts according to social class: (1) middle to superior, (2) average, and (3) poor. She clearly demonstrated that the highest incidence of handicap occurred in the poorest homes. This was one of the first studies relating social–environmental status factors to long-term outcome.

By 1940, there were 28 premature centers located in the United States, Hawaii, and the District of Columbia (Dunham & Bierman, 1940). In the succeeding years, a constantly increasing number of follow-up studies of varying duration and content have been published not only in the United States but around the world (Lubchenco, Horner, et al., 1963; Drillien, 1959; Kitchen, Yu, et al., 1982). Many initial followup studies were more often descriptive, retrospective, lacking control groups, with observations recorded over a brief period of time or at a single point in time. The importance of longitudinal, prospective, randomized, double-blind controlled studies with adequate patient populations emerged over time as the significance of unraveling the mysteries of therapeutic cause and effect (such as retinopathy of prematurity) led to renewed efforts to utilize the scientific method. Experimental epidemiologic studies with prospectively designed protocols began to appear in increasing numbers as the types of treatment modalities became more sophisticated, survival rates improved, and evidence of neurodevelopmental sequelae emerged.

Studies of a descriptive, observational nature, however, continue to be published in the 1980s as new populations of survivors emerge. These studies are of two types: either (1) passive monitoring of events or (2) active surveillance that includes a specific cohort and case control studies. During the 1960s and 1970s, pediatricians frequently reported descriptive, observational outcome data on low-birth-weight infants ≤1500 g. During the late 1970s and the 1980s, follow-up studies began to appear that focused on a variety of contemporary medical–social morbidities such as bronchopulmonary dysplasia, periventricular–intraventricular hemorrhage, special needs (home apnea monitors, home oxygen), maternal substance abuse, and teenage pregnancy.

1.4. Difficulties Encountered in Carrying Out Low-Birth-Weight Infant Follow-up Studies

Neonatal follow-up programs serve as a base for the assessment of high-risk, low-birth-weight infants and allow for the collection of morbidity statistics. A number of factors, including demographic variables, funding availability, staff training, and available assessment procedures, influence the direction of high-risk infant research among neonatal intensive care unit follow-up programs. Demographic variability relative to urban versus rural populations, transport versus inborn status, high socioeconomic versus low socioeconomic status, ethnic variability, percentage of teenage pregnancy, and substance abuse in the population will obviously influence the outcome data.

These variables in turn affect patient compliance for follow-up. A high attrition rate in a follow-up study will reduce the validity of the data. One factor that contributes to attrition is postneonatal mortality within a high-risk population, particularly relative to the improving neonatal survival of infants with severe chronic lung disease. A study was conducted at Women and Infants Hospital in Providence to assess the significant variables that resulted in parental noncompliance in returning to the Follow-up Clinic during the first year of life with a high-risk, low-birth-weight infant (birth weight 501 to 1500 g) born between 1/1/75 and 4/1/77. Adolescent pregnancy (maternal age ≤18 years), single marital status, and low socioeconomic status were identified as significant factors negatively affecting compliance (Vohr, Daniel, & Oh,

1981). The population stability of a specific geographic area also plays a role. The presence of universities, naval or army bases, and training centers results in a more transient population limiting the feasibility of long-term tracking studies.

Funding for follow-up programs remains a challenging problem for most tertiary care centers. The follow-up program service component, specifically, the identification of medical (cardiac, pulmonary, growth), neurological, developmental, and psychosocial disabilities that require further intervention or referral to appropriate community resources is expensive. A multidisciplinary staff is needed to carry out a comprehensive program and includes pediatrics, neonatology, psychology, neurology, speech and language disciplines, psychiatry, nursing, nutrition, social service, a coordinating secretary, and a statistician. Programs receive varying degrees of support from the core hospital, their state health departments, foundations, and to a limited extent, from third party payments. Competition for grant funding, particularly in the behavioral sciences, is an important consideration in attempting a longitudinal study of high-risk, low-birth-weight infants.

2. EVOLUTION OF ASSESSMENT TECHNIQUES

2.1. Introduction

Neurodevelopmental studies have become more sophisticated because of the greater detail and specificity of diagnostic techniques used in defining a child's neurological and developmental status. Early definitive assessments of neurological damage were made by autopsy evaluation (Towbin, 1970) and neonatal diagnoses in the nursery were made by clinical physical evaluation. The first manuscript to describe the motor and movement deficits that characterize cerebral palsy was published by Little in 1862. He related these abnormal findings to adverse perinatal events.

2.2. Assessment of Perinatal Risk Factors

A number of subsequent studies confirmed the association between adverse perinatal events, including low birth weight, perinatal asphyxia, intrauterine growth retardation and abnormal neonatal neurological signs, and later major motor deficits (Nelson & Ellenberg, 1979, 1981; Nelson & Broman, 1977). The positive relationship between multiple risk factors associated with pregnancy and subsequent neurologic deficit and mental retardation was first investigated in a comprehensive prospective study as part of a collaborative project (Berendes, 1966). It was Prechtl's work in 1967 that first suggested that nonoptimal conditions of pregnancy occurred in association with one another more commonly and that a cumulative tabulated risk score could be used as a prognostic tool. This concept of cumulative risk led to a large prospective study of 732 pregnancies in which 51 prenatal, 40 intrapartum, and 35 neonatal risk factors were analyzed to predict perinatal morbidity and mortality (Hobel, Hyvarinen, Okada, & Oh, 1973). This work led to a better understanding of the continuum of risk, to the interrelationships of risk factors, and to the use of prenatal, intrapartum, and neonatal risk scores as assessments that could serve as predictors of adverse neurodevelopmental outcome or indicators of similarities or dissimilarities between populations.

2.3. Central Nervous System Diagnostic Techniques

More recently, the development of real-time ultrasonography and computerized axial tomography as diagnostic techniques in the neonatal intensive care unit resulted in an accepted noninvasive method for evaluating fetal and premature infants' brains for intracranial hemorrhage, hydrocephalus, periventricular leukomalacia, and other complications (Grant et al., 1981; Sauerbrei, Digney, Harrison, & Cooperberg, 1981). Additional sophisticated brain imaging techniques include technetium scanning, positron emission tomography, and nucleic magnetic resonance scanning (Volpe, Perlman, Herscovitch, & Raichle, 1982; Delphy et al., 1982). With the advent of these techniques, more specific diagnostic labels could be given and the number of investigative studies, particularly of intraventricular hemorrhage in the low-birth-weight infant, have multiplied.

Another area of central nervous system assessment that has expanded the ability to assess infants' neurosensory function is the utilization of evoked potentials. The brain stem auditory evoked response (BAER) is a noninvasive method for evaluating the functional state of the peripheral auditory nerve and the brain stem auditory sensory pathway. Because of the increased risk of sensorineural hearing loss in specific populations of the neonatal intensive care unit, BAER has been used in a number of studies testing its ability to screen infants of various gestational ages for injury to the auditory pathways (Cox, Hack, & Metz, 1984; Shannon, Felix, Krumholz, Goldstein, & Harris, 1984). Hyperbilirubinemia has more recently been shown to produce changes in the BAER that are reversible (Perlman et al., 1983; Nakamura et al., 1985).

Transient abnormalities of the BAER may be indicative of a brain stem insult. Recent studies have shown a relationship between prolonged brain stem conduction time and apnea of prematurity (Henderson-Smart, Pettigrew, & Campbell, 1983).

Vision evoked response (VER) testing is likewise a noninvasive tool for the objective evaluation of the visual pathways from the photoreceptors to the occipital cortex. Recent studies have analyzed the relationships between neonatal vision responses, cerebral insult, and neurodevelopment (Barnet et al., 1980; Vohr & Garcia-Coll, 1987). Visual evoked responses in premature infants with hydrocephalus have demonstrated prolonged latencies, which reverse after shunt placement (Ehle & Sklar, 1979).

2.4. Gestational Age Assessment

Gestational age as determined by available clinical information, particularly the date of the mother's last menstrual period, may be unknown or inaccurate. Since medical, obstetric, and neonatal management, clinical course, neurological findings, and outcome are all determined by degree of fetal maturation, a method for assessing gestational age with an efficient standardized, reproducible test was needed as survival of low-birth-weight infants improved. Methods which evolved included assessments of neurologic findings, physical characteristics, or a combination of both. The first attempt to standardize a method used clinical and neurological findings and was published in 1955 (Saint-Anne-Dargassies, 1955). This was followed by a number of subsequent studies that expanded or modified the neurological assessment and added specific physical findings (Amiel-Tison, 1968; Farr, Mitchell, Neligan, & Parker, 1966; Usher, McLean, & Scott, 1966; Dubowitz, Dubowitz, & Goldberg, 1970; and Ballard, Novak, & Driver, 1979).

Assessment data must be interpreted with caution, since scores are less reliable in cases of maternal illness such as preeclampsia, chronic hypertension, or bleeding and neonatal illness such as perinatal asphyxia and respiratory distress syndrome, particularly if the infant is ventilator dependent, septic, or has suffered a periventricular–intraventricular hemorrhage. Also, as Dubowitz et al. (1970) and Ballard et al. (1979) demonstrated, reliability of the gestational age score is dependent on the age of the neonate when the test is administered. The optimal time for evaluating the infant is 30 to 42 hours of age. Ease of reproducibility, interobserver reliability, and duration of test administration time are important factors in a busy neonatal intensive care unit where the assessment is most often done by overworked house officers. The more simplified Ballard test takes a mean time of 3 minutes and 25 seconds to administer, compared with the Dubowitz mean time of 6 minutes and 54 seconds (Ballard et al., 1979). Assignment of gestational age has become a routine and required part of the neonatal evaluation in contemporary neonatal units.

2.5. Neurological Assessment

The method of determining and describing neurologic abnormality (or handicap) differs for the neonatal period to the first year of life, the preschool years, and adolescence. The extreme clinical neurobehavioral findings of an asphyxiated infant with seizures, hypotonia, and inability to suck do not require a standardized evaluation to identify the increased risk status. Early studies of neuromotor status simply differentiated normal and abnormal neurological status. Neurological abnormality implied major motor morbidities such as cerebral palsy (spastic diplegia, hemiplegia, quadriplegia, paraplegia, choreoathetosis, ataxia) or major sensory abnormalities (blindness secondary to retinopathy of prematurity and sensorineural deafness). The importance of defining more subtle neurological deviations, however, became apparent and a number of specific evaluation procedures were developed.

The Amiel-Tison neurological assessment (Amiel-Tison, 1968) has been successfully used at term and in the first year of life. The Dubowitz (Dubowitz & Dubowitz, 1981) neurological assessment is applicable to both preterm and term infants, has good interobserver reliability, and takes only 10 to 15 minutes to complete. It assesses motor tone, strength, reflexes, vision, hearing, and behavioral responses. The most widely used neurobehavioral assessment tool is the Brazelton Neonatal Behavioral Assessment Scale (Brazelton, 1984).

Establishing a diagnosis of specific motor abnormality in the first year of life, particularly in the premature infant, can be challenging. A number of investigators have shown that both increased and decreased tone patterns can be transient, and atypical findings at 6 to 12 months can completely resolve by 24 to 36 months. The neurological assessment during the first year continues, however, to be of benefit in identifying infants at greatest risk for future sequelae, and it has become apparent as high-risk infants have been followed for longer periods that infants with lesser degrees of perinatal morbidity also require serial neurobehavioral and developmental assessments for the purpose of identification, counseling, and referral. In the older child with minor motor findings, specific assessments of oral motor, fine motor, and gross motor performance are indicated (Riley, 1976; Touwen, 1979).

2.6. Cognitive Assessment

Early reports of cognitive (intellectual) development placed children in broad categories of either normal intelligence or mental retardation. The Stanford–Binet Intelligence Test (Terman & Merrill, 1973), which gives a global measure of intelligence, was first published in the United States in 1916, and has subsequently been utilized as an indicator of intellectual performance in a variety of low-birth-weight populations at 18 months of age or older. The demand subsequently developed for a method to evaluate development of the younger child. The Bayley Scales of Infant Development (Bayley, 1969) are presently the most common scales of sensorimotor function used for assessing infant performance and development between 2 months and 30 months of age. These scales divide the infant's performance into three separate areas yielding a Mental Developmental Index (MDI), a Psychomotor Developmental Index (PDI), and a series of behavioral scores. In 1967, Kohen-Raz published a method whereby the mental scale of the Bayley can be divided into five subscales of eye–hand coordination, manipulation, object relations, imitation–comprehension, and vocalization–socialization. Using these subscales of the Bayley is helpful in evaluating specific strengths and weaknesses of the infant relative to neurological findings.

An increasing number of longitudinal follow-up studies are using intelligence tests that give subscores and !herefore provide additional information for treatment or referral. The McCarthy Scales of Children's Abilities (McCarthy, 1972) have subscores for motor, verbal, quantitative, and memory skills in conjunction with a General Cognitive Index, thereby providing information on both global functioning and specific areas of skill. The McCarthy Scales have been used for testing children 2½ to 8½ years of age. Additional tests with both verbal and performance subscores are the Wechsler Preschool and Primary Scale of Intelligence (WPPSI) (Wechsler, 1974) for children 4 to 6½ years of age and the Wechsler Intelligence Scale for Children—Revised (WISC-R) (Wechsler, 1974) for children 6 to 16 years of age. Both of these tests contain subscales to assess performance variability. We have begun using a recently developed test, the Mullen Scales of Early Learning to assess learning patterns (Mullen, 1984). This test is divided into four major scales of visual and language learning and mental capacity: Visual Receptive Organization (VRO), which assesses visual discrimination, sequences, organization, and memory; Visual Expressive Organization (VEO), which assesses unilateral and bilateral hand skills such as folding, cutting, and writing; Language Receptive Organization (LRO), which assesses language comprehension, verbal/spatial awareness, and memory; and Language Expressive Organization (LEO), which assesses verbal ability. The Mullen subscales are intended for preschoolers of 15 to 68 months. A distinct advantage of this test is its ability to assess differences in receptive and expressive learning skills. Another test that is helpful in evaluating learning abilities of the school-age child is the Wide Range Achievement Test (WRAT) (Jastak & Jastak, 1978). The reading subscale gives an accurate assessment of reading level.

Recent studies (Vohr & Garcia-Coll, 1985a; Klein, Hack, et al., 1985) have shown that visual–perceptual–motor inefficiencies are increased in the low-birth-weight population. The Beery Visual Motor Integration Test (Beery & Buktenican, 1967) is easy to administer and provides a standard score and percentile rank. A variety of additional sensorimotor and cognitive assessments are available. With high-risk populations of motorically impaired, visually or hearing impaired children, standard tests must be modified (administering verbal portions to a blind child), or a test specifically designed for the disability must be administered. The Hiskey–Nebraska Test of Learning Aptitude (Hiskey, 1966) has norms available for the deaf child.

2.7. Psychosocial Assessment

The psychosocial characteristics of families of low-birth-weight infants have been addressed more systematically in follow-up studies as the recognition of the interplay between biological and social risk in determining developmental outcome has increased. Between 1920 and 1949, only 2 of 13 studies reviewed by Kopp and Krakow (1983) included any mention of the psychosocial characteristics of the families. Ethnic and socioeconomic backgrounds of families were mentioned as possible influences on performance of preterm infants in two early studies (Mohr & Bartelme, 1930; Shirley, 1938). These early findings have been corroborated in many subsequent studies that have assessed these factors (Drillien, 1964; Escalona, 1982; Vohr & Garcia-Coll, 1985b).

Socioeconomic status (SES) has been the variable used most frequently. It is determined by the education and/or occupation of the head of the household. Recent studies have used the Hollingshead Four Factor Index (1975), which takes into consideration both parents' educational and occupational levels (if they are both employed). Now modifications average both the mother's and father's education, even if the mother is not gainfully employed (e.g., Gutierrez, 1986).

However, various environmental variables are correlates, but not equivalents, of socioeconomic status (Sameroff, Seifer, Barocas, Zaz, & Greenspan, 1987). The association observed between SES and developmental outcome might not be a function of low SES, *per se,* but of the compounding effects of other environmental risk factors that are more often found in low SES groups. Among those to be considered are aspects of the caregiving environment and sources of stress and support for the parenting role. For example, patterns of mother–infant interaction are thought of as important mediators of both cognitive and socioemotional growth for both high- and low-risk populations (Ainsworth, Blehar, Waters, & Wall, 1978; Beckwith, Cohen, Kopp, Parmelee, & Marcy, 1976; Clarke-Stewart, 1973; Garcia-Coll, Vohr, Hoffman, & Oh, 1986; Lester, Hoffman, & Brazelton, 1985).

A variety of assessments are available that are based on standard laboratory procedures or naturalistic home settings, live observations, or coding of videotapes that employ either micro- or macroanalytic techniques (Bakeman & Brown, 1980; Beckwith et al., 1976; Clarke-Stewart, 1973; Field, 1977, 1979; Tronick, Als, & Brazelton, 1980). Feeding, face-to-face, teaching, or play situations are the most frequent contexts in which interactions are observed (Barnard et al., in press; Brazelton, Koslowski, & Main, 1974; Crnic, Ragozin, Greenberg, Robinson, & Basham, 1983; Levine, Garcia-Coll, & Oh, 1985). The choice of technique is dependent on the question being asked and logistics.

The caretaking environment encompasses not only the quality of the interactions with the main caregiver, but also other aspects of the home environment. The HOME Inventory [Home Observation for Measurement of the Environment (Caldwell, 1979)] is the most established instrument. The birth-to-3-years version consists of 45 items representing the following six subscales: (1) emotional and verbal responsiveness of the mother, (2) avoidance of restriction and punishment, (3) organization of the physical and temporal environment, (4) provision of appropriate play materials, (5) maternal involvement with the child, and (6) opportunities for daily variety in daily stimulation. Caldwell and other colleagues have presented a substantial amount of validity data on the birth-to-age-3-years scale (Elardo, Bradley, & Caldwell, 1975, 1977; Bradley & Caldwell, 1976). In addition, there have been other reports attesting to the validity of the infant version (Ramey, Mills, Campbell, & O'Brien, 1975; Wulbert, Inglis, Kriegsmann, & Mills, 1975).

Another area that is receiving increasing attention is the relationship between life stress and social support and the child's developmental outcome. Most studies have employed questionnaires that are administered to parents (primarily the mother) with concurrent measures of parent–infant interaction and/or the child's developmental status. In the area of life stress, parents are asked about the occurrence of a series of life events (e.g., a death in the family) and subjective ratings for the effects of each event. To assess social support, parents are asked specifically how much support (e.g., advice, child care) they are receiving from different sources (e.g., partner, friends, neighbors). Examples of questionnaires that have been used with high-risk populations are the Life Experience Survey (Sarason, Johnson, & Siegel, 1978) and the Social Support Interview (Crockenberg, 1981).

Psychosocial assessments of the infant itself have been used more infrequently, although there is an increased recognition of the importance of more subtle aspects of the child's competence and their relation to the infant's perinatal course. Escalona (1984), for example, suggests that the study of high-risk populations should include a measurement of the psychosocial domain, including the children's daily life and behavior patterns. There are also fewer standard instruments available for assessing the psychosocial functioning of infants and young children. Most of the measures of mother–infant interaction patterns mentioned above include interactive scores for the infant. Thus, not only are maternal responsivity, contingency, and sensitivity measured, but the infant's responsivity, irritability, and synchronicity to the mother can also be assessed.

Measuring the infant's quality of attachment to his or her mother using a device called the Strange Situation is one of the most standard psychosocial assessments utilized during the infancy period (Ainsworth et al., 1978; Bretherton & Waters, 1985). The Strange Situation consists of a series of eight episodes. Infants are observed in an unfamiliar playroom, where they are given an opportunity to explore toys as well as to interact with an unfamiliar adult in the presence and in the absence of the mother. The infant's classification as A (avoidant), B (secure), and C (resistant) is based primarily on his or her behavior during reunion with the mother (Ainsworth, Bell, & Stayton, 1971, 1972). The Strange Situation has been used primarily with 12- to 18-month-olds and attachment classifications have been related and validated against systematic and extensive correlations with maternal and infant behaviors in the home throughout the first year of life (Ainsworth et al., 1978; Main, Tomasini, & Tolan, 1979). Also, there is substantial accumulating evidence for the stability of attachment patterns, at least from 12 to 18 months (Connell, 1976; Main & Weston, 1981; Waters, 1978), and their correlation with subsequent cognitive development (Main, 1973; Matas, Arend, & Sroufe, 1978) and other social relationships (Waters, Wippman, & Sroufe, 1979; Londerville & Main, 1981; George & Main, 1979). Lack of stability or unpredictability have been associated in a predictable fashion with changing family life circumstances (Vaughn, Egeland, Sroufe, & Waters, 1979; Thompson, Lamb, & Estes, 1982).

The principal limitations of the Strange Situation procedure are that it is applicable only within a narrow age range and repeated assessments have to be spaced to prevent strong carryover effects, which makes it hard to investigate developmental changes in attachment. The procedure is also expensive to administer and score, and scoring is difficult to learn without formal training (Waters & Deane, 1985). Recently, a 100-item Q-sort for assessing attachment classification in 1- to 3-year-olds has been introduced (Waters & Deane, 1985). Data on adequate interobserver reliability has been published; however, other psychometric characteristics have not been addressed. More research is necessary before utility with high-risk populations can be ascertained.

Another aspect of the psychosocial development of infants is their temperament. The infant's temperamental characteristics have traditionally been assessed using parental reports (Bates, 1987). Several questionnaires are available for assessing infants and toddlers that vary in their psychometric properties (Hubert, Wachs, Peters-Martin, & Gandour, 1982). Some of the instruments available for younger infants are the Bates Infant Characteristics Questionnaire (Bates, Freeland, & Lounsbury, 1979), the Carey Infant Temperament Questionnaire (Carey & McDevitt, 1978), and the Infant Behavior Questionnaire (Rothbart, 1981), among others. For toddlers and children, the Toddler Temperament Scale (Fullard, McDevitt, & Carey, 1984), the Child Characteristics Questionnaire (Lee & Bates, 1985), the Behavioral Style Questionnaire (McDevitt & Carey, 1978), and the Middle Childhood Temperament Questionnaire (Hegvik, McDevitt, & Carey, 1982) are also available.

Recent research, however, has shown how parental characteristics (e.g., maternal personality, anxiety, etc.), measured before birth or concurrently, are associated with responses on this type of questionnaire (Bates et al., 1979; Vaughn, Deinard, & Egeland, 1980; Vaughn, Taraldson, Crichton, & Egeland, 1981). Therefore, parental reports of the infant or child's temperament can be difficult to interpret and might be conceptualized as a reflection of both parental and child characteristics.

Various methods have been developed using direct behavioral observations, rather than parental reports, to assess temperament characteristics of older infants, toddlers, and children during standardized laboratory situations (Garcia-Coll, Kagan, & Reznick, 1984; Kagan, Reznick, Clarke, Snidman, & Garcia-Coll, 1984; Matheny, Wilson, & Nuss, 1984; Wilson & Matheny, 1983). Recently, we have developed a standard laboratory observational paradigm that can be used with 3- and 7-month-old, high- or low-risk infants (Garcia-Coll et al., in press).

The assessment consists of the presentation of 19 visual, auditory, and tactile stimuli. The order of presentation is fixed and is designed to gradually increase the intensity and number of sensory modalities involved. The stimuli were chosen not only to sample various modalities, but also to cover various areas of responsiveness (e.g., reactions to social stimulation, caregiving activities, discrepant or novel stimulation). Several pilot studies were conducted to determine the order and nature of the stimuli to be presented and their adequacy in eliciting individual differences in the behavioral dimensions of interest. The procedure takes approximately 15 minutes, during which an experimenter presents each stimulus for 20 seconds to the infant, who is sitting on an infant chair. The infant's behavioral responses are coded later from videotapes or during the procedure by another observer.

The total frequency of each of the following behaviors is coded in response to each stimulus presentation: gross motor movements (startles, legs, arms, hands, head movements, and squirming or cuddling in reaction to being picked up); facial expressions coded as positive (smiling), neutral (staring), or negative (frowning); vocalizations (positive, negative, or crying), and subtle motor movements (eye widening, eye movements, blinking, increases in respiration). In addition, after each episode of crying, soothing interventions that are required to calm the infant are rated as (1) self-quiets, (2) examiner talks, (3) requires pacifier, (4) requires pick-up, (5) mother intervenes, and (6) unconsolable. Although still in the experimental stage, this procedure promises to be an alternative for measuring temperamental characteristics of high-risk infants.

3. NEURODEVELOPMENTAL FOLLOW-UP STUDIES

3.1. Biological Risk

An increased risk of subsequent neurological, cognitive, social–behavioral, or medical problems can result from specific biologic or environmental influences or a combination of these two factors. Biological risk factors can affect the neonate during the prenatal, perinatal, or postnatal periods. Prenatal risk factors include chronic maternal disorders such as hypertension, genetic disorders such as Trisomy 21, and congenital disorders such as fetal alcohol syndrome. The prenatal period extends from conception until the seventh month of gestation. Perinatal risk factors are significant between the seventh month of gestation and the first 28 days of life and include such conditions as asphyxia, low birth weight, respiratory distress, and intraventricular hemorrhage.

Postnatal risk factors are significant after 28 days and include infections, trauma, malnutrition, and apnea. The majority of studies of low-birth-weight infants have focused on perinatal risk factors.

Although innumerable risk factors have been studied, certain ones, either because of their prevalence or impact on outcome, have been reported more frequently. During the 1960s and 1970s, biological risk factors frequently reviewed included respiratory distress syndrome (Stahlman et al., 1973), hyperbilirubinemia (Stern & Denton, 1965), and intrauterine growth retardation (Fitzhardinge & Steven, 1972). During the 1970s and 1980s, studies began to focus on a variety of contemporary medical morbidities such as bronchopulmonary dysplasia (Vohr, Bell, & Oh, 1982), periventricular–intraventricular hemorrhage (Papile, Munsick-Bruno, & Schaefer, 1983), and infants with special medical needs such as home apnea monitors and home oxygen or those with short bowel syndrome (Tilson, 1980; Henderson-Smart, 1981; Zinman, Franco, & Pizzuti-Daechsel, 1985).

3.2. Social–Environmental Risk

Another source of risk, which was recognized in the past but is receiving renewed interest in the 1980s, is that of the low-birth-weight infant placed in a social high-risk environment. The initial model of development that guided research in the area was linear; i.e., it assumed that a particular perinatal event would have a specific developmental outcome. However, even early follow-up studies identified the role of socioeconomic factors in determining the outcome of low-birth-weight infants (Drillien, 1964; Werner & Smith, 1977). More recent studies have continued to provide evidence for the powerful role of the post-natal environment in mediating the effects of perinatal risk on developmental outcome (Escalona, 1982; Ross, Lipper, & Auld, 1985; Vohr & Garcia-Coll, 1985b). The evidence lends support to the transactional model of development proposed by Sameroff and Chandler (1975).

What aspects of the postnatal environment modify the effects of low birth weight on development? Socioeconomic status, the most consistent predictor of developmental outcome in high-risk and low-risk populations is a marker variable for an array of social factors. Most frequently, socioeconomic status is defined by maternal and paternal education and occupation (Hollingshead, 1975). However, lower class is associated with differences in parenting behavior (Tulkin, 1977), home environment (Tulkin & Kagan, 1972), attitudes about infants (Moss & Jones, 1977), and support or stresses that affect the parenting role.

Although some studies have isolated specific factors mediating the impact of low socioeconomic status on developmental outcome of low-birth-weight populations (Beckwith et al., 1976; Cohen & Beckwith, 1977; Siegel, 1982), future research should elucidate further the process behind this association. In addition, some subgroups have been identified that appear to be affected by a combination of both biological and social risk factors. Among those are maternal substance abuse and teenage pregnancy and childbearing.

3.2.1. Maternal Substance Abuse

Substance abuse in the United States is a current, serious problem affecting young people and potentially their offspring. Although alcohol remains the most common drug used by young people (66%), in one study 26% of high school seniors were found to use marijuana at least once a month, and 7% used cocaine once a month (Johnson, O'Malley, & Backman, 1985). The fetal alcohol syndrome/malformation syndrome was first described in the English language in 1973 (Jones, Smith, Ulleland, & Streissguth, 1973). Whereas numerous subsequent studies have investigated short- and long-term effects of alcohol on the fetus (Clarren & Smith, 1978; Majewski, 1981), more recently the focus has shifted to the detrimental effects of street drugs on pregnancy.

Cocaine is currently the leading street drug in the United States. Recent work has shown that 24% of mothers who are chronic cocaine users deliver before 37 weeks, 19% have infants suffering from intrauterine growth retardation, and 17% experience abruption (Pediatric Research, Abstract No. 1096, 1987). As pediatricians have become aware of the effects of cocaine on the neonate, multiple investigations have focused on both the immediate and long-term detrimental effects. The 1987 Program Issue of Pediatric Research contained 15 abstracts that studied the effects of cocaine on pregnancy and the infant (Pediatric Research, 1987). Preliminary findings indicate that there may be a persistence of visual–motor and oral–motor dysfunction identified in the neonatal period (Schneider & Chasnoff, 1987). The issue remains, however, as to the strength of the contribution of intrauterine insult versus postnatal environmental factors in this population.

3.2.2. Teenage Pregnancy and Childbearing

Infants born to adolescent mothers are known to be at risk for adverse perinatal and neonatal outcome. There is evidence suggesting that infants of very young adolescents, especially <15 years of age, are more likely to be low birth weight, of lower gestation, and small for gestational age (Hardy & Mellits, 1977; Field, Widmayer, Stringer, & Ignatoff, 1980). Less than optimal developmental outcome of these infants results from an interaction of such factors as a higher incidence of perinatal events with negative caretaking characteristics, less than adequate mother–infant interaction, lower socioeconomic background, and poorer home environment (Field et al., 1980; Field, Widmayer, Ignatoff, & Stringer, 1982). Experimental research involving a comprehensive early intervention approach has demonstrated that positive changes can be induced in the developmental outcome of infants of adolescent mothers.

The infant born to an adolescent mother represents an example of the interaction of biological and environmental risk affecting outcome. Because of its prevalence, teenage pregnancy remains a wide open area of research to further investigate interactive mechanisms, prevention, and intervention.

3.3. Low-Birth-Weight At-Risk Populations

This section will include primarily studies related to very-low-birth-weight infants (birth weight <1500 g). It will, however, address the subgroups of appropriate-for-gestational age (AGA) infants, small-for-gestational age (SGA) infants, and a variety of perinatal risk factors and morbidities. Because of the continuous interaction between perinatal risk factors and social and environmental factors, these influences will also be discussed.

3.3.1. Retrolental Fibroplasia

Infants born prematurely with immature lungs often manifest respiratory distress, irregular breathing, and apnea. Bakwin first reported on the use of oxygen administered by nasal tubing to premature infants to relieve cyanosis in 1923. He attributed anoxemia to the irregularities of breathing found in premature infants. It was not until 1942, however, that work was published on a group of 33 premature infants weighing <1984 g demonstrating that all the infants had irregular breathing on room air, and 23 of 28 placed in a high-oxygen environment developed regular breathing (Wilson, Long, & Howard, 1942). This study led to a general acceptance of the use of oxygen for premature infants. Simultaneously, the relationship between perinatal asphyxia, anoxia, and neurological insult became more fully established (Schreiber, 1938), providing yet another indication for oxygen use.

Retrolental fibroplasia (RLF) was first described as a disorder of prematurity in 1942 (Terry, 1942). Terry determined that the disorder developed in infants two to six months after birth and postulated it was caused by exposure to light. Premature nurseries across the country subsequently began to report cases of RLF and by 1949 it was felt to be the cause of one-third of blindness in preschool children (Reese, 1949). With an increasing awareness of the problem, innumerable studies were carried out looking for the cause of the disorder (Silverman, 1980).

The first clinical controlled prospective study to clearly demonstrate a relationship between hyperoxia and RLF was begun in 1951 at the Gallinger Municipal Hospital in Washington, D.C. (Patz, Hoeck, & De-laCruz, 1952). This and two subsequent controlled prospective studies confirmed the relationship and gradually resulted in more stringent recommendations for administration of oxygen to premature infants (Lanman, Guy, & Dancis, 1954; Kinsey, 1954).

The incidence of retrolental fibroplasia fell significantly. However, with the advent of increased survival of very-low-birth-weight infants receiving neonatal intensive care in the 1970s, the incidence of retrolental fibroplasia, now renamed retinopathy of prematurity, increased dramatically (Phelps, 1981). This has been associated with a revival of interest in investigations looking once again at additional etiologic factors (Hittner et al., 1981; Hillis, 1982; Phelps, 1982) and in neurodevelopmental morbidities experienced by infants and children with the disorder. School-age follow-up of children with retrolental fibroplasia born between 1945 and 1952 revealed that mental retardation ranged from 32% to 50% (Parmelee, Cutsforth, & Jackson, 1958; Parmelee, Fiske, & Wright, 1959; Genn & Silverman, 1964).

A recent study found that 14 (2.2%) of 645 survivors born between 1975 and 1981 with a birth weight of ≤1500 g developed stage III–IV retrolental fibroplasia in one or both eyes (Vohr & Garcia-Coll, 1985a). Mean birth weight was 985 g (<700 to 1500 g). Follow-up assessments over a five-year period showed that retrolental fibroplasia survivors have a significantly higher incidence of neurological abnormality (spastic cerebral palsy and seizure disorder), lower developmental quotients, increased requirements for special education, increased number of hospitalizations, and more maternal stress than controls matched for birth weight and perinatal morbidities. A total of 64% had developmental retardation. The only significant differences between the retrolental fibroplasia children and matched controls during the perinatal period were in the needs for supplemental oxygen and assisted ventilation ($p < .05$). The reason for the poor outcome is unclear in view of the overall improving outcome of infants in this weight category. Previous authors have noted a relationship between intraventricular hemorrhage and

retrolental fibroplasia, which may be contributing to the high incidence
of motor deficits in these children (Procianoy, Garcia-Prats, Hittner,
Adams, & Rudolph, 1981).

3.3.2. Bronchopulmonary Dysplasia

It is well known that respiratory distress syndrome (RDS) associated
with an immature surfactant system is a common condition in the premature infant, particularly those <1500 g and <32 weeks gestation.
Lung maturation progresses speedily throughout gestation, and therefore, infants who are born early are at an increased risk of respiratory
distress syndrome, also termed hyaline membrane disease. Early studies
focused on the clinical description of this abnormality, the radiographic
and clinical diagnosis, and the biochemical deficiencies contributing to
the disorder (Farrell & Avery, 1975; Gluck et al., 1971). As a direct result
of the development of neonatal intensive care units, however, with the
use of assisted ventilation for RDS, there was an improved survival of
very-low-birth-weight infants with RDS who developed chronic lung injury. Mechanical ventilation, initially with negative pressure ventilators
followed by more aggressive use of positive pressure ventilators, began
to be used fairly commonly for infants with respiratory distress syndrome or apnea in the mid to late 1960s (Stahlman, Hedvall, Lindstrom,
& Snell, 1982).

Early follow-up studies reporting outcome included infants with a
wide spectrum of gestational ages. Stahlman et al. evaluated pulmonary
function in 129 children born between 1961 and 1970 with a battery of
pulmonary function studies. Her results indicated only minor pulmonary sequelae in 12 children at 6 to 11 years, although residual pulmonary symptoms during the first year were related to positive pressure
ventilation. Likewise, early studies reporting neurodevelopmental outcome of infants with respiratory distress syndrome reported favorable
results (Mayes et al., 1985; Dinwiddie, Mellor, Donaldson, Tunstall, &
Russell, 1974; Johnson et al., 1974). Bennett, Robinson, and Sells (1982)
followed 161 low-birth-weight infants and found that birth weight and
gestation were both significantly related to cognitive performance at 12
months, and, whereas hyaline membrane disease affected developmental performance at 4 months, there was no evidence of effect at 12
months of age.

The continued improvement in survival of infants with a birth
weight <1500 g treated with assisted ventilation in the 1970s, however,
resulted in a reassessment of their quality of outcome. A two-year follow-
up of 73 infants born between 1970 and 1973 with a birth weight less

than 1501 g treated with positive pressure ventilation revealed a high incidence of sequelae. A total of 39% of boys and 18% of girls had major neurologic defects, and 48% of the children had Bayley scores <80 at 12 months of age (Fitzhardinge et al., 1976). A subsequent study reported the medical and neurodevelopmental status at one year of age of 38 infants born between 1976 and 1978 with a birth weight less than 1000 g. Twenty of the 38 infants required assisted ventilation and 14 (70%) of these infants developed bronchopulmonary dysplasia (Ruiz, LeFever, Hakanson, Clark, & Williams, 1981). There was an overall high incidence (45%) of developmental delay in the study population consisting of both ventilated and nonventilated infants. Developmental delay (DQ ≤ 84), however, related significantly to the need for mechanical ventilation, duration of oxygen therapy, and the diagnosis of bronchopulmonary dysplasia (BPD).

This pulmonary abnormality was first described by Northway, Rosan, and Porter (1967). Northway and colleagues originally described four radiographic stages that represented the evolution and increasing severity of this disorder. BPD was subsequently identified as developing in from 5% to 30% of patients admitted to intensive care units with RDS, although the incidence in very-low-birth-weight infants of 1000 ≤1500 g was even higher, ranging from 20% to 40% (Saigal, Rosenbaum, Stoskopf, & Sinclair, 1984; Rosenfield et al., 1984). These infants more often have prolonged hospitalizations because of the extended duration of assisted ventilation and oxygen supplementation required (Vohr, Bell, & Oh, 1982). They also have multiple secondary effects from the BPD, including failure to thrive, poor weight gain, rehospitalization for recurrent upper and lower respiratory tract infections, impaired pulmonary function, and neurodevelopmental sequelae (Vohr, Bell, & Oh, 1982; Weinstein and Oh, 1981; Mayes, Perkett, and Stahlman, 1983; Koops, Abman, & Accurso, 1984; Smyth, Tabachnik, Duncan, Reilly, & Levison, 1981). Pulmonary function testing in older BPD survivors has documented evidence of chronic air-flow limitation (Smyth et al., 1981). Whether pulmonary dysfunction persists in adult life is yet to be determined.

It has become apparent that more infants are being discharged from neonatal intensive care units with moderate degrees of lung injury requiring specialized discharge planning and long-term close medical management (Koops, Abman, & Accurso, 1984). Aside from the medical sequelae, these infants are at increased risk of significant neurodevelopmental handicap (Northway, 1979; Vohr et al., 1982). In a two-year follow-up of 21 infants (birth weight ≤1500 g) with bronchopulmonary dysplasia born in between 1975 and 1977 compared with 22 weight-matched controls with a maximum O_2 requirement of five days, major neurodevelopmental abnormalities were present in 11 of the 21 BPD children compared with 2 of the 22 controls. In addition, 4 of the BPD children were legally blind and had retinopathy of prematurity. Significant developmental delay was apparent at two years using the Bayley Mental Developmental Index (MDI). The mean MDI for BPD children was 65 ± 16 compared with 91 ± 26 for the control group.

A more recent study of 20 infants with respiratory distress syndrome and 17 infants with bronchopulmonary dysplasia all with a birth weight less than 2501 g born between 1980 and 1982 revealed similar trends for neurodevelopmental delays of BPD children despite the fact that these infants were larger at birth. The Bayley MDI for the BPD children at 2 years was 86 ± 13 and for the RDS children 106 ± 16 (Meisels, Plunkett, Roloff, Pasick, & Stiefel, 1986). This study is of particular interest since it excluded subjects with neuromuscular or sensory disorders, intraventricular hemorrhage > grade II, hydrocephalus, ROP, congenital malformations, metabolic disorders, hyperbilirubinemia, and intrauterine growth retardation. Families with significant psychosocial problems were likewise excluded. Regression analysis in this study revealed that BPD and RDS were better predictors of second-year outcome than birth weight and gestational age. The data contrasted with previous studies that did not have limiting factors defining their populations. It remains apparent that infants with respiratory distress and bronchopulmonary dysplasia represent serious at-risk populations.

Research efforts have continued to focus on preventing or ameliorating the disorder. The administration of vitamin E during acute respiratory distress syndrome has been less effective than originally proposed (Ehrenhranz, Bonta, Arlow, & Warshaw, 1978). Although a deficiency of surfactant in the pulmonary system resulting in an abnormal surface tension and subsequent atelectasis was first described by Avery and Mead in 1959, it was not until 20 years later that the first promising animal and human studies began to appear demonstrating the positive effects of various phospholipids in altering lung pressure/volume dynamics (Ikegami, Silverman, & Adams, 1979; Fujiwara et al., 1980). Numerous studies have been published recently supporting the administration of human or bovine surfactant to ameliorate the course of RDS in LBW infants (Ikegami et al., 1987; Hallman et al., 1983; Edwards et al., 1985; Merritt et al., 1986; Gitlin et al., 1987; Enhorning et al., 1985; Shapiro et al., 1985). Results presently indicate that if exogenous surfactant is administered early in the course of hyaline membrane disease, it can reduce the amount of respiratory support needed (Gitlin et al., 1987) and improve gas exchange significantly (Enhorning et al., 1985).

Sustained and long-term effects of exogenous surfactant administration, however, remain uncertain.

The potential amelioration of RDS in very-low-birth-weight infants remains an important issue. Because of the large number of current ongoing clinical studies testing surfactant administration in the very-low-birth-weight infant, it is imperative that studies be conducted evaluating the neurodevelopmental outcome status of surfactant-treated infants versus randomly assigned controlled infants of similar gestation and birth weight. These surfactant-treated babies represent an at-risk population of infants who have survived because of contemporary fetal medicine and neonatology management. Future studies must look further at preventive therapies, treatment modalities, and outcome, which will require collaboration of the perinatologist, neonatologist, and follow-up team.

3.3.3. Intraventricular Hemorrhage

Periventricular–intraventricular hemorrhage (IVH) is the most common cause of mortality and morbidity identified in premature infants in neonatal intensive care units (Valdes-Dapena & Arey, 1970; Leech, 1974; Ahman, Lazzara, Dykes, Brann, & Schwartz, 1980). Early published studies looking at the incidence of this condition were based on autopsy findings or clinical signs, and since symptoms were inexact, clinical investigation tended to identify only infants with large intraventricular bleeds.

Two major developments took place: the improved survival of very-low-birth-weight infants (≤1500 g birth weight and ≤32 weeks gestation) (Rawlings et al., 1971; Williams & Chen, 1982; Paneth et al., 1982; Kitchen, Yu, et al., 1982; and Hack et al., 1983) and the advent of computerized tomography (CT) (Rumack, McDonald, O'Meara, Sanders, & Rudikoff, 1978; Burstein, Papile, & Burstein, 1977) and cranial ultrasound (Johnson, Rumack, Mannes, & Appareti, 1981; Babcock & Han, 1981).

The increased incidence of IVH in prematures can be attributed in part to developmental changes that occur in the germinal matrix between 28 and 36 weeks. The germinal matrix of 28 weeks is loosely organized, friable, and has a rich capillary bed. Involution and transformation to a more avascular area occurs by 36 weeks (Volpe, 1981). Infants of very low birth weight, therefore, because of the very nature of their cerebral germinal matrix, are most vulnerable to periventricular IVH. This has resulted in multiple studies looking at etiology, pathogenesis, prevention, and outcome.

The first work describing the incidence. extent, and evolution of IVH in 46 infants <1500 g based on CT brain scan was published in 1978 (Papile, Burstein, Burstein, & Koffler, 1978). The incidence of IVH in this study was 43% (20/46). CT scan data from this study were developed into a grading system for defining the severity of a bleed as follows: Grade I—isolated subepidermal hemorrhage, Grade II—intraventricular hemorrhage without ventricular dilatation, Grade III—intraventricular hemorrhage with ventricular dilatation, and Grade IV—intraventricular hemorrhage with parenchymal involvement. This grading system or modifications of it have been used in multiple subsequent studies of IVH (Kuban & Teele, 1984). Two important results of this study were the realization that the incidence of IVH in low-birth-weight survivors was greater than realized and that 78% of the low-birth-weight infants <1500 g with IVH had no clinical signs of IVH.

Because of the significant mortality and morbidity associated with the disorder, multiple studies have been conducted attempting to identify etiologic factors. These studies have focused on identifying prenatal, perinatal, and postnatal factors that contribute to IVH. Results of early studies assessing the effects of mode of delivery and labor on IVH have been, at times, conflicting (Kosmetatos, Dinter, Williams, Lourie, & Berne, 1980; Bada, Korones, Magill, & Anderson, 1982; Bada, Korones, Anderson, Magill, & Wong, 1984). A recent prospective study that assessed the impact of mode of delivery on IVH in 151 low-birth-weight infants (<1500 g) who had serial cranial ultrasounds during the first five days of life found no relationship between mode of delivery (or multiple obstetric variables) and IVH. Risk factors that contributed significantly were birth weight, gestation, and low Apgar scores. This study divided the timing of IVH into early (first 24 hours—55%) and late (after 24 hours—24%) assuming that obstetrical factors contribute primarily to IVH in the first 24 hours.

A second recent prospective study of 112 low-birth-weight infants <1500 g demonstrated that fetal distress, defined as suspicious or ominous fetal heart rate tracings and acidosis as determined by umbilical cord arterial blood pH <7.20, was significantly more common in infants with intraventricular/subependymal hemorrhage (Strauss, Kirz, Mondanlou, and Freeman, 1985). This study, likewise, found no relationship between mode of delivery, presentation, duration of labor, or antepartum complications and IVH. Confirmation of this data is of great importance and emphasizes the constant need for collaboration between perinatologist and neonatologist in the aggressive management of fetal distress. Neonatal factors including acute asphyxia and hemodynamic changes associated with pneumothorax have been shown to have a relationship to IVH (Hill, Perlman, & Volpe, 1982).

Prevention and treatment have become a focus of numerous studies. Preventive measures shown to have probable beneficial effects on IVH include the early administration of vitamin E, a naturally occurring antioxidant that protects the endothelial cell (Chiswick et al., 1983; Speer et al., 1984), and the utilization of muscle paralysis on infants receiving mechanical ventilation for respiratory distress syndrome to minimize or eliminate fluctuating cerebral blood-flow velocity (Perlman, Goodman, Kreusser, & Volpe, 1985). A prospective controlled study that attempted to prevent post hemorrhage hydrocephalus from developing in preterm infants with Grade III–IV IVH by administering serial intermittent lumbar punctures was unsuccessful (Anwar, Kadam, Hiatt, & Hegyi, 1985). Other investigators have evaluated the effects of various medications including phenobarbitone and indomethacin in an attempt to identify medical means to reduce the incidence of IVH (Morgan, Massey, & Cooke, 1982; Maher, Lane, Ballard, Piecuch, & Clyman, 1985). Clinical approaches have changed as additional management factors including rapid volume expansion, mask ventilation, and hyperosmolarity were identified as contributing to intraventricular hemorrhage (Goldberg, Chung, Goldman, & Bancalari, 1980; Pape, Armstrong, & Fitzhardinge, 1976; Thomas, 1976).

As survival of very-low-birth-weight infants with IVH continues to improve and prevention or amelioration of the problem remains limited, their neurodevelopmental outcome has become an important issue. One of the first follow-up studies (mean age 24 months) consisted of a cohort of 15 infants (mean birth weight 1.7 kg) with grades of IVH ranging from I to IV identified on CT scan (Krishnamoorthy, Shannon, DeLong, Todres, & Davis, 1979). Neurological outcome correlated with degree of IVH and 100% of infants with Grade IV IVH had severe neuromotor abnormalities. Papile, Munsick-Bruno, and Shaefer (1983) later studied 260 infants with a birth weight <1501 g for the effects of IVH on outcome. The study population was biased in that subjects with known risk factors contributing to IVH were enrolled. The results, however, indicate that infants with IVH are at increased risk for neurodevelopmental sequelae and the incidence of sequelae is related to the severity of IVH. Major handicaps were present in 11 percent of infants with no IVH, 9% of infants with Grade I IVH, 11% of infants with Grade II IVH, and 58% of infants with Grade III–IV IVH. An important contribution of Papile's large cohort study was the knowledge that infants with Grade I–II IVH had a prognosis similar to those low-birth-weight infants with no IVH. Her study also found no difference in outcome between subjects with or without hydrocephalus, in contrast to findings previously reported (Fitzhardinge, Flodmark, Fitz, & Ashby, 1982).

Conflicting results in studies of outcome of posthemorrhagic hydrocephalus may well be related to the fact that the majority of low-birth-weight infant survivors with ventriculomegaly have normal pressure hydrocephalus that resolves spontaneously (Hill & Volpe, 1981). Persistence of major neurocognitive abnormalities at 3 years of age has been identified in 41% of a group of low-birth-weight infants with IVH, indicating long-term morbidities (Williamson et al., 1983). Another factor contributing to conflicting outcome data includes the birth weight and gestational age ranges of the study infants. One study with a more optimistic outcome for IVH consisted of 131 infants with birth weights <1800 g with no gestational age restriction (Shinnar et al., 1982). Finally, improved scanning techniques have resulted in the identification of ischemic brain lesions (Sinka, Sims, Davies, & Chiswick, 1985; Szymonowicz, Yu, Bajuk, & Astbury, 1986; Guzzetta, Shackelford, Volpe, Perlman, & Volpe, 1986). A recent study reported the results of 75 infants <2000 g birth weight who were identified as having ultrasonographic evidence of periventricular intraparenchymal echodensities (IPE) (Guzzetta et al., 1986). This study indicates that the extent of ischemic involvement determines neurologic outcome, and that infants with extensive IPE who survive have a poor neurologic and cognitive outcome. The increasing survival of very-low-birth-weight infants with IVH and IPE means more survivors with the worst severity of insult and sequelae. Numerous additional investigations aimed at preventing and treating this neonatal morbidity can be anticipated.

3.3.4. Infants <800 Grams Birth Weight

Survival data first available in the 1940s showed that survival of infants ≤1000 g ranged from 0% to 9% (Dunham, 1948) and subsequent neurodevelopmental outcome for these rare infant survivors was grim (Lubchenco, Horner, et al., 1963). Aggressive prenatal and neonatal intervention with vigorous resuscitation and ventilatory support has resulted in the improved survival of these infants cared for in neonatal units. This dramatic change in survival for infants ≤800 g during two time periods, 1975 to 1977 (incomplete neonatal care) and 1977 to 1979 (complete neonatal care), at the Children's Hospital of Buffalo is reflected in survival data that changed from 4% to 44%. Other neonatal units have likewise begun to have increasing numbers of these tiny babies survive.

Because of the previous grim outlook for these infants (100% handicap), the question of quality of survival was again raised, and four follow-up studies were recently published evaluating neurodevelopmental outcome (Britton, Fitzhardinge, & Ashby, 1981; Buckwald, Zorn, and Egan, 1984; Bennett, Robinson, & Sells, 1983; Hirata et al., 1983) (see Table 2). Although neonatal survival has improved, it varies among the centers from 20% to 47%. The study population samples vary from 16 to 54, and the age of follow-up varies from 6 months to 7 years. It is, therefore, not surprising that the incidence of major handicap varies from 16% to 49%. The point has been made, however, that these infants are surviving in increasing numbers, and there is a trend for improving neurodevelopmental outcome with aggressive neonatal care.

3.3.5. Infants with Intrauterine Growth Retardation

The first case report of a full-term infant who was malnourished at birth was published in 1947 (McBurney, 1947). It was not until 1953, however, that data were published that led to questioning whether all low-birth-weight infants were indeed premature. Critical clinical observations of neurologic status and reflexes indicated that some low-birth-weight infants were more mature than expected (Soderling, 1953). This was termed "pseudoprematurity." Finally, in 1963 data were published indicating intrauterine growth retardation was a common entity in the low-birth-weight population (Gruenwald, 1963).

The development of standardized intrauterine growth charts in the 1960s resulted in a method for establishing birth weights specific for age with the subsequent differentiation of infants below the 10th percentile of weight for gestation (small for gestational age—SGA), between the 10th and 90th percentile (appropriate for gestational age—AGA), and

TABLE 2. Follow-up of Infants <800 g

Study	Birth dates	Survival	Evaluated	Age evaluation	Neurodevelopmental handicap (%)
Dunham (1948)	1943–1945	0%	—	—	—
Britton et al. (1981)	1974–1977	25%	37	18 mo	49%
Bennett et al. (1982)	1977–1980	20%	16	6–36 mo	19%
Hirata et al. (1983)[a]	1975–1980	47%	22	≤7 yr	16%
Buckwald et al. (1984)	1977–1981	44%	54	12 mo	35%

[a] <750 g.

greater than the 90th percentile (large for gestational age—LGA) (Lubchenco, Hansman, Dressler, & Boyd, 1963). Terms also used for the SGA infant were "small for date" and "intrauterine growth-retarded infant." Relative impaired fetal growth of infants with a birth weight above the 10th percentile can be estimated using the Ponderal Index. This index describes the relationship between weight and crown–heel length. It is calculated as follows: weight (g) ÷ length (cm)^3 × 100.

Dr. Lubchenco's meticulous analysis of growth parameters for gestational age led to further understanding of this method of assessing growth. Another important distinguishing factor of types of intrauterine growth retardation (IUGR) is whether the infant has asymmetric or symmetric growth retardation. Infants with symmetric growth retardation have head circumference and length and weight measurements all falling below the 10th percentile on the intrauterine growth curve. These infants are at greater risk for subsequent sequelae. The etiology of their IUGR more often is secondary to congenital infections, fetal anomolies, chromosomal abnormalities, or chronic maternal abnormalities including alcohol or substance abuse. Decreased substrate availability that is constant throughout the three trimesters of pregnancy will result in decreased weight and length and a Ponderal Index above the 10th percentile, or symmetric growth retardation. Decreased substrate availability beginning after the 27th week affects primarily weight and results in asymmetric growth retardation. Recently, advances in real-time ultrasound techniques have led to the establishment of normative values for fetal growth including biparietal diameter measurements that facilitate diagnosing IUGR *in utero* (Hadlock, Deter, & Harrist, 1982; O'Brien & Queenan, 1981).

The need to diagnose IUGR has been an important issue because of the unique problems these infants experience in the neonatal period and their at times poorer neurodevelopmental and growth outcome. Since 15% to 20% of pregnancies have inaccurate dates by maternal history, the need for appropriate prenatal and neonatal diagnostic techniques for gestational age assessment was obvious. It was, therefore, through the combined investigative efforts of Lubchenco (1967) in the area of fetal growth and Dubowitz (1970) and others with the development of methodology for clinical neonatal gestational age assessments that both full-term and preterm IUGR infants could be identified at birth.

Studies of low-birth-weight infants with IUGR initially did not differentiate between infants with symmetric and asymmetric growth retardation. Drillien in 1970 documented a high incidence of poorer outcome in growth-retarded infants with associated birth defects. These infants more often have symmetric growth retardation. Investigative studies subsequently focused to a greater extent on infants with growth retardation secondary to maternal substrate deficiency. These infants more often have asymmetric growth retardation and are at risk for a host of perinatal morbidities including fetal distress, neonatal asphyxia, hypoglycemia, polycythemia, difficulties with thermoregulation, and hypocalcemia (Minkowski et al., 1977; Cornblath, Wybregt, Baens, & Klein, 1964; Humbert, Abelson, Hathaway, & Battaglia, 1969; Tsang, Gigger, Oh, & Brown, 1975; Lee, Younger, & Babson, 1966).

Another methodologic problem with studies of IUGR has been study populations based on weight criteria alone, thus combining low-birth-weight term infants with low-birth-weight preterm infants. Likewise, severity of growth retardation, type of perinatal care, neonatal complications, socioeconomic level, age of assessment, and criteria for growth retardation all have contributed to heterogenicity of study populations and, at times, conflicting data (Bard, 1978; Fitzhardinge & Steven, 1972; Lugo & Cassady, 1971; Villar, Smeriglio, Martorell, Brown, & Klein, 1984).

Numerous studies have been published examining the different growth problems found in subgroups of IUGR infants and their "catch-up" growth patterns (Fitzhardinge & Steven, 1972a; Villar et al., 1984; Vohr & Oh, 1983; Hack, Merkatz, Gordon, Jones, & Fanaroff, 1982; Harvey, Prince, Burton, Parkinson, & Campbell, 1982). The relationship between growth at critical time periods and subsequent neurodevelopmental outcome has been shown to be important. Harvey et al. (1982) published a unique five-year follow-up study of 51 SGA children born at >37 weeks gestation whose intrauterine growth had been monitored by serial ultrasonic cephalometry. He identified that children whose head growth slowed prior to 26 weeks gestation, as monitored by serial biparietal diameter measurements, had significantly lower McCarthy Test results for perceptual performance, quantitative performance, motor performance, and General Cognitive Index when compared to AGA controls. Of significance, however, was the fact that they also performed significantly better than SGA infants without ultrasound evidence of similar head growth slowing. This study demonstrates the important link between fetal growth and long-term outcome, and the importance of collaboration between the perinatologist and the follow-up team.

The Hack et al. 1982 comprehensive study of 192 very-low-birth-weight SGA infants identified the importance of postnatal growth on outcome. Both the AGA and SGA infants who did not "catch up" in weight by eight months of age had lower Bayley mental developmental indices, a higher rate of neurosensory impairment, and smaller head circumference. SGA infants who demonstrated good postnatal growth did not differ from controls.

We followed 21 preterm <37 weeks gestation SGA infants (birth weight <1500 g) to five years of age. Developmental test scores for SGA children were delayed when compared to AGA children at 1 to 3 years of age but did not differ at 4 and 5 years of age (Vohr & Oh, 1983). Linear regression analysis of the relationship between a modified Hollingshead SES score and developmental quotient was not significant at one year but had become significant at five years. These data again point out that SES factors can play a role in overcoming the effects of prematurity and intrauterine growth retardation. The overall developmental outcome in this population was good. Head circumference measurements in the SGA infants did not differ from the AGA controls at one year indicating a "catch-up" phenomenon, a favorable sign. These findings are consistent with an analysis of the growth data of the large population of children participating in the National Collaborative project, which indicated a positive correlation between head circumference at 1 year and IQ at 4 years (Nelson & Deutschberger, 1970). Investigations of the relationships between growth, nutrition, and neurodevelopmental outcomes will continue until such a time that IUGR can be treated and prevented *in utero*.

3.4. Low-Birth-Weight Infant Survivors: Toddler to School Age

The fact that low-birth-weight survivors are at increased risk of major neurodevelopmental sequelae such as cerebral palsy, hydrocephalus, seizure disorders, and mental retardation was identified in early studies documenting their outcome (Drillien, 1959; Lubchenco, Horner, et al., 1963). Although the incidence of major sequelae in early studies ranged from 50% to 100%, it dropped significantly (10% to 18%) in the 1960s, the early intensive care era (Hack, Fanaroff, & Merkatz, 1979; Stewart, Reynolds, & Lipscomb, 1981). Despite the trend for overall improving neurodevelopmental outcome, studies following low-birth-weight children to early childhood (1.5 to 3 years) continue to report variability in the percentage of survivors and of surviving infants manifesting major neurologic deficits. As shown in Table 3, the incidence of major sequelae for infants under 1500 g ranges from 7.4% to 16.8%, and for infants under 1250 g from 14% to 30%.

Although social environmental differences play a role, factors relating to patient management obviously affect both survival and morbidity. Study populations are currently described as Inborn (I), which includes maternal transports because of a high-risk pregnancy, and Outborn (O),

TABLE 3. Survival and Major Neuromotor Morbidity in Low-Birth-Weight Infants

Author	I/O[a]	Year of birth	Birth weight (g)	Percent survival	Survivors	Age (yr)	Major neurologic deficit	
							N	(%)
Rawlings et al. (1971)	I + O	1966–1969	<1500	46%	72	2.3	5	(7.4)
Saigal et al. (1982)	I + O	1973–1978	<1500	63%	184	3	30	(16.8)
Kitchen et al. (1982)	I	1977–1978	<1500	54%	91	2	16	(9.6)
Kumar et al. (1980)	I	1974–1977	<1251	45%	50	1.5–4	7	(14.0)
Pape et al. (1978)	O	1974	<1001	47%	43	1.5	13	(30.0)
Walker et al. (1985)	I + O	1971–1981	<1000	32%	68	2.5	11	(16.0)

[a] I = inborn; O = outborn.

which includes high-risk infants born at secondary-level hospitals or at home and transported into a neonatal intensive care unit at variable time intervals after delivery with or without a transport team. It has previously been shown that the outborn high-risk infant has an immediate disadvantage because of absent or less sophisticated immediate intensive care efforts including resuscitation, assisted ventilation, and temperature control. The pattern of referral from the secondary-level hospital likewise contributes to outcome depending on whether all high-risk infants, only the sickest infants, or only infants felt to have a chance of survival are transported.

Another factor affecting mortality and morbidity is the aggressiveness of management of critically ill infants or very-low-birthweight infants with serious complications such as BPD and IVH. In one report, intensive care was either not instituted or withdrawn in 18 of 294 live births (16%) of infants with a birth weight <1500 g (Saigal et al., 1982). In another early report of morbidities in infants less than 1000 grams, intensive care was withdrawn electively in 56% of cases (Stewart, Turcan, Rawlings, & Reynolds, 1977). If only the sickest infants are transported to the tertiary care center and the subsequent management is aggressive, the incidence of handicaps can be expected to be higher.

Studies that have followed children longitudinally behond three years of age have identified an increased prevalence of learning disabilities, language delays, and attention and behavior abnormalities in the low-birth-weight infant (Lubchenco, Horner et al., 1963; Wiener, Rider, & Opel, 1965, Drillien, 1967). These learning disabilities and cognitive dysfunctions have been identified in both low-birth-weight infants with major motor deficits and infants with a "normal neurological" status (Klein, Hack, Gallagher, & Fanaroff, 1985; Vohr & Garcia-Coll, 1985b), indicating the possibility of a continuum of central nervous system insult from very mild (soft clinical signs) to the most severe (spastic quadriplegia with seizures and retardation). A recent pathologic study of the brains of 16 premature infants who died in the first month of life identified significant abnormal neurologic findings of varying severity in multiple areas of gray and white matter including cortical and basal brain structures. Sites of the lesions were consistent with areas that control a variety of learning skills (Fuller, Guthrie, & Alvord, 1983). The study has its limitations in that the analysis was done on infants who expired. However, the fact that there was a spectrum of neuropathological change suggests that similar lesions exist in infants who survive. Various scanning techniques can now be utilized to support these findings.

Wiener et al. (1968) followed a large cohort of 500 low-birth-weight children (<2501 g) and 492 full-term controls. Of the original cohort 822 received extensive neurodevelopmental evaluations at 8 to 10 years of age. The low-birth-weight children had impaired function on 10 subtests of the Wechsler Intelligence Scale for Children including information, comprehension, arithmetic, similarities, digit span, vocabulary, picture completion, block design, object assembly, and digit symbol, and on the WRAT reading test. The degree of impairment correlated with lower birth weight and associated neurological deficit.

Hunt, Tooley, and Harven (1982) followed a cohort of 102 children with a birth weight <1500 g until 11 years of age. The incidence of learning disabilities likely to interfere with classroom performance was 37%. Problems identified were difficulties with language comprehension and visual motor integration. Of significance was the fact that the majority of children who manifested learning problems had IQs in the normal range.

Klein et al., (1985) evaluated 46 children with a birth weight <1500 g born in 1976 who had normal intelligence at 5 years of age and compared them with classmate-matched control children. No differences were found between the two groups in IQ. This study again documented the effects of social and environmental factors on cognitive function. In both the low-birth-weight and control groups, IQ correlated with social class and material education. The low-birth-weight infants performed significantly poorer on tests of spatial relations and visual–motor integration. Difficulties in visual–motor function performance by low-birth-weight survivors have now been documented by a number of investigators (Fitzhardinge & Ramsey, 1973; Francis-Williams & Davies, 1974; Vohr & Garcia-Coll, 1985b).

Another area of disability, impaired speech and language performance, has been documented in the low-birth-weight infant by a number of investigators (Hunt et al., 1982; Largo, Molinari, Comenale, Weber, & Dric, 1986; Hubatch, Johnson, Kistler, Burns, & Moneha, 1985; Wright, Thislethwaite, Elton, Wilkinson, & Forfar, 1983). A recent Swiss study (Largo et al., 1986) identified language delay present in both the neurologically abnormal and neurologically normal subgroups of 114 high-risk preterm infants with a mean gestation of 33 weeks. We followed 50 low-birth-weight (<1500 g) infants for two years with neurological and language assessments. Receptive or expressive language delay was present in 28% of the children. We found that neurologic status at 8 months, SES, and gestational age all correlated with degree of language delay at 2 years of age (Vohr, Garcia-Coll, and Oh, in press).

Finally, the increased incidence of soft or suspect neurological findings including fine and gross motor coordination deficits, balancing inefficiencies, and hyperactivity have been documented (Lubchenco, Horner et al., 1963; Vohr & Garcia-Coll, 1985b; Nichel, Bennett, & Lamson, 1982; Black, Brown, & Thomas, 1977). The neurological findings may be of a relatively minor nature in that they do not interfere with activities of daily living. It has become apparent that low-birth-weight infants manifest a multiplicity of learning difficulties that predispose them to academic difficulties in spite of normal intelligence. Drillien (1967) reported on low-birth-weight infant survivors of the pre-intensive-care era (1948–1956) and found that 50% of survivors were placed in special schools for the handicapped and another 25% required special education service. Similarly, Nichel et al. (1982) identified that 64% of children with a birth weight <1000 g born between 1960 and 1972 were in special education placement at a mean age of 10.6 years.

We have followed a cohort of 42 infants (birth weight <1500 g) born in 1975 for seven years (Vohr & Garcia-Coll, 1985b). A total of 54% of the sample required special education or resource help at 7 years. The sample included subgroups of children who were normal, suspect, or abnormal neurologically at one year of age. In the abnormal group, 88% of the children, in the suspect group 50%, and in the normal group 28% were receiving additional educational resource help or were in special education. Children from families with the lowest socioeconomic status were more likely to require comprehensive special education services.

The following questions can still be asked. Do the learning disabilities manifested in low-birth-weight survivors significantly affect academic and work performance in adolescence and in adult life? What modifications can be made in perinatal care to diminish the insults experienced by the central nervous system that are associated with learning problems? And can interventions in the realm of enrichment programs or massive social programs diminish the effects of central nervous system insults on functional outcome?

3.5. Low-Birth-Weight Infants with Chronic Medical Needs

The increased perinatal survival of high-risk infants has resulted in a new population of infants with chronic medical or neurological disorders who are ready for hospital discharge. This heterogeneous group of infants has dependencies on a variety of therapeutic modalities such as nasogastric feeding, gastrostomy feeding, hyperalimentation, home oxygen, home assisted ventilation, cardiorespiratory monitor, frequent suctioning, and recurrent cardiopulmonary resuscitation. Although, fortunately, there are small numbers of these infants, advances in medical management, surgical technique, and improved nutrition have all contributed to their long-term survival.

Consider the "short bowel syndrome" (Tilson, 1980). Infants with severe necrotizing enterocolitis and intestinal atresias that result in surgical bowel resection make up the majority of this population. These infants suffer from the effects of malabsorption, malnutrition, prolonged hospitalization, and failure to thrive. Neurodevelopmental follow-up of these infants indicates a difficult clinical course with signs of overall improvement by 30 months of age (Bohane, Haka-Ikso, Biggar, Hamilton, & Gall, 1979).

Another example is persistent apnea at a time when the infant is otherwise ready for discharge. Apnea and periodic breathing are the most common respiratory control disturbances that occur in premature infants (Henderson-Smart, 1981). Recent work has indicated that apnea of prematurity may be related to prematurity of the central nervous system (Henderson-Smart et al., 1983), although the issue of immaturity versus insult remains unclear. There are as yet a limited number of studies examining the long-term effects of persistent apnea and the need for a home apena monitor. One focus has been on the psychosocial effects of a home apnea monitor on the family (McElroy, Steinschneider, Weinstein, 1986; Vohr, Chen, Garcia-Coll, & Oh, in press). These studies indicate that mothers of infants who require electronic surveillance for a specific medical abnormality experience great stress.

The increased survival of low-birth-weight infants with severe bronchopulmonary dysplasia has resulted in a population of infants with oxygen dependence at the time of hospital discharge. Such infants represent a challenge for home management (Zinman, Franco, & Pizzuti-Daechsel, 1985; Solimano, Smyth, Mann, Albersheim, & Lockitch, 1986) and are known to be at risk for multiple long-term morbidities (Vohr, Bell et al., 1982). Home management of these infants is a complex issue requiring comprehensive parent education and long-term follow-up to address the medical, neurological, and psychosocial issues. Here is yet another example of biological risk coupled with chronic environmental risk.

4. BEHAVIORAL FOLLOW-UP STUDIES

4.1. Neonatal Behavior

Various studies have examined the behavior of the preterm and low-birth-weight infant after medical stabilization or just before discharge from the hospital at various conceptional ages (29 to 44 weeks). Most studies have employed the Neonatal Behavioral Assessment Scales (NBAS) (Brazelton, 1973), although this tool was not initially designed

for use with high-risk infants. In comparison to full-term healthy infants, preterm infants have been found to have lower scores on motoric
responses (Werner, Bartlett, & Siqueland, 1982) and on state control
and regulation (Telzrow, Kang, & Mitchell, 1982). In addition, multivariate studies have found gestational age and birth weight to be significantly related to response decrement, orientation, and motor organization scores (Lester, Emory, Hoffman, & Eitzman, 1976; Sepkoski,
Garcia-Coll, & Lester, 1982).

Thus prematurity and low birth weight affect the newborn's behavioral organization. However, these studies fail to evaluate the processes
by which prematurity and/or low birth weight affects the infant's behaviors. Preterm infants are not only less mature but also more susceptible
to a variety of respiratory, metabolic, and other disorders that require
prolonged hospitalization. Thus the morbidity status places the infant in
very different environmental conditions during the neonatal period.
Another question that remains is the stability of these behavioral observations and their long-term consequences, if any.

In a recent study (Holmes et al., 1982), the differential effects of
gestational age, degree of illness, and length of hospitalization on neonatal behavior were examined. Four groups of infants were compared:
(1) preterm infants (with a mean birth weight of 2096 ± 617 g and
gestational age of 33 ± 2 weeks) residing in an intensive care nursery
(ICN), (2) sick full-term infants residing in an ICN, (3) full-term infants
with prolonged hospitalizations due to maternal illness, and (4) healthy
full-term infants with less than five days of hospitalization. Infants with
perinatal illness (full-term and preterm) performed significantly poorer
on interactive and motoric processes. No significant effects of prematurity were found in any of the behavioral dimensions assessed. The
findings would suggest that degree of illness is a powerful influence on
the neonate's behavior. Because of the small sample size ($N = 44$) and
the inclusion of preterm infants who are not representative of the very-
low-birth-weight infant (≤1500 g), the findings have to be interpreted
cautiously.

However, several other studies have confirmed the effects of perinatal illness on the behavior of premature infants. DiVitto and Goldberg (1979) found that lower ratings for social interactive and motoric
processes were associated with shorter gestational age and greater degree of illness. Sostek, Quinn, and Davitt (1979) compared preterm and
full-term infants in the following categories: healthy, ill without central
nervous system (CNS) involvement, and ill with CNS involvement (e.g.,
seizures, intracranial hemorrhage, spina bifida). Motoric processes were
poorer for prematures than full-terms and also differed according to

diagnostic category: motoric processes were poorest for the ill and CNS group, intermediate for the ill babies, and best for the healthy newborns. In addition, prematures had more marked physiologic responses to stress (excessive startles, tremors, and poor skin color liability) than all full-term groups except the ill group.

In another study with a large sample of preterm infants ($N = 227$, with mean birth weight of 1753 g and gestational age of 33 weeks), the effects of perinatal illness have also been confirmed (Sostek, Davitt, & Renzi, 1982). Even when gestational age was covaried, infants with more perinatal complications scored lower on the response decrement items. Thus the presence and severity of postnatal illness is a strong influence on neonatal behavior.

Other studies suggest that specific medical complications might have differential effects on the newborn's behavior. Preterm infants with Respiratory Distress Syndrome (RDS) were compared with postmature and normal term infants (Field et al., 1978). The preterm infants with RDS were typically floppy, hypotonic, difficult to arouse and to maintain alert, and had weak reflexes, flat affect, and a raspy cry, although they rarely cried. Consequently, they scored lower on interactive and motoric processes, in comparison with the full-term healthy infants. In a more recent study (Anderson et al., unpublished manuscript), we have documented the effects of prematurity as well as the presence and degree of intraventricular hemorrhage (IVH) on neonatal behavior. Four groups of infants were compared: preterm infants with no IVH, preterm infants with IVH I–II, preterm infants with IVH III–IV, and full-term healthy controls. All preterm infants (with or without IVH) scored lower on regulation of state and had a higher number of deviant reflexes. The presence of an IVH (Grade I–II, or III–IV) was associated in addition with lower scores on range of state. A Grade III–IV IVH was also associated with lower motoric and orientation scores. Thus, lower levels of arousal, immature motoric processes, and poor visual orientation differentiated the preterm infants with IVH from preterms without this perinatal complication. These behavioral characteristics may represent early manifestations of visual–perceptual and motoric problems documented in follow-up studies of infants with IVH (Bozynski et al., 1984; Palmer, Dubowitz, Levene, & Dubowitz, 1982; Gaiter, 1982).

Thus, presence, severity, and nature of perinatal illness are important factors in the behavioral characteristics of preterm infants. Although Brazelton's (1973) original formulation of the uses of the NBAS did not include low-birth-weight and other high-risk infants, the revision of this scale (Brazelton, 1984) provides guidelines for its use with these populations. As in the original formulation, Brazelton emphasizes the need to examine the neonate's performance on repeated examinations over several days in the neonatal period. This notion might be more critical with low-birth-weight infants in the process of recovery from perinatal illness.

In a recent study (Lester, Hoffman, & Brazelton, unpublished manuscript), the patterns of change in neonatal behavior were measured and compared in two groups: term and preterm infants born between 26 and 34 weeks of gestation with birth weight ranging from 680 to 2440 g. The infants were tested on the NBAS at 40, 42, and 44 weeks postconceptual age. Full-term infants had higher levels of performance (average scores of the three exams) on orientation, motor and range, and regulation of state scores than preterm infants. Full-term infants also had a narrower range (the difference between the highest and lowest scores) across the three examinations on orientation and state range and regulation. These findings emphasize the need for repeated examinations, since a wider range in performance reflects the variability to be expected in the behavioral responses of preterm infants during the early postnatal period.

Additional studies using other techniques have corroborated some of the findings obtained with the BNBAS and have found other behavioral deficits in preterm and low-birth-weight infants. As stated above, orientation responses of preterm infants are less optimal than those displayed by full-term infants as measured with the NBAS. Riese (1983) reported that preterm twins were less responsive to visual following of bull's-eye and showed less auditory orienting to rattle, bell, voice, and face and voice and alertness during presentation of orienting items.

Other studies of visual responses in low-birth-weight infants report difficulty in maintaining alert, eyes-open states for presenting stimuli as well as less mature patterns of visual preferences (Miranda, 1976). Poorer performance of preterm infants on visual tasks seems to reflect, in part, their developmental immaturity, since when equating them on postconceptual age with full-term infants their pattern preferences are very similar (Fantz, Fagan, & Miranda, 1976). However, in two studies (Kopp, Sigman, Parmelee, & Jeffrey, 1975; Sigman, Kopp, Littman, & Parmelee, 1977), preterm infants tested at 40 weeks postconceptual age looked longer at simple checkerboard stimuli than full-term infants. The authors interpreted this to indicate a more passive, obligatory attention indicating inability to actively control visual fixations. A more recent study (Spungen, Kurtzberg, & Vaughan, 1985) also found that the visual behavior of low-birth-weight infants was more often marked by long, continuous looking at the same pattern, in contrast with shorter, more discrete and rapidly decrementing looks by full-term infants. These authors speculate that aside from reflecting developmental immaturity, the longer looking in preterm infants may also reflect slower information processing, and thus, the longer fixation times might be functionally appropriate behaviors for these infants.

Behavioral responsivity or the infant's reaction to a standard stimulus has also been assessed during the neonatal period in preterm and low-birth-weight infants. Frequently, preterm infants have been characterized as hyporesponsive. Rose, Schmidt, and Bridger (1976) observed a lack of cardiac responding among preterm infants, even to the strongest stimulus. In a subsequent study (Rose, Schmidt, Riese, & Bridger, 1980), the hyporesponsivity was replicated in both cardiac and behavioral measures during quiet and active sleep. However, using stronger stimuli, Field and other colleagues (Field, Dempsey, Hatch, Ting, & Clifton, 1979) have found the magnitude of cardiac responding to auditory and tactile stimulation to be comparable to that observed in full-term infants. Aside from pointing out the importance of the stimulus intensity, higher birth weight and lower prestimulus heart rate seem to be associated with larger cardiac accelerations (responses similar to those found in full-term infants).

However, other studies have characterized preterm infants as hyperresponsive. The study of Field et al. (1979) reported that the preterm infant was unable to habituate to repeated presentations of stimuli. Lack of habituation in the preterm neonate has been found in other laboratories (Eisenberg, Coursin, & Rupp, 1966; Martinius & Papousek, 1970; Rose et al., 1976), as with the BNBAS (Sepkoski et al., 1982). In another study, which examined the preterm's responses to social stimulation (visual, auditory, tactile, and combined auditory and tactile social stimulation), preterm infants were found to be more motorically active and less visually responsive when tactually stimulated (McGehee & Eckerman, 1983). The preterm infant was able to visually orient to a partner but unable to control erratic body movements, gasps and grunts, or frequent shifts in state. The authors suggest that the heightened arousal of the preterm infant could result from hyperresponsivity to stimulation or from heightened sensitivity to stimulation.

Again, all these studies have failed to account for the effects of perinatal illness on the behavioral responses measured. Krafchuk, Tronick, and Clifton (1983) have compared both behavioral and cardiac responses to sound in low-risk (healthy, full-term), moderate-risk (healthy preterm), and high-risk (sick preterm) infants at 36 to 38 weeks of conceptual age. Prematurity was related to higher baseline heart rate and lack of habituation. Degree of illness was related to hyporesponsivity including fewer startles, and increased signs of physiological stress (i.e., more color changes). The investigators characterize preterm infants as both hypo- and hyperreactive, suggesting that they have elevated sensory thresholds as a protective mechanism, but lower response thresholds for making defense reactions to stimuli that are strong enough to pass the sensory threshold. Some preterm infants show both hypo- and hyperresponsivity to stimulation, cannot or do not readily habituate, and have reaction patterns that are more global and diffuse. These characteristics produce an infant who is less available to stimulation but more reactive once a response is initiated. The stability of these observations as an individual difference characteristic is still an open empirical question.

Another aspect of the behavioral repertoire of preterm infants that has been studied during the neonatal period is the characteristics of their cry and soothability. Preterm infants tend to have shorter crying episodes (Lester & Zeskind, 1978) or cry less often (Field et al., 1978; Sostek et al., 1979; Riese, 1984). In addition, acoustic features of the cry have been related to prematurity. Michelsson (1980) reported that the more immature the neonate, the more high-pitched the signals; moreover, the maximum pitch was significantly increased in all prematures irrespective of gestational age. Lester and Zeskind (1978) reported that poor performance on the NBAS plus a low Ponderal Index and short gestation were associated with infant cries of short duration, high fundamental frequency, high maximum frequency, and fewer harmonics in the cry sound. Because of the small sample size, these results should be regarded as preliminary.

However, their importance is indicated by a recent report in which acoustic characteristics of the cry measured at 40 weeks conceptual age in full-term and preterm infants were related to developmental outcome at 18 months and 5 years of age (Lester, 1987). Measures of the frequency characteristics of the cry (i.e., fundamental frequency and the first format) and measures of the amplitude and duration of the cry were significant predictors of developmental outcome. These findings were based on small sample sizes and warrant further investigation.

4.2. Infancy

Several lines of research have looked at the effects of prematurity, low birth weight, and, less often, perinatal illness on behavioral characteristics during the infancy period. Because of the initial behavioral characteristics (e.g., lower visual and auditory orientation) that preterm infants display, they have been characterized as potential "poor" social partners (DiVitto & Goldberg, 1979; Masi & Scott, 1983; McGehee & Eckerman, 1983). Several reports have indeed demonstrated that the preterm infant's interactive capacities are less competent than those displayed by full-term infants during the first few months of life. During interactions with their mothers, preterm infants are less alert, less active, and less responsive than full-term infants during the neonatal period and throughout the first few months of infancy (Bakeman & Brown, 1980; DiVitto & Goldberg, 1979; Field, 1977, 1980).

Although initially mothers of preterm infants are less actively involved with their infants (DiVitto & Goldberg, 1979; Leifer, Leidermen, Barnett, & Williams, 1972), by 4 months mothers of preterm infants stimulate their infants more than mothers of full-term infants do (Bakeman & Brown, 1980; Field, 1977). By this age, preterm infants display more gaze aversion and inattention than full-term infants suggesting that greater maternal activity represents overstimulation for these infants (Field, 1977). In addition, the rhythms of their interactions are different: higher levels of mother–infant synchronicity are found in term dyads than in preterm dyads at both 3 and 5 months of age (Lester et al., 1985). Also, term infants more often led the interaction at both ages. Thus, not only do the behaviors between preterm and full-term infants and their mothers differ, but also the temporal quality of their interactions reflects less synchronicity.

Similar findings have been reported during the second half of the first year of life. In a recent study (Malatesta, Grigoryev, Lamb, Albin, & Culver, 1986), groups of preterm and full-term infants were compared at 2½, 5, and 7½ months of age (corrected age). Preterm infants were found to spend less of their face-to-face interaction in eye contact with their mothers across all ages. In addition, mothers of preterm infants failed to match their infant's surprise and sadness responses and tended to ignore their infant's angry expressions. The authors speculate that these maternal responses are partly influenced by each mother's infant's responses and might have important impjications in the socialization of emotions in preterm infants.

In another longitudinal study, Crawford (1982) reports on the spontaneous interactions observed during two-hour home observations between preterm or full-term infants and their mothers at 6, 8, 10, and 14 months of age. Preterm infants vocalized less, played less, and were more fretful than full-term infants of the same chronological age, but looked at objects and their environment more. These differences with the exception of fewer vocalizations disappeared by 14 months. Mothers of preterm infants demonstrated more caretaking and behavior toward their infants; however, by 14 months these differences disappeared. These findings suggest that at least in some aspects of maternal–infant interactions, preterm infants and their mothers behaved increasingly like full-term infants as the infants get older.

However, research involving laboratory structured observations reveals that other behavioral differences between mothers of preterm and mothers of full-term infants persist longer than the differences in their infants' behavior. Crnic and his colleagues (Crnic et al., 1983) assessed mother–infant interactions at 4, 8, and 12 months of age. Unlike Crawford (1982), they found that preterm infants were less active and less responsive than full-term infants; the infants vocalized and smiled less frequently, averted their gaze and bodies more frequently, and showed less positive general affective tone. This pattern was observed not only at 4 months of age, replicating the findings of several previous investigations, but it was also apparent at 8 and 12 months of age. In fact, differences between mean scores were greater at 8 and 12 months for two infant measures (vocalizations and affect). Mothers of preterm infants were more active and stimulating with their infants during early interactions, and many of these maternal behaviors persisted throughout the first year.

Only one study has assessed mother–infant interactions in preterm and full-term infants beyond the first year of life. Barnard, Bee, and Hammond (1984) observed preterm and term infants during teaching interactions with their mothers at 4, 8, and 24 months of age. Mothers of preterm infants were high in positive, sensitive, well-paced interactions at 4 months of age, but then declined in these areas at 8 and 24 months relative to the mothers of term infants. This pattern was in contrast with that displayed by their infants: preterm infants were least involved and responsive at four months and showed substantial increases in involvement over the next 20 months relative to the term infants. These findings suggest that the differences observed in interaction patterns between mothers of preterm and term infants do not disappear completely by 24 months even when the preterm infants have largely "caught up" in their level of participation in the interaction.

Research with other populations suggests that early patterns of mother–infant interaction relate to the child's social–emotional development, especially their attachment classification (Ainsworth et al., 1978; Main et al., 1979). It has been postulated that these early interactional patterns of preterm infants and their mothers might be related to insecure or avoidant attachment classifications. However, studies so far have found that the behavior of preterm infants in the Ainsworth Strange Situation at one year (corrected age) is not different from that displayed by full-term infants (Bakeman & Brown, 1980; Field et al., 1979). The percentage of securely attached infants found among preterm infants is similar to that observed in normative studies of full-term dyads (Rode, Chang, Niau, Fisch, & Scroufe, 1981; Frodi & Thompson, 1985; Goldberg, Perotta, Minde, & Corter, 1986). These findings suggest that the early responses of preterm infants and their mothers might be adaptive to the behavioral repertoire of these infants, and the development of a secure attachment might be possible from these early interactions.

Another possibility is that there are other consequences of these early interactions. Beckwith and her colleaues (Beckwith et al., 1976; Cohen & Beckwith, 1979) made naturalistic observations in the home when the infants were 1, 3, and 8 months of age and related them to 9- and 24-months test performances. The infant's and caregiver's readiness to engage at one month of age in positive social interactions with each other as in mutual gaze, mutual smiling, social play, and talking appeared to be very significant in test performance at 2 years of age. The low level of social interactions during the first year among preterm infants and their mothers was predictive of lowered infant competence at age 2. Since the correlations were smaller or different in nature at nine months of age, these findings suggest the need for longer-term follow-up.

Fewer studies have assessed other behavioral characteristics of preterm infants during the infancy period. One area of research has been the infant's visual responses to familiar and novel stimuli. Although total attention time to a variety of stimuli is similar by 4 months of age, full-term infants show a novelty preference not demonstrated by preterm infants (Sigman & Parmelee, 1974). Other investigations have noted deficits in immediate recognition memory among preterm infants relative to the performance of full-term infants. Rose, Gottfried, and Bridger (1979) reported poorer performances in visual recognition of objects at 6 and 12 months (corrected age) in preterm infants than in full-term infants. In addition, Rose (1980) found inferior performances on tests of visual recognition at 28 weeks (corrected age) by preterm infants.

However, in this particular study and in another previous study with 8-month old infants (Sigman, 1976), it has been shown that with a longer familiarization process, preterm infants showed similar preferences for the novel stimulus. Both studies suggest that preterm infants are capable of storing and retrieving information, but that they take longer to process the information than full-term infants. This might be compounded by the fact that preterm infants show longer latencies to examine (focused visual inspection) resulting in less examination time of the stimulus (Russ, 1986).

Again, the degree of perinatal illness, although not examined in these studies, might be an important factor in the infant's exploratory capacities. Ruff, McCarton, Kurtzberg, and Vaughan (1984) reported no differences between preterm and full-term 9-month-old infants in their exploration of novel objects. However, high-risk preterm infants fingered, rotated, and transferred the objects less than either the full-term or low-risk preterms. The data suggest that earlier medical and neurobehavioral history are strong determinants of the preterm infant's manipulative exploration of objects.

Other research using the framework of infant temperament has compared preterm and full-term infants in their temperamental characteristics during the infancy period. Since preterm infants differ in their behavioral characteristics during the neonatal period, it has been hypothesized that they would have different temperamental characteristics during the infancy period. Most studies have used parental reports, which are subject to different biases (Bates et al., 1979; Vaughn et al., 1980, 1981). These studies have found consistently that parents of preterm infants tend to rate their infant's temperaments as more difficult during the first year of life (Medoff-Cooper, in press; Medoff-Cooper & Schraeder, 1982; Schraeder & Medoff-Cooper, 1983; Spungen & Farran, 1986). However, direct behavioral observations were not done, and the findings might be more a reflection of parents' experiences or attitudes.

In a recent study, we have found that preterm infants showed less positive responses and less overall activity level in response to stimulation (Garcia-Coll et al., 1988). Thus the diminished responsiveness previously identified in preterm infants during the perinatal period (McGehee & Eckerman, 1983; Rose et al., 1976) is still present at 3 months corrected age. In addition, infants who had intraventricular hemorrhages Grade I–II were less sociable and more difficult to sooth. These findings are consistent with the clinical literature on neurological syndromes, which has noted a relationship between mild brain insult and exaggerated negative responses to stimulation (Schaeffer, 1968; Sarnat & Sarnat. 1976; Robertson & Finer, 1985). Our findings emphasize the importance of dividing preterm and low-birth-weight infants into subgroups according to their perinatal course in order to identify the relative contribution of prematurity, low birth weight, and perinatal illness in the development of behavioral characteristics.

4.3. Long-Term Follow-up

Fewer studies have examined the behavioral characteristics of preterm and low-birth-weight infants beyond the infancy period. Early studies, which were either retrospective or employed unsystematic measures, suggested that prematurely born children were more irritable, were poor sleepers, and lacked concentration and attention (Benton,

1940). Knobloch, Rider, Harper, and Pasamanick, (1956) and Lilienfeld, Pasamanick, and Rogers (1955) also found that a higher percentage of prematurely born children were reported by their teachers to show disorganized, hyperactive, and confused behaviors at 2 years of age. These findings were repeated in a large-scale study conducted in England (Douglas, 1960). In a recent study conducted in Australia (Astbury, Orgill, Bajuk, & Yu, 1985), early attentional deficits have also been reported; 34% of infants with a birth weight <1500 g showed symptoms of Attention Deficit Disorder (e.g., difficulty in complying with situational demands during psychological testing including too much activity, little sustained attention, and inhibition of impulsive behavior).

The important role of the environment in the behavioral development of prematurely born children is suggested by Drillien (1964), who undertook the first truly comprehensive follow-up study of premature infants. Teachers' and observers' reports of behavior maladjustment were associated with low birth weight, low SES, "problematic mothers," and life stress. Early birth seemed to have made some children more vulnerable to the difficulties within their particular environment.

Perinatal illness is also a contributing factor. Werner and her colleagues (Werner, Bierman, & French, 1971; Werner & Smith, 1977,) found that prematurity alone did not contribute to serious mental health problems at age 10 or 18. On the other hand, children who had suffered moderate or severe perinatal stress (e.g., asphyxia, respiratory distress syndrome) regardless of their birth weight had a higher rate of serious mental health problems than did the total cohort. Field and her colleagues (Field, Dempsey, & Shuman, 1979) reported behavioral data on premature infants surviving respiratory distress syndrome at 4 years of age. More behavioral and minimal brain dysfunction symptoms were found among the prematurely born than the controls.

Needless to say, large-scale longitudinal studies of the high-risk populations of the 1980s that assess behavioral development from infancy into childhood are needed. These studies should go beyond just documenting full-term/preterm low-birth-weight comparisons, and they should look at the processes by which prematurity, perinatal illness, and social-environmental factors affect behavior development.

5. SUMMARY AND CONCLUSIONS

The low-birth-weight graduate of a neonatal intensive care unit, because of his or her history, is automatically considered "at risk." Yet because of the heterogenicity of this population and its constantly changing character over time, the degree of risk for further morbidity is often unclear. The model for neurological, cognitive, and behavioral development is complex with the interaction of biological, social–environmental, recovery, and relapse factors producing results that cannot be easily predicted.

The research of the last 25 to 35 years has resulted in a clearer picture of normal child development, improved medical, diagnostic, and treatment techniques, and more sophisticated and standardized testing procedures for evaluating the neurobehavioral and cognitive status of normal and at-risk infant and children. Physicians and psychologists have become better observers and recorders and have taken greater initiatives in developing innovative approaches to early childhood research.

There has been an increased awareness of such factors as the continuum of development and the plasticity of the central nervous system for recovery. The value of a single observation in time to determine outcome has dropped as the importance of sequential and longitudinal observations and assessments has become substantiated.

5.1. A Schema for Follow-up Studies

Collaboration of professionals in a multidisciplinary evaluation and diagnostic team for comprehensive longitudinal assessments has become the contemporary format for more sophisticated follow-up research studies incorporating technical, medical, behavioral, neurological, developmental, and social–environmental components. The fact that the outcome of low-birth-weight infants is based on a continuum of events rather than any single biological, social, or behavioral event emphasizes the importance of repetitive assessments of varying magnitude at specific critical time periods. As shown in Table 4, this format requires the collaboration of multiple professionals including the perinatologist, neonatologist, social worker, pediatrician, the follow-up evaluation team, and a variety of resources within the community. Participation of any single professional may occur during specific time intervals or over a prolonged period. It is an ambitious, time-consuming, and expensive undertaking to plan and complete prospective long-term studies. Clearly, with continued attempts to plan and successfully carry out both short-term and longitudinal studies, we will continue to learn more about the etiology, prevention, and treatment of morbidities found in low-birth-weight infants.

We can conclude that there is still a great deal we do not know about the development of high-risk infants. The impact of perinatal, neonatal, and early childhood events on subsequent functioning at school age and

TABLE 4. A Schema for Follow-up Studies

Timing	Fetal	Neonatal	First year/2–7 years	Adolescent / School age adult
Assessor	Perinatologist	Neonatologist Social worker	Pediatrician Neurologist Physical therapist Educator	Psychologist Ophthalmologist Audiologist Social worker Statistician
Assessment	Hypoxia, acidosis, biochemical derangements, growth, hydrocephalus, chromosomal	Physiological, biochemical growth parameters, neurological behavior	Neurological, developmental, behavioral, temperament, visual, auditory, educational status	
Technique/ Treatment	Amniocentesis, ultrasound, CT, stress test, non-stress test	Comprehensive NICU Management Brazelton	EEG, ultrasound, NMR, neurological exam, ABR, VER, ophthalmological, audiological, SES, and life stress/social support assessment observation	

in the adult and the further development of prevention, intervention, and treatment methodologies will continue to be important areas for investigation.

Acknowledgments

The authors wish to acknowledge the assistance of Jeannine Nadeau and Kathy Daigneault in the preparation of this manuscript.

6. REFERENCES

Ahman, P. A., Lazzara, A., Dykes, F. D., Brann, A. W., Jr., & Schwartz, J. F. (1980). Intraventricular hemorrhage in the high risk preterm infant: Incidence and outcome. *Annals of Neurology, 7*, 118–124.

Ainsworth, M. D. S., Bell, S. M., & Stayton, D. J. (1971). Individual differences in strange situation behavior of one-year olds. In H. R. Schaffer (Ed.), *The origins of human social relations.* London: Academic Press.

Ainsworth, M. D. S., Bell, S. M., & Stayton, D. J. (1972). Individual differences in the development of some attachment behaviors. *Merrill-Palmer Quarterly, 18*, 123–143.

Ainsworth, M. D. S., Blehar, M. C., Waters, E., & Wall, S. (1978). *Patterns of attachment: A psychological study of the Strange Situation.* Hillsdale, NH: Erlbaum.

Amiel-Tison, C. (1968). Neurological examination of the maturity of newborn infants. *Archives of Diseases of Childhood, 43*, 89–93.

Anderson, L., Garcia-Coll, C., Vohr, B. R., Emmons, L., Brann, B., Shaul, P. W., Mayfield, S. R., & Oh, W. *Behavioral characteristics and early temperament of preterm infants with intraventricular hemorrhage during the neonatal period.* Unpublished manuscript submitted 1987.

Anwar, M., Kadam, S., Hiatt, I. M., & Hegyi, T. (1985). Serial lumbar punctures in prevention of post hemorrhagic hydrocephalus in preterm infants. *Journal of Pediatrics, 107*, 446–450.

Astbury, J., Orgill, A. A., Bajuk, B., & Yu, V. Y. H. (1985). Neonatal and neurodevelopmental significance of behavior in very low birthweight-children. *Early Human Development, 11*, 113–121.

Avery, M. E., & Mead, J. (1959). Surface properties in relation to atelectasis and hyaline membrane disease. *American Journal of Disease in Children, 97*, 517–523.

Babcock, D. S., & Han, B. K. (1981). The accuracy of high resolution real-time ultrasonography of the head in infancy. *Radiology, 139*, 665–676.

Bada, H. S., Korones, S. B., Anderson, G. D., Magill, H. L., & Wong, S. P. (1984). Obstetric factors and relative risk of neonatal germinal layer/intraventricular hemorrhage. *American Journal of Obstetrics and Gynecology, 148*, 798–804.

Bada, H. S., Korones, S. B., Magill, H. L., & Anderson, G. D. (1982). Influence of the mode of delivery on the recurrence of intraventricular hemorrhage. *Pediatric Research, 16*, 275, Abstract No. 1181.

Bakeman, R., & Brown, J. (1980). Early interaction: Consequences for social and mental development at three years. *Child Development, 51*, 437–447.

Bakwin, H. (1923). Oxygen therapy in premature babies with anoxemia. *American Journal of Diseases of Children, 25*, 157.

Ballard, J. L., Novak, K. K., & Driver, M. (1979). A simplified score for assessment of fetal maturation of newly born infants. *Journal of Pediatrics, 95,* 769–774.

Bard, H. (1978). Neonatal problems of infants with intrauterine growth retardation. *Journal of Reproductive Medicine, 21,* 359–364.

Barnard, K. E., Bee, H. L., & Hammond, M. A. (1984). Developmental changes in maternal interactions with term and preterm infants. *Infant Behavior and Development, 7,* 101–113.

Barnard, K. E., Hammond, M. A., Booth, C. L., Bee, H. L., Mitchell, S. K., and Spieker, S. J. (in press). Measurement and meaning of parent-child interaction. In F. Morrison, C. Lord, & D. Keating (Eds.), *Applied developmental psychology: Volume 3.* San Diego: Academic Press.

Barnet, A. B., Friedman, S. L., Weiss, I. P., Ohlrich, E. S., Shanks, B., & Lodge, A. (1980). VER development in infancy and early childhood. A longitudinal study. *Electroencephalography and Clinical Neurophysiology, 49,* 476–489.

Bates, J. (1987). Temperament in infancy. In J. D. Osofsky (Ed.), *Handbook of infant development* (2nd ed.). New York: Wiley.

Bates, J. E., Freeland, C. A., & Lounsbury, M. L. (1979). Measurement of infant difficultness. *Child Development, 50,* 794–803.

Bayley, N. (1969). *Manual for the Bayley Scales of Infant Development.* New York: The Psychological Corp.

Beckwith, L., Cohen, S. E., Kopp, C. B., Parmelee, A. H., & Marcy, T. G. (1976). Caregiver-infant interaction and early cognitive development in preterm infants. *Child Development, 47:* 579–587.

Beery, K. E., & Buktenican, N. A. (1967). *Developmental test of visual-motor integration.* Chicago: Follett.

Bennett, F. C., Robinson, N. M., & Sells, C. J. (1982). Hyaline membrane disease. Birth weight and gestational age. *American Journal of Diseases of Children, 136,* 888–891.

Bennett, F. C., Robinson, N. M., & Sells, C. J. (1983). Growth and development of infants weighing less than 800 grams at birth. *Pediatrics, 71,* 319–323.

Benton, A. L. (1940). Mental development of prematurely born children. *American Journal of Orthopsychiatry, 10,* 719–746.

Berendes, H. W. (1966). The structure and scope of the collaborative project on cerebral palsy, mental retardation, and other neurological and sensory disorders of infancy and childhood. In S. S. Chipman, A. M. Lillienfeld, B. G. Greenberg, & J. F. Donnelly (Eds.), *Research, methodology and needs in perinatal studies.* Springfield, IL: Charles C Thomas.

Black, B., Brown, C., & Thomas, D. (1977). A follow-up of 58 preschool children less than 1500 grams birth weight. *Australian Paediatrics Journal, 13,* 265–270.

Bohane, T. D., Haka-Ikso, K., Biggar, W. D., Hamilton, J. R., & Gall, D. G. (1979). A clinical study of young infants after small intestinal resection. *Journal of Pediatrics, 94,* 552–558.

Bozynski, M. E., Nelson, M. N., Genaze, D., Rosati-Skertich, C., Chilcote, W. S., Ramsey, R. G., O'Donnell, K. J., & Meier, W. A. (1984). Intracranial hemorrhage and neurodevelopmental outcome at one year in infants weighing 1200 grams or less: Prognostic significance of ventriculomegaly at term gestational age. *American Journal of Perinatology, 1*(4), 325–330.

Bradley, R., & Caldwell, B. (1976). The relation of infants' home environments to mental test performance at fifty-four months: A follow-up study. *Child Development, 47,* 1172–1174.

Brazelton, T. B. (1973). Neonatal behavioral assessment scale. In *Clinics in Developmental Medicine,* No. 50. Philadelphia: Lippincott.

Brazelton, T. B. (1984). Neonatal behavioral assessment scale (2nd ed.). In *Clinics in Developmental Medicine*, No. 88. Philadelphia: Lippincott.

Brazelton, T. B., Koslowski, B., & Main, M. (1974). The origins of mother-infant interaction. In M. Lewis & L. A. Rosenblum (Eds.), *The effect of the infant on its caregiver.* New York: Wiley.

Bretherton, I., & Waters, E. (1985). Growing points of attachment theory and research. *Monographs of the Society for Research in Child Development, 50*(1–2, Serial No. 209).

Britton, S. B., Fitzhardinge, P. M., & Ashby, S. (1981). Is intensive care justified for infants weighing less than 801 grams at birth? *Journal of Pediatrics, 99,* 937–943.

Buckwald, S., Zorn, W. A., & Egan, E. (1984). Mortality and follow-up data for neonates weighing 500–800 grams at birth. *American Journal of Diseases of Children, 138,* 779–782.

Burstein, J., Papile, L., & Burstein, R. (1977). Subependymal germinal matrix and intraventricular hemorrhage in premature infants: Diagnoses by CT. *American Journal of Roentgenology, 128,* 971–976.

Caldwell, B. M. (1979). *Home observation for measurement of the environment (HOME).* Little Rock: University of Arkansas, Center for Early Development and Education.

Carey, W. B., & McDevitt, S. (1978). Revision of the infant temperament questionnaire. *Pediatrics, 61,* 735–739.

Chiswick, M. L., Johnson, M., Woodhall, C., Gowland, M., Davis, J., Toner, N., & Sims, D. G. (1983). Protective effect of Vitamin E (DL-alpha-tocopherol) against intraventricular hemorrhage in premature babies. *British Medical Journal, 287,* 81–84.

Clarke-Stewart, K. A. (1973). Interactions between mothers and their young children: Characteristics and consequences. *Monographs of the Society for Research in Child Development, 38*(5–6, Serial No. 153).

Clarren, S. K., & Smith, D. W. (1978). The fetal alcohol syndrome. *New England Journal of Medicine, 298,* 1063–1067.

Cohen, S. E., & Beckwith, L. (1977). Caregiving behaviors and early cognitive development are related to ordinal position in preterm infants. *Child Development, 48,* 152–157.

Cohen, S. E., & Beckwith, L. (1979). Preterm infant interaction with the caregiver in the first year of life and competence at age two. *Child Development, 50,* 767–766.

Cohen, S. E., Parmalee, A. H., Beckwith, L., & Sigman, M. (1986). Cognitive development in preterm infants: Birth to 8 years. *Developmental and Behavioral Pediatrics, 7,* 102–110.

Commey, J. O., & Fitzhardinge, P. M. (1979). Handicap in the preterm small-for-gestational age infant. *Journal of Pediatrics, 94*(5), 779–786.

Connell, D. B. (1976). *Individual differences in attachment: An investigation into stability, implications and relationships to structure of early language development.* Unpublished doctoral dissertation. University of Syracuse.

Cornblath, M., Wybregt, S. H., Baens, G. S., & Klein, R. I. (1964). Symptomatic neonatal hypoglycemia. Studies of carbohydrate metabolism in the newborn infant, VIII. *Pediatrics, 33,* 388–402.

Cox, L. C., Hack, M., & Metz, D. A. (1984). Auditory brain stem response abnormalities in the very low birth weight infant: Incidence and risk factors. *Ear and Hearing, 5,* 47–51.

Crawford, J. W. (1982). Mother-infant interaction in premature and full term infants. *Child Development, 53,* 957–962.

Crnic, K. A., Ragozin, A. S., Greenberg, M. T., Robinson, N. M., & Basham, R. B. (1983). Social interaction and developmental competence of preterm and full-term infants during the first year of life. *Child Development, 54,* 1199–1210.

Crockenberg, S. B. (1981). Infant irritability, mother responsiveness, and social support influences on the security of mother-infant attachment. *Child Development, 52,* 857–865.

Delphy, D. T., Gordon, R. E., Hope, P. L., Parker, D., Reynolds, E. O. R., Shaw, D., & Whitehead, M. D. (1982). Noninvasive investigations of cerebral ischemia by phosphorus nuclear magnetic resonance. *Pediatrics, 70,* 310–313.

Dinwiddie, R., Mellor, D. H., Donaldson, S. H. C., Tunstall, M. E., & Russell, G. (1974). Quality of survival after artificial ventilation of the newborn. *Archives of Diseases of Childhood, 49,* 703–710.

DiVitto, B., & Goldberg, S. (1979). The effects of newborn medical status on early parent-infant interaction. In T. M. Field, A. M. Sostek, S. Goldberg, & H. H. Shuman (Eds.), *Infants born at risk.* New York: Spectrum.

Douglas, J. W. B. (1960). "Premature" children at primary school. *British Medical Journal, 1,* 1008–1013.

Drillien, C. M. (1959). Physical and mental handicaps in the prematurely born. *Journal of Obstetrics and Gynaecology of the British Community, 66,* 721.

Drillien, C. M. (1964). *The growth and development of the prematurely born infant.* Edinburgh: Livingstone.

Drillien, C. M. (1967). The incidence of mental and physical handicaps in school age children of very low birth weight, II. *Pediatrics, 39,* 238–247.

Drillien, C. M. (1970). The small-for-date infant etiology and prognosis. *Pediatric Clinics of North America, 17,* 9–24.

Dubowitz, L. M., Dubowitz, V., & Goldberg, C. (1970). Clinical assessment of gestational age in the newborn infant. *Journal of Pediatrics, 77,* 1–10.

Dubowitz, V., & Dubowitz, L. (1981). The neurological assessment of the preterm and full term newborn infant. *Clinics in Developmental Medicine, 79,* 10–44.

Dunham, E. C. (1948). *Premature infants* (Children's Bureau Publication). Washington, D.C.: U.S. Government Printing Office, *325,* 42–43.

Dunham, E. C., & Bierman, J. M. (1940). Care of premature infants. *Journal of the American Medical Association, 115,* 658–662.

Edwards, D. K., Hilton, S. W., Merritt, T. A., Hallman, M., Mannino, F., & Boynton, B. R. (1985). Respiratory distress syndrome treated with human surfactant: Radiographic findings. *Radiology, 15,* 329–334.

Ehle, A., & Sklar, F. (1979). Visual evoked potentials in infants with hydrocephalus. *Neurology, 29,* 1541–1544.

Ehrenhranz, R. A., Bonta, B. W., Arlow, R. C., & Warshaw, J. B. (1978). Amelioration of bronchopulmonary dysplasia after vitamin E administration. *New England Journal of Medicine, 299,* 564–569.

Eisenberg, R. B., Coursin, D. B., & Rupp, N. R. (1966). Habituation to an acoustic pattern as an index of differences among human neonates. *Journal of Auditory Research, 6,* 239–248.

Elardo, R., Bradley, R., & Caldwell, B. (1975). The relation of infants home environments to mental test performance from six to thirty-six months: A longitudinal analysis. *Child Development, 46,* 71–76.

Elardo, R., Bradley, R., & Caldwell, B. (1977). A longitudinal study of the relation of infants' home environments to language development at age three. *Child Development, 48,* 595–603.

Enhorning, G., Shennen, A., Possmayer, F., Dunn, M., Chen, C. P., & Milligan, J. (1985). Prevention of neonatal respiratory distress syndrome by tracheal instillation of surfactant: A randomized clinical trial. *Pediatrics, 76,* 45–153.

Escalona, S. K. (1982). Babies at double hazard: Early development of infants at biologic and social risk. *Pediatrics, 70*(5), 670–676.

Escalona, S. K. (1984). Social and other environmental influences on the cognitive and personality development of low birthweight infants. *American Journal of Mental Deficiency, 88*(5), 508–512.

Fantz, R. L., Fagan, J. F., & Miranda, S. (1976). Early visual selectivity as a function of pattern variables, previous exposure, age from birth and conception, and expected cognitive deficit. In L. B. Cohen & P. Salapatek (Eds.), *Infant perception: From sensation to cognition: Vol. 1*. New York: Academic Press.

Farr, V., Mitchell, R. G., Neligan, G. A., & Parker, J. M. (1966). The definition of some external characteristics used in the assessment of gestational age in the newborn infant. *Developmental Medicine and Child Neurology, 8*, 507–511.

Farrell, P. M., & Avery, M. E. (1975). State of the art: Hyaline membrane disease. *American Review of Respiratory Disease, 111*, 657–688.

Field, T. M. (1977). Effects of early separation, interactive deficits, and experimental manipulation on mother-infant interaction. *Child Development, 48*, 763–771.

Field, T. M. (1979). Interaction patterns of preterm and term infants. (1979). In T. M. Field, A. M. Sostek, S. Goldberg, & H. H. Shuman (Eds.), *Infants born at risk*. New York: Spectrum.

Field, T. M. (1980). Interactions of preterm and term infants with their lower- and middle-class teenage and adult mothers. In T. M. Field, S. Goldberg, D. Stern, & A. Sostek (Eds.), *High-risk infants and children: Adult and peer interactions*. New York: Academic Press.

Field, T. M., Dempsey, J. R., Hatch, J., Ting, G., & Clifton, R. K. (1979). Cardiac and behavioral responses to repeated tactile and auditory stimulation by preterm and term neonates. *Developmental Psychology, 15*, 406–416.

Field, T. M., Dempsey, J., & Shuman, H. H. (1979). Developmental assessments of infants surviving the respiratory distress syndrome. In T. M. Field, A. Sostek, S. Goldberg, & H. H. Shuman (Eds.), *Infants born at risk*. New York: Spectrum.

Field, T. M., Hallock, N., Ting, G., Dempsey, J., Dabiri, C., & Shuman, H. H. (1978). A first year follow-up of high risk infants: Formulating a cumulative risk index. *Child Development, 49*, 119–131.

Field, T. M., Widmayer, S. M., Ignatoff, E., & Stringer, S. (1982). Developmental effects of an intervention for preterm infants of teenage mothers. *Infant Mental Health Journal, 1*, 19–27.

Field, T. M., Widmayer, S. M., Stringer, S., & Ignatoff, E. (1980). Teenage, lower-class, black mothers and their preterm infants: An intervention and developmental follow-up. *Child Development, 51*, 426–436.

Fitzhardinge, P. M., Flodmark, O., Fitz, C. R., & Ashby, S. (1982). The prognostic value of computed tomography of the brain in asphyxiated preterm infants. *Journal of Pediatrics, 100*, 476.

Fitzhardinge, P. M., Pape, K., Arstihaitis, M., Boyle, M., Ashby, S., Rowley, A., Netley, C., & Swyer, P. R. (1976). Mechanical ventilation of infants of less than 1501 grams birth weight: Health, growth, and neurologic sequelae. *Journal of Pediatrics, 88*, 531–541.

Fitzhardinge, P. M., & Ramsey, M. (1973). The improving outlook for the small prematurely born infant. *Developmental Medicine and Child Neurology, 15*, 447–459.

Fitzhardinge, P. M., & Steven, E. M. (1972a). The small-for-date infant. I. Later growth patterns. *Pediatrics, 49*, 671–681.

Fitzhardinge, P. M., & Steven, E. M. (1972b). The small-for-date infant. II. Neurological and intellectual sequelae. *Pediatrics, 50*, 50–57.

Francis-Williams, J., & Davies, P. A. (1974). Very low birth weight and later intelligence. *Developmental Medicine and Child Neurology, 16,* 709–728.

Frodi, A., & Thompson, R. (1985). Infants' affective responses in the strange situation: Effects of prematurity and of quality of attachment. *Child Development, 56,* 1280–1290.

Fujiwara, T., Chida, S., Watabe, Y., Maeta, H., Morita, T., & Abe, T. (1980). Artificial surfactant therapy in hyaline membrane disease. *Lancet, 1,* 55–59.

Fullard, W., McDevitt, S. C., & Carey, W. B. (1984). Assessing temperament in one to three year old children. *Journal of Pediatric Psychology, 9,* 205–217.

Fuller, P. W., Guthrie, R. D., & Alvord, E. C. (1983). A proposed neuropathological basis for learning disabilities in children born prematurely. *Developmental Medicine and Child Neurology, 25,* 214–231.

Gaiter, J. L. (1982). The effects of intraventricular hemorrhage on Bayley developmental performance in preterm infants. *Seminars in Perinatology, 6,* 305–316.

Garcia-Coll, C. T., Emmons, L., Vohr, B. R., Ward, A. M., Brann, B. S., Shaul, P. W., Mayfield, S. R., & Oh, W. (March, 1988). Behavioral responsiveness in preterm infants with intraventricular hemorrhage (IVH). *Pediatrics.*

Garcia-Coll, C. T., Kagan, J., & Reznick, J. S. (1984). Behavioral inhibition in young children. *Child Development, 55,* 1005–1019.

Garcia-Coll, C. T., Vohr, B. R., Hoffman, J., & Oh, W. (1986). Maternal and environmental factors affecting developmental outcome of infants of adolescent mothers. *Journal of Developmental and Behavioral Pediatrics, 7*(4), 230–236.

Genn, M. M., & Sulverman, W. A. (1964). The mental development of ex-premature children with retrolental fibroplasia. *Journal of Nervous and Mental Diseases, 138,* 79–86.

George, C., & Main, M. (1979). Social interactions of young abused children: Approach, avoidance, and aggression. *Child Development, 50,* 306–318.

Gitlin, J. D., Soll, R. F., Parad, R. B., Horbar, J. D., Feldman, H. A., Lucey, J. F., & Taeusch, H. W. (1987). Randomized controlled trial of exogenous surfactant for the treatment of hyaline membrane disease. *Pediatrics, 79,* 31–37.

Gluck, L. K., Kulovich, V. M., Borer, R. C., Jr., Brenner, P. H., Anderson, G. G., & Spellacy, W. N. (1971). Diagnosis of the respiratory distress syndrome by amniocentesis. *American Journal of Obstetrics and Gynecology, 109,* 440–445.

Goldberg, R. N., Chung, D., Goldman, S. L., & Bancalari, E. (1980). The association of rapid volume expansion and intraventricular hemorrhage in the preterm infant. *Journal of Pediatrics, 96,* 1060–1063.

Goldberg, S., Perrotta, M., Minde, K., & Corter, C. (1986). Maternal behavior and attachment in low-birthweight twins and singletons. *Child Development, 57,* 34–46.

Grant, I. G., Borts, F. T., Schelliuger, D., McCullough, D. C., Sivasubramanian, K. N., & Smith, Y. (1981). Real-time ultrasonography of neonatal intraventricular hemorrhage and comparison with computed sonography. *Radiology, 139,* 687–691.

Gruenwald, P. (1963). Chronic fetal distress and placental insufficiency. *Biology Neonate, 5,* 215–265.

Gutierrez, S. M. (1986). *Determinants of complexity in Mexican-American and Anglo-American mothers' conceptions of child development.* Unpublished doctoral dissertation, University of Illinois, Chicago.

Guzzetta, F., Shackelford, G. D., Volpe, S., Perlman, J. M., & Volpe, J. J. (1986). Periventricular intraparenchymal echodensities in the premature newborn: Critical determinant of neurologic outcome. *Pediatrics, 78,* 995–1006.

Hack, M., Caron, B., Rivers, A., & Fanaroff, A. A. (1983). The very low birth weight infant: The broader spectrum of morbidity during infancy and early childhood. *Development and Behavior Pediatrics, 4,* 243–249.

Hack, M., Fanaroff, A. A., & Merkatz, K. R. (1979). The low birth weight infants: Evolution of a changing outlook. *New England Journal of Medicine, 301,* 1162.

Hack, M., Merkatz, I. R., Gordon, D., Jones, P. K., & Fanaroff, A. A. (1982). The prognostic significance of postnatal growth in very low birth weight infants. *American Journal of Obstetrics and Gynecology, 143,* 693–699.

Hadlock, F. P., Deter, R. L., & Harrist, R. B. (1982). Fetal biparieta diameter. A critical re-evaluation of the relation to menstrual age by means of real-time ultrasound. *Journal of Ultrasound Medicine, 1,* 97.

Hallman, M., Merritt, A. T., Schneider, H., Epstein, B. L., Mannino, F., Edwards, D. K., & Gluck, L. (1983). Isolation of human surfactant from amniotic fluid and a pilot study of its efficacy is respiratory distress syndrome. *Pediatrics, 71,* 473–482.

Hardy, J. B., & Mellits, E. G. (1977). Relationships of low birth weight to maternal characteristics of age, parity, education, and body size. In D. M. Reed & F. H. Stanley (Eds.), *The epidemiology of prematurity.* Baltimore: Urban and Schwarenberg.

Harvey, D., Prince, J., Burton, J., Parkinson, C., & Campbell, S. (1982). Abilities of children who were small-for-gestational age babies. *Pediatrics, 69,* 296–300.

Hegvick, R. L., McDevitt, S. C., & Carey, W. B. (1982). The middle childhood temperament questionnaire. *Journal of Developmental and Behavioral Pediatrics, 3,* 197–200.

Henderson-Smart, D. J. (1981). The effect of gestational age on the incidence and duration of recurrent apnea in newborn babies. *Austrian Pediatric Journal, 17,* 273–276.

Henderson-Smart, D. J., Pettigrew, A. G., & Campbell, D. J. (1983). Clinical apnea and brain stem neural function in preterm infants. *New England Journal of Medicine, 308*(7), 353–357.

Hess, J. H. (1953). Experiences gained in a thirty year study of prematurely born infants. *Pediatrics, 11,* 425–434.

Hill, A., Perlman, J. M., & Volpe, J. J. (1982). Relationship of pneumothorax to occurrence of intraventricular hemorrhage in the premature newborn. *Pediatrics, 69,* 144–149.

Hill, A., & Volpe, J. J. (1981). Normal pressure hydrocephalus in the newborn. *Pediatrics, 68,* 623–629.

Hillis, A. (1982). Vitamin E in retrolental fibroplasia. *New England Journal of Medicine, 306,* 867.

Hirata, T., Epcar, J. T., Walsh, A., Mednick, J., Harris, M., McGinnis, M. S., Sehring, S., & Papedo, G. (1983). Survival and outcome of infants 501–570 grams: A six-year experience. *Journal of Pediatrics, 102,* 741–748.

Hiskey, M. S. (1966). *Manual, Hiskey-Nebraska test of learning aptitude.* Lincoln, NE: Union Colley Press.

Hittner, H. M., Godio, L. B., Rudolph, A. J., Adams, J. M., Garcia-Prats, J. A., Friedman, A., Kautz, J. A., & Monaco, W. A. (1981). Retrolental fibroplasia: Efficacy of vitamin E in a double-blind clinical study of preterm infants. *New England Journal of Medicine, 305,* 1365–1371.

Hobel, C. J., Hyvarinen, M. A., Okada, D. M., & Oh, W. (1973). Prenatal and intrapartum high risk screening. I. Prediction of the high-risk neonate. *American Journal of Obstetrics and Gynecology, 117,* 1–9.

Hollingshead, A. B. (1975). *Four factor index of social status.* New Haven, CN: Unpublished manuscript.

Holmes, D. L., Nagy, J. N., Slaymaker, G., Sosnoroski, R. J., Prinz, S. M., & Pasternak, J. F. (1982). Early influences of prematurity, illness, and prolonged hospitalization on infant behavior. *Developmental Psychology, 18*(5), 744–750.

Hubatch, L. M., Johnson, C. J., Kistler, D. J., Burns, W. J., & Moneha, W. (1985). Early language abilities of high risk infants. *Journal of Speech and Hearing Disorders, 50,* 195–207.

Hubert, N. C., Wachs, T. D., Peters-Martin, P., & Gandour, J. (1982). The study of early temperament: Measurement and conceptual issues. *Child Development, 53,* 571–600.

Humbert, J., Abelson, H., Hathaway, W. E., Battaglia, F. C. (1969). Polycythemia in small for gestational age infants. *Journal of Pediatrics, 75,* 812–819.

Hunt, J. V., Tooley, W. H., & Harven, D. (1982). Learning disabilities in children with birth weights ≤1500 grams. *Seminars in Perinatology, 6,* 266–273.

Ikegami, M., Agata, Y., Eldaky, T., Hallman, M., Berry, D., & Jobe, A. (1987). Comparison of four surfactants: In vitro surface properties and responses of preterm lambs to treatment at birth. *Pediatrics, 79,* 38–46.

Ikegami, M., Silverman, J., & Adams, F. (1979). Restoration of lung pressure-volume characteristics with various phospholipids. *Pediatric Research, 13,* 777–780.

Jastak, J. F., & Jastak, S. (1978). *The wide range achievement test: Manual of instructions.* Wilmington, DE: Jastak Associates.

Johnson, J. D., Malachowski, N. C., Grobstein, R., Welse, D., Daily, W. J. R., & Sunshine, P. (1974). Prognosis for children surviving with the aid of mechanical ventilation in the newborn period. *Journal of Pediatrics, 84,* 272–276.

Johnson, L. D., O'Malley, R. P., & Backman, J. G. (1985). *Use of licit and illicit drugs by America's high school students 1975–1984* (National Institute on Drug Abuse) (DHHS Publication No. ADM 85-1394). Washington, DC: U.S. Government Printing Office.

Johnson, M. L., Rumack, C. M., Mannes, E. J., & Appareti, K. E. (1981). Detection of neonatal intracranial hemorrhage utilizing real-time and static ultrasound. *Journal of Clinical Ultrasound, 9,* 427–433.

Jones, K. L., Smith, D. W., Ulleland, C. N., & Streissguth, A. P. (1973). Pattern of malformation in offspring of chronic alcoholic mothers. *Lancet, 1,* 1267–1271.

Kagan, J., Reznick, J. S., Clarke, C., Snidman, N., & Garcia-Coll, C. (1984). Behavioral inhibition to the unfamiliar. *Child Development, 55,* 2212–2225.

Kinsey, V. E. (1954). *Report of the American Academy of Opthamology and Otolaryngology.* New York: September 22.

Kitchen, W. H., Lissenden, J. U., Yu, V. Y. H., & Bajuk, B. (1982). Collaborative study of very low birth weight infants: Outcome of 2 year old survivors. *Lancet, 1,* 1457–1460.

Kitchen, W. H., Yu, V. Y., Orgill, A., Ford, G. W., Rickards, A., Astbury, J., Ryan, M. M., Russo, W., Lissenden, J. U., & Bayuk, B. (1982). Infants born before 29 weeks gestation: Survival and morbidity at two years of age. *British Journal of Obstetrics and Gynaecology, 89,* 887–891.

Klein, N., Hack, M., Gallagher, J., & Fanaroff, A. A. (1985). Preschool performance of children with normal intelligence who were very low birth weight infants. *Pediatrics, 75,* 531–537.

Knobloch, C., & Kanoy, R. C. (1982). Hearing and language development in high risk and normal infants. *Applied Research in Mental Retardation, 3,* 293–301.

Knobloch, H., Rider, R., Harper, P., & Pasamanick, B. (1956). Neuropsychiatric sequelae of prematurity: A longitudinal study. *Journal of the American Medical Association, 161,* 581–585.

Kohen-Raz, R. (1967). Scalogram analysis of some developmental sequences of infant behavior as measured by the Bayley Scales of Mental Development. *Genetic Psychology Monographs, 76,* 3–21.

Koops, B. L., Abman, S. H., & Accurso, F. J. (1984). Outpatient management and follow-up of bronchopulmonary dysplasia. *Clinical Perinatology, 11,* 101–122.

Kopp, C. B., & Krakow, J. B. (1983). The developmentalist and the study of biological risk. A view of the past with an eye toward the future. *Child Development, 54,* 1086–1108.

Kopp, C. B., Sigman, M., Parmelee, A. H., & Jeffrey, W. E. (1975). Neurological organization and visual fixation in infants at 40 weeks conceptual age. *Developmental Psychobiology, 8,* 165–170.

Kosmetatos, N., Dinter, C., Williams, M. L., Lourie, H., & Berne, A. S. (1980). Intracranial hemorrhage in the premature: Its predictive features and outcome. *American Journal of Diseases of Children, 134,* 855–859.

Krafchuk, E. E., Tronick, E. Z., & Clifton, R. K. (1983). Behavioral and cardiac responses to sound in preterm neonates varying in risk status: A hypothesis of their paradoxical reactivity. In T. M. Field & A. Sostek (Eds.), *Infants born at risk: Physiological, perceptual, and cognitive processes.* New York: Grune & Stratton.

Krishnamoorthy, K. S., Shannon, D. C., DeLong, G. R., Todres, I. D., & Davis, K. R. (1979). Neurologic sequelae in the survivors of neonatal intraventricular hemorrhage. *Pediatrics, 64,* 233–237.

Kuban, K., & Teele, R. L. (1984). Rationale for grading intracranial hemorrhage in premature infants. Pediatrics, 74, 358–363.

Kumar, S. P., Anday, E. K., Sachs, L. M., Ting, R. X., & Delivoria-Papadopoulos, M. (1980). Follow-up studies of very low birth weight infants (1250 grams or less) born and treated within a perinatal center. *Pediatrics, 66,* 438–444.

Lanman, J. T., Guy, L. P., & Dancis, J. (1954). Retrolental fibroplasia and oxygen therapy. *Journal of the American Medical Association, 155,* 223–226.

Largo, R. H., Molinari, L., Comenale, P. L., Weber, M., & Dric, G. (1986). Language development of term and preterm children during the first five years of life. *Developmental Medicine and Child Neurology, 28,* 333–335.

Lee, C., & Bates, J. (1985). Mother-child interaction at age two years and perceived difficult timperament. *Child Development, 56,* 1314–1325.

Lee, M. H., Younger, E. W., & Babson, S. G. (1966). Thermal requirements of undergrown human neonates. *Biology of the Neonate, 10,* 288.

Leech, R. W., & Kohnen, P. (1974). Subependymal intraventricular hemorrhages in the newborn. *American Journal of Pathology,*

Leifer, A. D., Leiderman, P. H., Barnett, C. R., & Williams, J. A. (1972). Effects of mother–infant separation on maternal attachment behavior. *Child Development, 43,* 1203–1218.

Lester, B. M. (1987). Developmental outcome prediction from acoustic cry analysis in term and preterm infants. *Pediatrics 80*(4), 529–534.

Lester, B. M., Emory, E. K., Hoffman, S. L., & Eitzman, D. V. (1976). A multivariate study of the effects of high-risk factors on performance on the Brazelton Neonatal Assessment Scale. *Child Development, 47,* 515–517.

Lester, B. M., Hoffman. J., & Brazelton, T. B. *A model for assessing patterns of change in neonatal (NBAS) behavior.* Unpublished manuscript.

Lester, B. M., Hoffman, J., & Brazelton, T. B. (1985). The rhythmic structure of mother-infant interaction in term and preterm infants. *Child Development, 56,* 15–27.

Lester, B. M., & Zeskind, P. S. (1978). Brazelton Scale and physical size correlates of neonatal cry features. *Infant Behavior and Development, 1,* 393–402.

Levine, L., Garcia-Coll, C., & Oh, W. (1985). Determinants of mother–infant interaction in adolescent mothers. *Pediatrics, 75,* 23–29.

Lilienfeld, A. M., Pasamanick, B., & Rogers, M. (1955). Relationship between pregnancy experience and the development of certain neuropsychiatric disorders in children. *American Journal of Public Health, 15,* 637–645.

Little, W. J. (1862). On the influence of abnormal parturition, difficult labor, premature birth, asphyxia neonatorum, on the mental and physical condition of the child, especially in relation to deformities. *Transactions of Obstetrics Society*, London, *3*, 293.

Londerville, S., & Main, M. (1981). Security of attachment, compliance and maternal training methods in the second year of life. *Developmental Psychology, 17*, 289–299.

Lubchenco, L. O., Hansman, C., & Boyd, E. (1966). Intrauterine growth in length and head circumference as estimated from live births at gestational ages from 26 to 42 weeks. *Pediatrics, 37*, 403–408.

Lubchenco, L. O., Hansman, C., Dressler, M., & Boyd, E. (1963). Intrauterine growth as estimated from liveborn birth-weight data at 24 to 42 weeks of gestation. *Pediatrics, 32*, 793–800.

Lubchenco, L. O., Horner, F. A., Reed, L. H., Hix, I. E., Jr., Metcalf, D., Cohig, R., Elliott, H. C., & Boug, M. (1963). Sequelae of premature birth. Evaluation of premature infants of low birth weights at 10 years of age. *American Journal of Diseases of Children, 106*, 101–115.

Lugo, G., & Cassady, G. (1971). Intrauterine growth retardation. Clinico-pathologic findings in 233 consecutive infants. *American Journal of Obstetrics and Gynecology, 109*, 615–622.

McBurney, R. D. (1947). The undernourished full term infant: A case report. *West Journal of Surgery, 55*, 363–370.

McCarthy, D. (1972). *Manual for the McCarthy Scales of Children's Abilities*. New York: The Psychological Corp.

McCormick, M. C., Shapiro, S., & Starfield, B. H. (1985). The regionalization of perinatal services: Summary of the evaluation of national demonstration program. *Journal of the American Medical Association, 253*, 799–804.

McDevitt, S. C., & Carey, W. B. (1978). The measurement of temperament in 3–7 year old children. *Journal of Child Psychology and Psychiatry, 19*, 245–253.

McElroy, E., Steinschneider, A., & Weinstein, S. (1986). Emotional and health impact of home monitoring of mothers: A controlled perspective study. *Pediatrics, 78*, 780–786.

McGehee, L. J., & Eckerman, C. O. (1983). The preterm infant as a social partner: Responsive but unreadable. *Infant Behavior & Development, 6*, 461–470.

Maher, P., Lane, B., Ballard, R., Piecuch, R., & Clyman, R. I. (1985). Does indomethacin cause extension of intracranial hemorrhages: A preliminary study. *Pediatrics, 75*, 497–500.

Main, M. (1973). *Play, exploration and competence as related to child–adult attachment*. Unpublished doctoral dissertation, Johns Hopkins University.

Main, M., Tomasini, L., & Tolan, W. (1979). Differences among mothers of infants judged to differ in security. *Developmental Psychology, 15*, 472–473.

Main, M., & Weston, D. R. (1981). The quality of the toddler's relationship to mother and to father: Related to conflict behavior and the readiness to establish new relationships. *Child Development, 52*, 932–940.

Majewski, F. (1981). Alcohol embryopathy: Some facts and speculations about pathogenesis. *Neurobehavioral Toxicology and Teratology, 3*(2), 129–144.

Malatesta, C. Z., Grigoryev, P., Lamb, C., Albin, M., & Culver, C. (1986). Emotion socialization and expressive development in preterm and fullterm infants. *Child Development, 57*, 316–330.

Martinius, J., & Papousek, H. (1970). Responses to optic and exteroceptive stimuli in relation to state in the human newborn. *Neuropaediatrie, 1*, 452–460.

Masi, W. S., & Scott, K. G. (1983). Preterm and full-term infants' visual responses to mothers' and strangers' faces. In T. M. Field & A. Sostek (Eds.), *Infants born at risk*. New York: Grune & Stratton.

Matas, L., Arend, R. A., & Sroufe, L. A. (1978). Continuity of adaptation in the second year: The relationship between quality of attachment and later competence. *Child Development, 49,* 547–556.

Matheny, A. P., Wilson, R. S., & Nuss, S. M. (1984). Toddler temperament: Stability across settings and over ages. *Child Development, 55,* 1200–1211.

Mayes, L. C., Kirk, V., Haywood, N., Buchanan, D., Hedvall, G., & Stahlman, M. T. (1985). Changing cognitive outcome in preterm infants with hyaline membrane disease. *American Journal of Diseases of Children, 139,* 20–24.

Mayes, L., Perkett, E., & Stahlman, M. T. (1983). Severe bronchopulmonary dysplasia: A retrospective review. *Acta Paediatrica Scandinavica, 72*(2), 225–229.

Medoff-Cooper, B. (in press). Temperament in very low birth weight infants. *Nursing Research.*

Medoff-Cooper, B., & Schraeder, B. (1982). Developmental trends and behavioral styles in very low birth weight infants. *Nursing Research, 31,* 69–72.

Meisels, S. J., Plunkett, J. W., Roloff, D. W., Pasick, P. L., & Stiefel, G. S. (1986). Growth and development of preterm infants with respiratory distress syndrome and bronchopulmonary dysplasia. *Pediatrics, 77,* 345–352.

Merritt, T. A., Hallman, M., Bloom, B. T., Berry, C., Benirischke, K., Sahn, D., Key, T., Edwards, D., Jarvenpaa, A. L., Pohjavuori, M., Kankaanpaa, K., Kunnas, M., Paatero, H., Rapola, J., & Jaaskelainen, J. (1986). Prophylactic treatment of very premature infants with human surfactant. *New England Journal of Medicine, 315,* 785–790.

Michelsson, K. (1980). *Cry analyses of symptomless low birth weight neonates and of asphyxiated newborn infants.* Academic dissertation, Department of Paediatrics, University of Oulu, Helsinki, Finland.

Minkowski, A., Amiel-Tison, C., Cukier, F., Dreyfus-Brisac, C., Relier, J. P., & Bethmann, H. (1977). Long-term follow-up and sequelae of asphyxiated infants. In L. Gluck (Ed.), *Intrauterine asphyxia and the developing brain.* Chicago: Year Book Medical Publishers.

Mirada, S. B. (1976). Visual attention in defective and high risk infants. *Merrill-Palmer Quarterly, 22:* 201–228.

Mohr, G. J., & Bartelme, P. (1930). Mental and physical development of children prematurely born. *American Journal of Diseases of Childhood, 40,* 1000–1015.

Morgan, M. E. I., Massey, R. F., & Cooke, R. W. I. (1982). Does phenobarbitone prevent periventricular hemorrhage in very low birth weight babies: A controlled trial. *Pediatrics, 70,* 186–189.

Moss, H. A., & Jones, S. J. (1977). Relations between maternal attitudes and maternal behavior as a function of social class. In P. H. Leiderman, S. R. Tulkin, & A. Rosenfeld (Eds.), *Culture and infancy: Variations in the human experience.* New York: Academic Press.

Mullen, E. M. (1984). *Mullen Scales of Early Learning.* Providence: TOTAL Child, Inc.

Nakamura, H., Takada, S., Shimabuku, R., Matsuo, M., Matsuo, T., & Negishi, H. (1985). Auditory nerve and brain stem responses in newborns with hyperbilirubinemia. *Pediatrics, 75*(4), 703–708.

Nelson, R. B., & Broman, S. H. (1977). Perinatal risk factors in children with serious motor and mental handicaps. *Annals of Neurology, 2,* 371–377.

Nelson, K. B., & Deutschberger, J. (1970). Head size at one year as a predictor of four year IQ. *Developmental Medicine and Child Neurology, 12,* 487.

Nelson, K. B., & Ellenberg, J. H. (1979). Neonatal signs as predictors of cerebral palsy. *Pediatrics, 64,* 225–232.

Nelson, K. B., & Ellenberg, J. H. (1981). Apgar scores as predictors of chronic neurological disability. *Pediatrics, 68,* 36–44.

Nichel, R. E., Bennett, F. C., & Lamson, F. N. (1982). School performance of children with birth weight of 1000 grams or less. *American Journal of Diseases of Children, 136,* 105–110.

Noble-Jamieson, Lukeman, D., Silverman, M., & Davies, P. A. (1982). Low birth weight children at school age: Neurological, psychological and pulmonary function. *Seminars in Perinatology, 6,* 266–273.

Northway, W. H. (1979). Observations on bronchopulmonary dysplasia. *Journal of Pediatrics, 95,* 815–818.

Northway, W. H., Rosan, R. C., & Porter, D. Y. (1967). Pulmonary disease following respirator therapy of hyaline membrane disease. *New England Journal of Medicine, 276,* 357–368.

O'Brien, G. D., & Queenan, J. T. (1981). Growth of the ultrasound fetal femur length during normal pregnancy. Part I. *American Journal Obstetrics and Gynecology, 141,* 833–837.

Palmer, P., Dubowitz, L. M. S., Levene, M. I., & Dubowitz, V. (1982). Developmental and neurological progress of preterm infants with intraventricular haemorrhage and ventricular dilatation. *Archives of Diseases in Childhood, 57,* 748–753.

Paneth, N., Kiely, J. L., Phil, M., Wallenstein, S., Marcus, M., Pakter, J., & Susser, M. (1982). Neonatal intensive care and neonatal mortality in low birth weight infants. *New England Journal of Medicine, 307,* 149–155.

Pape, K. E., Armstrong, D. L., & Fitzhardinge, P. M. (1976). Central nervous system pathology associated with mask ventilation in the very low birthweight infant: A new etiology for intracerebellar hemorrhages. *Pediatrics, 58,* 473–483.

Pape, K. E., Buncic, R. J., Ashby, S., & Fitzhardinge, P. M. (1978). The status of two years of low birth weight infants born 1974 with birth weights of less than 1001 grams. *Journal of Pediatrics, 92,* 253–260.

Papile, L. A., Burstein, L., Burstein, R., & Koffler, H. (1978). Incidence and evolution of subependymal and intraventricular hemorrhage: A study of infants with birth weights less than 1500 grams. *Journal of Pediatrics,92*(4), 529–534.

Papile, L. A., Munsick-Bruno, G., & Shaefer, A. (1983). Relationship of cerebral intraventricular hemorrhage and early childhood neurologic handicaps. *Journal of Pediatrics, 103*(2), 273–280.

Parmelee, A. H., Cutsforth, M. G., & Jackson, C. L. (1958). Mental development of children with blindness due to retrolental fibroplasia. *American Journal of Diseases of Children, 96,* 641–654.

Parmelee, A. H., Fiske, C. E., & Wright, R. H. (1959). The development of 10 children with blindness as a result of retrolental fibroplasia. *American Journal of Diseases of Children, 98,* 198–220.

Patz, A., Hoeck, L. E., & DeLaCruz, E. (1952). Studies on the effect of high oxygen administration in retrolental fibroplasia: Nursery observations. *American Journal of Opthamology, 35,* 1248–1253.

Pediatric Research. (1987, April). *21*(4), Abstracts 68, 317, 344, 364, 384, 387, 402, 530, 1096, 1112, 1113, 1114, 1126, 1191, 1364.

Perlman, M., Fainmesser, P., Sohmer, H., Tamari, H., Wax, Y., & Pevsmer, B. (1983). Auditory nerve-brainstem evoked responses in hyperbilirubinemic neonates. *Pediatrics, 72,* 658–664.

Perlman, J. M., Goodman, S., Kreusser, K. L., & Volpe, J. J. (1985). Reduction in intraventricular hemorrhage by elimination of fluctuating cerebral bloodflow velocity in preterm infants with Respiratory Distress Syndrome. *New England Journal of Medicine, 312,* 1353–1357.

Phelps, D. L. (1981). Retinopathy of prematurity: An estimate of vision loss in the United States—1979. *Pediatrics, 67,* 924–925.

Phelps, D. L. (1982). Vitamin E and retrolental fibroplasia. *Pediatrics, 70,* 420–425.

Prechtl, H. F. R. (1967). Neurological sequelae of prenatal and perinatal complication. *British Medical Journal, 4,* 763.

Procianoy, R. S., Garcia-Prats, J. A., Hittner, H. M., Adams, J. M., & Rudolph, A. J. (1981). An association between retinopathy of prematurity and intraventricular hemorrhage in very low birth weight infants. *Acta Paediatrics Scandinavia, 70,* 473–477.

Ramey, C., Mills, R., Campbell, F., & O'Brien, C. (1975). Infants' home environments: A comparison of high-risk families and families from the general population. *American Journal of Mental Deficiencies, 80,* 40–42.

Rawlings, G., Stewart, A., & Reynolds, E. O. R. (1971). Changing prognosis for infants of very low birth weight. *Lancet, 1,* 516–519.

Reese, A. B. (1949). Persistence and hyperplasia of primary vitreous, retrolental fibroplasia—two entities. *Archives of Opthamology, 41,* 527–552.

Riese, M. C. (1983). Behavioral patterns in full-term and preterm twins. *Acta Geneticae Medicae et Gemellologiae* (Roma), *32,* 209–220.

Riese, M. L. (1984). Within-pair differences in newborn twins: Effects of gender and gestational age on behavior. *Acta Geneticae Medicae et Gemellologiae* (Roma), *33,* 159–164.

Riley, G. D. (1976). *Motor problems inventory.* Los Angeles: Western Psychological Services.

Robertson, C., & Finer, N. (1985). Term infants with hypoxic-ischemic encephalopathy: Outcome at 3 and 5 years. *Developmental Medicine and Child Neurology, 27,* 473–484.

Rode, S. S., Chang, P., Niau, P., Fisch, R. O., & Scroufe, L. A. (1981). Attachment patterns in infants separated at birth. *Developmental Psychology, 17,* 188–191.

Rose, S. A. (1980). Enhancing visual recognition memory in preterm infants. *Developmental Psychology, 16,* 85–92.

Rose, S. A., Gottfried, A. W., & Bridger, W. H. (1979). Effects of haptic cues on visual recognition memory in full-term and preterm infants. *Infant Behavior and Development, 2,* 55–67.

Rose, S., Schmidt, K., & Bridger, W. H. (1976). Cardiac and behavioral responsivity to tactile stimulation in premature and full-term infants. *Developmental Psychology, 12,* 311–320.

Rose, S. A., Schmidt, K., Riese, M. L., & Bridger, W. H. (1980). Effects of prematurity and early intervention on responsivity to tactile stimuli: A comparison of preterm and full term infants. *Child Development, 51,* 416–425.

Rosenfield, W., Evans, H., Concepcion, L., Jhaveri, R., Schaeffer, H., & Friedman, A. (1984). Prevention of bronchopulmonary dysplasia by administration of bovine superoxide dismutase in preterm infants with respiratory distress syndrome. *Journal of Pediatrics, 105,* 781–785.

Ross, G., Lipper, E. G., & Auld, P. A. M. (1985). Consistency and change in the development of premature infants weighing less than 1501 grams at birth. *Pediatrics, 76(6),* 885–891.

Rothbart, M. K. (1981). Measurement of temperament in infancy. *Child Development, 52,* 659–578.

Ruff, H. A. (1986). Attention and organization of behavior in high-risk infants. *Developmental and Behavioral Pediatrics, 7,* 298–301.

Ruff, H. A., McCarton, C., Kurtzberg, D., & Vaughan, H. G., Jr. (1984). Preterm infants' manipulative exploration of objects. *Child Development, 55,* 1166–1173.

Ruiz, M. P. D., LeFever, J. A., Hakanson, D. O., Clark, D. A., & Williams, M. L. (1981). Early development of infants of birth weight less than 1000 grams with reference to mechanical ventilation in newborn period. *Pediatrics, 68,* 330–335.

Rumack, C. M., McDonald, M. M., O'Meara, O. P., Sanders, B. B., & Rudikoff, J. C. (1978). CT detection and course of intracranial hemorrhage in premature infants. *American Journal of Radiology, 131,* 493–497.

Saigal, S., Rosenbaum, P., Stoskopf, B., & Melner, R. (1982). Follow-up of infants 501–1500 grams birth weight delivered to residents of a geographically defined region with perinatal intensive care facilities. *Journal of Pediatrics, 100,* 606–613.

Saigal, S., Rosenbaum, P., Stoskopf, B., & Sinclair, J. C. (1984). Outcome in infants 501–1000 grams birth weight delivered to residents of the McMaster health region. *Journal of Pediatrics, 105,* 969–976.

Saint-Anne-Dargassies, S. (1955). La maturation neurologique du premature. *Revue Neurologique* (Paris), *93,* 331–340.

Sameroff, A. J., & Chandler, M. J. (1975). Reproductive risk and the continuum of caretaking casualty. In F. D. Horowitz (Ed.), *Review of child development research.* Chicago: University of Chicago Press.

Sameroff, A. J., Seifer, R., Barocas, R., Zaz, M., & Greenspan, S. (1987). Intelligence quotient scores of 4-year-old children: Social-environmental risk factors. *Pediatrics, 79,* 343–350.

Sarason, I. G., Johnson, J. H., & Siegel, J. M. (1978). Assessing the impact of life changes: Development of the life experiences survey. *Journal of Consulting and Clinical Psychology, 46,* 932–946.

Sarnat, H. B., & Sarnat, M. S. (1976). Neonatal encephalopathy following fetal distress. *Archives of Neurology, 33,* 696–705.

Sauerbrei, E. E., Digney, M., Harrison, P. B., & Cooperberg, P. L. (1981). Ultrasonic evaluation of neonatal intracranial hemorrhage and its complications. *Radiology, 139*(3), 677–685.

Schaeffer, A. (1968). Disorders related to the birth process. In R. E. Cooke (Ed.), *The biologic basis of pediatric practice.* New York: McGraw-Hill.

Schneider, J., & Chasnoff, I. (1987). Motor assessment of cocaine-exposed infants. *Pediatric Research, 21,* 184A, Abstract 68.

Schraeder, B., & Medoff-Cooper, B. (1983). Temperament and development in VLBW infants: The second year. *Nursing Research, 32,* 231–335.

Schreiber, F. (1938). Apnea of the newborn and associated cerebral injury; Clinical and statistical study. *Journal of the American Medical Association, 111,* 1263–1269.

Sepkoski, C., Garcia-Coll, C., & Lester, B. M. (1982). The cumulative effects of obstetric risk variables on newborn behavior. In L. P. Lipsitt and T. M. Field (Eds.), *Infant behavior and development: Perinatal risk and newborn behavior.* Norwood, NJ: Ablex.

Shannon, D. A., Felix, J. K., Krumholz, A., Goldstein, P. J., & Harris, K. C. (1984). Hearing screening of high risk newborns with brain stem auditory evoked potentials: A follow-up study. *Pediatrics, 73,* 22–26.

Shapiro, D. L., Notter, R. H., Morin, F. C., Deluga, K. S., Golub, L. M., Sinkin, R. A., Weiss, K. I., & Cox, G. (1985). Double-blind randomized trial of a calf lung surfactant extract administered at birth to very premature infants for prevention of respiratory distress syndrome. *Pediatrics, 76,* 593–599.

Shinnar, S., Molteni, R., R. A., Gammon, K., D'Souza, B. J., Altman, J., & Freeman, J. M.

(1982). Intraventricular hemorrhage in the premature infant: A changing outlook. *New England Journal of Medicine, 306,* 1464–1467.

Shirley, M. (1938). A behavior syndrome characterizing prematurely born children. *Child Development, 10,* 115–128.

Siegel, L. S. (1982). Reproductive, perinatal, and environmental factors as predictors of the cognitive and language development of preterm and full term infants. *Child Development, 53,* 963–973.

Sigman, M. (1976). Early development of preterm and full term infants: Exploratory behavior in eight month olds. *Child Development, 47,* 606–612.

Sigman, M., Kopp, C. B., Littman, B., & Parmelee, A. H. (1977). Infant visual attentiveness in relation to birth condition. *Developmental Psychology, 13,* 431–437.

Sigman, M., & Parmelee, A. H. (1974). Visual preferences of four-month-old premature and full-term infants. *Child Development, 45,* 959–965.

Silverman, W. A. (1980). *Retrolental fibroplasia. A modern parable.* New York: Grune & Stratton.

Sinka, S. K., Sims, D. G., Davies, J. M., & Chiswick, M. L. (1985). Relation between periventricular haemorrhage and ischemic brain lesions diagnosed by ultrasound in very preterm infants. *Lancet, 1,* 1154–1155.

Smith, G. F., & Vidyasagar, D. (1983). *Historical review and recent advances in neonatal and perinatal medicine: Vol. II.* Mead Johnson Nutritional Division, Evansville, Indiana.

Smyth, J. A., Tabachnik, E., Duncan, W. J., Reilly, B. J., & Levison, H. (1981). Pulmonary function and bronchial hyperreactivity in long-term survivors of bronchopulmonary dysplasia. *Pediatrics, 68,* 336–340.

Soderling, B. (1953). Pseudomaturity. *Acta Pediatrica, 942,* 520–524.

Solimano, A. J., Smyth, J. A., Mann, T. K., Albersheim, S. G., & Lockitch, G. (1986). Pulse oximetry advantages in infants with bronchopulmonary dysplasia. *Pediatrics, 78,* 844–849.

Sostek, A. M., Davitt, M. K., & Renzi, J. (1982). Factor analysis of behavioral assessments of preterm neonates. In L. P. Lipsitt & T. M. Field (Eds.), *Infant behavior and development: Perinatal risk and newborn behavior.* Norwood, NJ: Ablex.

Sostek, A. M., Quinn, P. O., & Davitt, M. K. (1979). Behavior, development and neurologic status of premature and full-term infants with varying medical complications. In T. M. Field, A. M. Sostek, S. Goldberg, and H. H. Shuman (Eds.), *Infants born at risk.* New York: Spectrum.

Speer, M. E., Blifeld, C., Rudolph, A. J., Chadda, P., Holbein, M. E. B., & Hittner, H. M. (1984). Intraventricular hemorrhage and vitamin E in the very low birth weight infant: Evidence for efficacy of early intramuscular vitamin E administration. *Pediatrics, 74,* 1107–1112.

Spungen, L. B., & Farran, A. C. (1986). Effect of intensive care unit exposure on temperament in low birth weight preterm infants. *Journal of Developmental and Behavioral Pediatrics, 7,* 288–292.

Spungen, L. B., Kurtzberg, D., & Vaughan, H. G. (1985). Patterns of looking behavior in full term and low birth weight infants at 40 weeks post conceptional age. *Journal of Developmental and Behavioral Pediatrics, 6*(5), 287–294.

Stahlman, M., Hedvall, G., Dolanski, E., Faxelius, A., Burke, H., & Kirk, V. (1973). A six year follow-up of clinical hyaline membrane disease. *Pediatric Clinics of North America, 20,* 433–446.

Stahlman, M., Hedvall, G., Lindstrom, D., & Snell, J. (1982). Role of hyaline membrane disease in production of later childhood. Lung abnormalities. *Pediatrics, 69,* 572–576.

Stern, L., & Denton, R. L.(1965). Kernicterus is small premature infants. *Pediatrics, 35*, 483–485.

Stewart, A. L., & Reynolds, E. O. R. (1974). Improved prognosis for infants of very low birth weight. *Pediatrics, 54*, 724–735.

Stewart, A. L., Reynolds, E. O. R., & Lipscomb, A. P. (1981). Outcome for infants of very low birth weight. Survey of world literature. *Lancet, 11*, 1038–1941.

Stewart, A. L., Turcan, D. M., Rawlings, G., & Reynolds, E. O. R. (1977). Prognosis for infants weighing 1000 grams or less at birth. *Archives of Diseases of Childhood, 52*, 97.

Strauss, A., Kirz, D., Mondanlou, H. D., & Freeman, R. K. (1985). Perinatal events and intraventricular/subependymal hemorrhage in the low birth weight infant. *American Journal of Obstetrics and Gynecology, 151*, 1022–1027.

Szymonowicz, W., Yu, V. Y. H., Bajuk, B., & Astbury, J. (1986). Neurodevelopmental outcome of periventricular haemorrhage and leukomalacia in infants 1250 grams or less at birth. *Early Human Development, 14*, 1–7.

Telzrow, R. W., Kang, R. R., & Mitchell, S. K. (1982). An assessment of the behavior of the preterm infant at 40 weeks conceptual age. In L. Lipsitt & T. M. Field (Eds.), *Infant behavior and development:* Perinatal risk and newborn behavior. Norwood, NJ: Ablex.

Terman, L. M., & Merrill, M. A. (1973). Stanford-Binet intelligence scale: Manual for the third revision—Form L-M. Boston: Houghton Mifflin.

Terry, T. L. (1942). Extreme prematurity and fibroblastic overgrowth of persistent vascular sheath behind each crxstalline lens; preliminary report. *American Journal of Opthamology, 25*, 203.

Thomas, D. B. (1976). Hyperosmolality and intraventricular haemorrhage in premature babies. *Acta Paediatrica Scandinavica, 65*, 429–432.

Thompson, R. A., Lamb, M. R., & Estes, D. (1982). Stability of infant-mother attachment and its relationship to changing life circumstances in an unselected middle-class sample. *Child Development, 53*, 144–148.

Tilson, M. D. (1980). Pathophysiology and treatment of short bowel syndrome. *Surgical Clinics of North America, 60*, 1273–1284.

Touwen, B. C. L. (1979). Examination of the child with minor neurological dysfunction. *Clinics in Developmental Medicine, 71*, 1–141.

Towbin, A. (1970). Central nervous system damage in the human fetus and newborn infant. *American Journal of Diseases of Children, 119*, 529–542.

Tronick, E., Als, H., & Brazelton, T. (1980). Monadic phases: A structural descriptive analysis of infant–mother face-to-face interaction. *Merrill-Palmer Quarterly, 26*, 3.

Tsang, R. C., Gigger, M., Oh, W., & Brown, D. R. (1975). Studies in calcium metabolism in infants with intrauterine growth retardation. *Journal of Pediatrics, 86*(6), 936–941.

Tulkin, S. R. (1977). Social class differences in maternal and infant behavior. In P. H. Leiderman, S. R. Tulkin, & A. Rosenfeld, (Eds.), *Culture and infancy: Variations in the human experience.* New York: Academic Press.

Tulkin, S. R., & Kagan, J. (1972). Mother-child interaction in the first year of life. *Child Development, 43*, 31–41.

Usher, R.,McLean, F., & Scott, K. E. (1966). Judgement of fetal age. II. Clinical significance of gestational age and an objective method for its assessment. *Pediatric Clinics of North America, 13*, 835–862.

Valdes-Dapena, M. A., & Arey, J. B. (1970). The cause of neonatal mortality: An analysis of 501 autopsies on newborn infants. *Journal of Pediatrics, 77*, 366–375.

Vaughn, B. E., Deinard, A., & Egeland, B. R. (1980). Measuring temperament in pediatric practice. *Journal of Pediatrics, 96*, 510–514.

Vaughn, B., Egeland, B., Sroufe, L. A., & Waters, E. (1979). Individual differences in infant–mother attachment at twelve and eighteen months: Stability and change in families under stress. *Child Development, 50,* 971–975.

Vaughn, B. E., Taraldson, B. J., Crichton, L., & Egeland, B. (1981). The assessment of infant temperament: A critique of the Carey Infant Temperament Questionnaire. *Infant Behavior and Development, 4,* 1–17.

Villar, J., Smeriglio, V., Martorell, R., Brown, C. H., & Klein, R. E. (1984). Heterogeneous growth and mental development of intrauterine growth retarded infants during the first three years of life. *Pediatrics, 74,* 783–791.

Vohr, B. R., Bell, E. F., & Oh, W. (1982). Infants with bronchopulmonary dysplasia: Growth patterns and neurologic and developmental outcome. *American Journal of Diseases of Children, 136*(5), 443–447.

Vohr, B. R., Chen, A., Garcia-Coll, C., & Oh, W. (in press). Mothers of preterm and full term infants on home apnea monitors. *American Journal of Diseases of Children.*

Vohr, B., Daniel, P., & Oh, W. (1981). Analysis of perinatal variables affecting compliance to a follow-up program. *Pediatric Research,* Abstract No. 697, p. 558.

Vohr, B. R., & Garcia-Coll, C. T. (1985a). Increased morbidity in low birth weight survivors with severe retrolental fibroplasia. *Journal of Pediatrics, 106,* 287–291.

Vohr, B. R., & Garcia-Coll, C. T. (1985b). Neurodevelopmental and school performance of very low birth weight infants: A seven year longitudinal study. *Pediatrics, 76*(3), 345–350.

Vohr, B. R., & Garcia-Coll, C. (1987). Serial brainstem vision evoked response (VER) as a marker of neurological abnormality in low birth weight infants. *Pediatric Research, 21,* 404A, Abstract No. 1391.

Vohr, B. R., & Oh, W. (1983). Growth and development in preterm infants small-for-gestational age. *Journal of Pediatrics, 103,* 941–945.

Vohr, B. R., Oh, W., Rosenfeld, A. G., & Cowett, R. M. (1979). The preterm small-for-gestational age infant: A two year follow-up study. *American Journal of Obstetrics and Gynecology, 133*(4), 425–431.

Vohr, B. R., Garcia-Coll, C., & Oh, W. (in press). Language development at 2 years of age in low birth weight infants.

Volpe, J. J. (1981). Neurology of the newborn. In *Major Problems in Clinical Pediatrics.* Philadelphia: W. B. Saunders.

Volpe, J. J., Perlman, J. M., Herscovitch, P., & Raichle, M. E. (1982). Positron emission tomography in the assessment of regional cerebral blood flow in the newborn. *Annals of Neurology, 12,* 225–226.

Walker, D. J., Feldman, A., Vohr, B. R., & Oh, W. (1984). Cost benefit analysis of neonatal intensive care for infant weighing less than 1000 grams at birth. *Pediatrics, 74,* 20–25.

Walker, D. J., Vohr, B. R., & Oh, W. (1985). Economic analysis of regionalized neonatal care for very low birth weight infants in the State of Rhode Island. *Pediatrics, 76,* 69–74.

Waters, E. (1978). The reliability and stability of individual differences in infant–mother attachment. *Child Development, 49,* 483–494.

Waters, E., & Deane, K. E. (1985). Defining and assessing individual differences in attachment relationships: A methodology and the organization of behavior in infancy and early childhood. In I. Bretherton & E. Waters (Eds.), *Growing points of attachment theory and research. Monographs of the Society for Research in Child Development, 50*(1–2, Serial No. 209).

Waters, E., Wippman, J., & Sroufe, L. A. (1979). Attachment, positive affect, and competence in the peer group: Two studies in construct validation. *Child Development, 50,* 821–829.

Wechsler, D. (1974a). *WPPSI Wechsler Preschool and Primary Scale of Intelligence.* New York: The Psychological Corp.

Wechsler, D. (1974b). *Wechsler Intelligence Scale for Children Revised WISC-R.* New York: The Psychological Corp.

Weinstein, M. R., & Oh, W. (1981). Oxygen consumption in infants with bronchopulmonary dysplasia. *Journal of Pediatrics, 99,* 958–961.

Werner, E. E., Bierman, J. M., & French, F. E. (1971). *The children of Kauai. A longitudinal study from the premature period to age ten.* Honolulu: University Press of Hawaii.

Werner, E. E., & Smith, R. S. (1977). *Kauai's children come of age.* Honolulu: University Press of Hawaii.

Werner, J. S., Barlett, A. W., & Siqueland, E. R. (1982). Assessment of preterm and full term infant behavior. In L. P. Lipsitt & T. M. Field (Eds.), *Infant behavior and development: Perinatal risk and newborn behavior.* Norwood, NJ: Ablex.

Wiener, G., Rider, R. V., & Opel, W. C. (1965). Correlates of low birth weight psychological status at six to seven years of age. *Pediatrics, 35,* 434–444.

Wiener, G., Rider, R. V., Opel, W. C., & Harper, P. A. (1968). Correlates of low birth weight. *Pediatric Research, 2:*110–118.

Williams, R. L., & Chen, P. M. (1982). Identifying the sources of the recent decline in perinatal mortality rates in California. *New England Journal of Medicine, 306,* 207–214.

Williamson, W. D., Desmond, M. D., Wilson, G. S., Murphy, M. A., Rozelle, J., & Garcia-Prats, J. A. (1983). Survival of low birth weight infants with neonatal intraventricular hemorrhage. *American Journal of Diseases of Childhood, 137,* 1181–1184.

Wilson, J. L., Long, S. B., & Howard, P. J. (1942). Respiration of premature infants; Response to variations of oxygen and to increased carbon dioxide in inspired air. *American Journal of Diseases of Children, 63,* 1080–1085.

Wilson, R. S., & Matheny, A. P. (1983). Assessment of temperament in infant twins. *Developmental Psychology, 19,* 172–183.

Wulbert, M., Inglis, S., Kriegsmann, E., & Mills, B. (1975). Language delay and associated mother–child interactions. *Developmental Psychology, 11,* 61–70.

Wright, N. E., Thislethwaite, D., Elton, R. A., Wilkinson, E. M., & Forfar, J. O. (1983). The speech and language development of low birth weight infants. *British Journal of Disorders of Communication, 18,* 187–196.

Zinman, R., Franco, I., & Pizzuti-Daechsel, R. (1985). Home oxygen delivery system for infants. *Pediatric Pulmonology, 1,* 325–327.

## 2

Mothers, Infants, and the Development of Cognitive Competence

MARC H. BORNSTEIN

1. INTRODUCTION

Before children are old enough to enter formal social learning situations, like school, or even informal ones, like play groups, nearly all of their experiences stem directly from interactions they have with their primary caretakers. To put it another way, caretakers are responsible for virtually all of infants' early experiences. What is the nature of caretaker-provided experience in the first year? What are the concurrent and predictive effects of infants' experiences?

This chapter addresses the related issues of the nature and the effects of experience in the infant's first year. The following section defines a threefold taxonomy of interpersonal parenting activities—including the nurturant, social, and didactic—and illustrates some effects on infants of each of these categories of caretaking. In the past, much emphasis has been placed on social forms of parenting; this chapter stresses a comparison of social and didactic.

The next section of the chapter reviews some elements of a research program designed to examine the short- and long-term consequences of different styles of social and didactic caretaking in infancy. The studies

Marc H. Bornstein • Child and Family Research, National Institute of Child Health and Human Development, Bethesda, Maryland 20892, and Department of Psychology, New York University, New York, New York 10003.

focus on mother as principal caretaker, although it is an open empirical question whether father, grandparent, sib, or any significant other in the infant's life could serve the same functions equally well. These studies also focus on the first year of life, although it is an open empirical question whether the same or different effects obtain beyond infancy. In addition, these studies focus on cognitive development broadly construed, although it is an open empirical question whether such experiences may also substantially affect the course of socioemotional development.

Finally, theoretical mechanisms of action and temporal models according to which the effects of early experiences are thought to operate are discussed and additional data sets are brought to bear on the evaluation of these mechanisms and models with respect to social and didactic forms of caretaking.

To forecast some of the main conclusions, research and theory concur in suggesting that certain maternal activities constitute experiences for infants that have both immediate and protracted consequences in children's cognitive growth across the first years of life.

2. THREE CATEGORIES OF CARETAKING: A TYPOLOGY AND THEIR CHARACTERISTICS

Three conceptually distinct categories of caretaker–child interactions can be identified: nurturant, social, and didactic. Together, these categories aggregate to encompass much (though not all) of caretakers' everyday behaviors. Caretakers show considerable interindividual variability as well as considerable intraindividual consistency when engaging in these several kinds of caretaking (Bornstein, 1987a). In this section, I define each category, provide concrete examples of each, discuss their psychometric adequacy, and illustrate each with respect to the early mental development of the child. Of course, this taxonomy does not reflect a unique or exhaustive classification: The scheme omits purely material forms of caretaking, the main categories subsume many different subactivities, and these categories are not mutually exclusive. Nonetheless, this system of distinctions has emerged as invested with considerable practicable significance for child rearing as well as substantial heuristic value for developmental study.

2.1. Defining Categories of Caretaking

There are three main categories of caretaking with which I am concerned. *Nurturant caretaking* meets the physical needs of the infant to ensure well-being, including feeding, cleaning, grooming, and the like. In most species, parents are nurturant of their offspring, especially during the earliest stages of the infant's postnatal life; indeed, solicitousness toward the young may be requisite to their survival and well-being and, of much importance, may "gate" the infant's taking advantage of the two other main forms of caretaking. *Social caretaking* includes the physical and verbal strategies parents use to express feelings toward infants and to engage their young in primarily emotional exchanges. Rocking, kissing, and tactile comforting, smiling, nonverbal vocalizing, and maintaining playful face-to-face contact, as well as game play illustrate some commonly observed types of social interactions. Finally, *didactic caretaking* includes physical or verbal strategies parents use in stimulating and arousing their offspring, in focusing infants' attention on properties, objects, or events in the environment, in introducing, mediating, and interpreting the external world, and in provoking or providing opportunities to observe, to imitate, and to learn. Social and didactic categories of caretaking often contrast with one another in the following sense: The locus of interaction in social caretaking is usually "dyadic," whereas the locus of interaction in didactic caretaking is usually "extradyadic."

Psychometric considerations dictate that to possess construct validity the categories of caretaking distinguished here need to be internally consistent, to show a degree of discriminant validity, and to be stable at least in the short term. The criterion of internal consistency applies where a caretaking category is composed of different items; to meet this criterion items in a category must covary. That is, individuals should perform about the same on the different items that go to make up the category, some individuals performing each item relatively infrequently and other individuals performing each item relatively frequently. Thus, for example, mothers who are more social should not only rock their infants more but should tend to comfort them more and smile at them more, and mothers who are less social should not only rock their infants less but should tend to comfort them less and smile at them less.

Relatedly, discriminant validity requires that, if caretaking categories are to be considered independent, different categories must assess distinct characteristics of the caretaker. That is, to meet the criterion of discriminant validity performance of social caretaking items must not strictly covary with performance of didactic caretaking items. Thus, for example, if mothers who regularly rock, comfort, and smile at their infants also regularly focus their infants' attention, interpret the external world, and provide opportunities to imitate, there will be no way to distinguish the social and didactic forms of caretaking as separate constructs. Of course, independence of categories need not be absolute; a moderate degree of overlap is acceptable if anticipated by theory. However, a high degree of overlap indicates that constructs are redundant and vitiates both their independence (Allen & Yen, 1979; Nunnally, 1978) and explanatory power (Cohen & Cohen, 1983).

The criterion of short-term consistency dictates that to find its utility as a meaningful construct a psychological phenomenon must be repeatable across occasions spaced reasonably close together in time. Thus, for example, if mothers widely varied in their performance of social and didactic activities from day to day, these caretaking constructs may possess momentary psychological integrity but it would not be possible to look to them to characterize infants' experiences. Satisfaction of these several criteria is prerequisite to evaluating the concurrent or predictive validity of categories of caretaking for some developmental outcome like cognitive growth.

Insufficient attention has been paid to the companion issues of internal consistency and discriminant validity in studying caretaking and in evaluating the effects of different modes of caretaking in development. If the collection of caretaking activities categorized together is not reasonably homogeneous, those that are mutually related and affect development may be mixed with others that are unrelated and not effective, thereby attenuating potential influences in development. And, if the collection of caretaking activities categorized together is heterogeneous, it will not be possible to identify which category of caretaking actually influences development. Historically, categories of caretaking have often been defined pluralistically. For example, Bradley, Caldwell, and Elardo (1979) found that "maternal involvement" at 6 months positively influenced infants' Bayley Scale scores at 12 and at 24 months, but they defined involvement to include "active encouragement of developmental advancement plus the structuring of experiences to promote social involvement and intellectual challenge" (p. 247). Which caretaking activity or activities actually contributed to the assessed effects?

The separate categories of social and didactic caretaking are each usually constructed of several individual items that are then collected together and used to evaluate relations to mental development in the infant and toddler. Work in my laboratory has shown that identifiably separate but significantly intercorrelated items can be collected within each of these categories (e.g., physical and verbal didactic encouragement of attention) to yield only marginally overlapping categories of social versus didactic caretaking (e.g., didactic encouragement versus face-to-face social play). Thus, social and didactic categories of caretaking interaction may be distinguished as psychometrically coherent but reasonably distinct entities.

Beyond internal consistency and discriminant validity, evidence at least of short-term stability is basic to validating caretaking categories. Although adult caretakers vary considerably among themselves in terms of the range of activity they perform within each kind of caretaking, and the caretaker–child relationship is dynamic and transactional in nature, caretakers seem to be reasonably consistent in a variety of categories of interaction, at least over short temporal periods necessary to establish psychometric stability.

Several studies have examined stability of maternal and paternal activities toward older infants and young children. Clarke-Stewart (1973), Bradley et al. (1979), Russell (1983), Beckwith and Cohen (1983), Bates and his colleagues (Olson, Bates, & Bayles, 1984; Pettit & Bates, 1984), and Belsky and his colleagues (e.g., Belsky, Gilstrap, & Rovine, 1984; Belsky, Goode, & Most, 1980) have all documented significant degrees of stability in parental activities toward infants in the first two years of life. My own research has specifically assessed maternal social and didactic activities repeatedly over the first year: Short-term day-to-day and week-to-week assessments reveal generally significant, if sometimes only moderate, levels of stability in caretaking (Bornstein, 1985; Bornstein & Ruddy, 1984; Bornstein & Tamis-LeMonda, 1987b; Ruddy & Bornstein, 1982), although it is normally to be expected that long periods between assessments will result in attenuated stability values. Notably, however, Dunn, Plomin, and Nettles (1988) found that mothers were consistent in a range of caretaking activities over a period of 1½ years as their first- and second-born toddlers each reached 12 months of age. Establishing the stability of modes of caretaking is essential since, as elaborated below, caretaker interactions may exert a profound influence in development because of their cumulative nature.

The stability of caretaking can be expected to vary with many factors, over and above the test–retest interval between assessments; among the most notable of these are the age, developmental status, and temperament of the child. Independent of how "fixed" in their ways caretakers may be, having a new baby, or a baby who changes, or a baby with particular traits each might differentially influence caretaking. For example, Belsky, Gilstrap et al. (1984) found that mothers and fathers alike were less consistent over the 2-month period of their infants' growth from 1 to 3 months than they were over the 6-month period of their infants' growth from 3 to 9 months. Over the longer course of child development, caregiving requirements dramatically change; thus, categories of caretaking cannot be expected to remain stable (Maccoby, 1980). Finally, individual differences among babies can play a formative role in shaping social interactions. For example, Bates, Olson, Pettit, and

Bayles (1982) found that temperamentally "difficult" babies demand and receive more attention than do temperamentally "easy" babies.

2.2. Illustrating the Effects of Categories of Caretaking

Astute psychological observers from Plato (*ca.* 355 B.C./1970) through J. S. Mill (1873/1924) have commented on and speculated about the lasting effects of young children's early experience. However, systematic scrutiny of the differential effects of child-rearing practices from the beginning of life did not begin until the late 1950s (e.g., Sears, Maccoby, & Levin, 1957), and studies of infancy did not mature until the 1960s (see Lamb & Bornstein, 1987). These late starts combined disadvantageously with the necessarily longitudinal nature of research in the field of developmental assessment and prediction when it came to placing an evaluation of specific caretaking experiences for children's mental achievement.

In the 1970s, an important direction of research finally emerged in developmental psychology whose goals were the identification, specification, and operationalization of caretaker interaction patterns that might influence children's development, especially their mental growth (see Bornstein, 1987a; The Consortium for Longitudinal Study, 1983; Gottfried, 1984; Wachs & Gruen, 1982). This movement had its roots in publications that documented differential effects of diverse child-rearing practices such as institutionalization, adoption, social class, and culture, although it found prominent contemporary focus in observational and experimental studies of caretaking in normal intact families. What long-term effects have nurturant, social, and didactic modes of caretaking, especially for children's cognitive development?

By itself, nurturance seems to have few if any direct implications for mental development in the child (e.g., Clarke-Stewart & Apfel, 1979). For example, Clarke-Stewart (1973) found that mothers' attending to their 9-month-olds' physical needs could be distinguished conceptually from a complex of their other activities, including expressed affection, verbal interaction, stimulation, responsivity, and the age appropriateness of their actions, and that the latter constellation at 9 months, not solicitousness, predicted children's cognitive competence at 18 months. As suggested, nurturance could nonetheless serve as an important prerequisite to other patterns of caretaking, for surely in its absence these other forms of caretaking have no opportunity to take effect.

Purely social caretaking practices may influence growth in a variety of ways—even as Harlow (Harlow & Harlow, 1966) observed long ago—and some seem specifically to relate to children's mental development.

Longitudinal research has suggested that generally warm, sensitive, affectionate, nonrestrictive parental care is positively associated with cognitive growth in children (e.g., Beckwith, Cohen, Kopp, Parmelee, & Marcy, 1976; Ramey, Farran, & Campbell, 1979; Solkoff & Matusak, 1975; Solkoff, Sumner, Weintraub, & Blase, 1969; Yarrow, Rubenstein, & Pedersen, 1975), and evaluative review indicates that the absence of social caretaking interactions early in life can be deleterious to mental development (Rutter, 1979). Two recent studies illustrate that affectively positive caretaking interactions may play a role in the mental development of the child. Bee, Barnard, Eyres, Gray, Hammond, Spietz, Snyder, and Clark (1982) found that maternal attentiveness and mood during feeding when infants were 4 and also 12 months of age significantly, if inconsistently, predicted children's 3-year language performance and 4-year IQ. Likewise, Olson et al. (1984) found that mothers' affectionately touching, rocking, holding, and smiling at their 6-month-olds significantly, if moderately, predicted a composite measure of cognitive/language competence in the same children at 2 years (a further interpretation of Olson et al. is reviewed below).

On the basis of research strategies adopted to establish causal links between caretaking and mental growth in early childhood, clear evidence is emerging that specific didactic interactions exert identifiable influences on cognitive development beginning in infancy. In one experiment, for example, Riksen-Walraven (1978) implemented two types of training programs among mothers of 9-month-old infants: Some mothers received instructions on the importance of encouraging their children to attend visually to characteristics of the environment, and other mothers were instructed about the importance of responding contingently to their infants' signals. After three months, Riksen-Walraven found that mothers trained on responsivity had 1-year-olds who demonstrated higher levels of exploratory competence, whereas mothers trained on sensory stimulation had toddlers who habituated more efficiently. Likewise, Belsky and his co-workers (1980) studied the effects of caretakers' didactic interactions on infants' engaging their environment; they did so first in a correlational way and afterward in an experimental way. In one study, Belsky et al. observed that mothers who stimulated their babies didactically had babies who explored in play more competently. In a second study, Belsky et al. observed that infants whose mothers were reinforced in their attempts to stimulate didactically scored significantly higher in exploratory competence than did infants whose mothers were treated neutrally.

In overview, certain caretaking interactions are thought to have identifiable implications for children's mental development, and they

have generally been found to meet basic psychometric criteria of construct validity, including internal consistency, discriminant validity, and
short-term stability. In the next section, I look empirically at specific
relations between social and didactic caretaking on the one hand and on
the other a variety of infant and child competences important in the first
years of life.

3. STUDIES OF SOCIAL AND DIDACTIC CARETAKING IN RELATION TO CHILDREN'S COGNITIVE COMPETENCE

How does the infant's experience with different kinds of caretaking
affect the growth of cognition? This important developmental question
has two sets of answers. The first is in terms of *specificity of effects;* namely,
which experiences affect which kinds of development and when? In this
section, I review several sets of experimental studies that provide data on
the first answer. The second answer is in terms of *process;* namely, by
what mechanisms and according to what schedule do experiences affect
development? Response to this interpretation of the question is provided in the section following this one.

To assess the roles of two main categories of caretaking on early
mental development, several colleagues and I have conducted different
sets of studies. The first concerned the role of maternal social and didactic caretaking in 3-month-olds' perceptual–cognitive competence. The
second and third concerned the selectivity of maternal caretaking modes
for 2- and 5-month-olds' exploratory competence and for 13-month-
olds' language and play competence, respectively. The fourth concerned
the predictive validity of categories of caretaking in the middle of the
infant's first year for childhood intellectual competence evaluated years
later. To evaluate their generalizability, we have replicated some of these
effects in a second culture, specifically among Oriental families in Japan.

The general conduct of basic observations of mothers and infants in
these studies was standardized so as to render results of the studies
directly comparable. Of course, procedural details changed with experiment, depending, for example, on the specific purpose of the study, and
to maximize age appropriateness of the individual measures. Observations of mothers and infants followed established methods (Bornstein,
1985; Bornstein & Ruddy, 1984). Trained, reliable observers visited
mothers and their infants at home when the mother and infant were
alone, and when the infant was sated, rested, and alert. Mothers were
asked to behave in their usual manner and to disregard the observer's
presence insofar as possible. Observation periods averaged approx-

imately 1 hour after warm-up. Observations were divided into time-sampling intervals, for example 60 seconds (Seitz, 1988): a 30-second "on" observation period followed by a 30-second "off" period, during which observers recorded the occurrence or nonoccurrence of selected mother and infant activities. Maternal activities that were recorded always included social and didactic interactions that used either physical or verbal means to elaborate on a topic of interaction already introduced or to introduce a new topic of interaction. Infant activities minimally included visual exploration, coded either as dyadic (looking at mother) or as extradyadic (looking at a property, object, or event in the environment), vocalization of nondistress or distress, and tactual exploration.

3.1. Caretaking and Perceptual–Cognitive Competence

Our first study asked what role, if any, mothers' social and didactic caretaking strategies may play in very young infants' perceptual–cognitive sensitivity. Specifically, we examined maternal correlates of 3-month-olds' ability to distinguish among facial expressions (Kuchuk, Vibbert, & Bornstein, 1986).

The ability to understand affective expressions by reading facial features has long been considered essential to successful interpersonal communication and is thought to be a skill that begins to develop within the context of early infant–caretaker interaction (e.g., Bowlby, 1969; Spitz & Wolf, 1946; Stern, 1974). Infants still in the first four months of life have been shown to discriminate among categories of facial expression (Barrera & Maurer, 1981; Field, Woodson, Greenberg, & Cohen, 1982; La Barbera, Izard, Vietze, & Parisi, 1976; Young-Browne, Rosenfeld, & Horowitz, 1977); indeed, this ability has been demonstrated in newborns and so may be universal and inborn (e.g., Ekman, 1972; Field et al., 1982; Izard, 1971). However, infants' sensitivity to variation within a category of facial expression may have multiple determinants. Provocatively, Barrera and Maurer (1981b) observed that 3-month-olds find it easier to discriminate among facial expressions worn by their own mothers than among the same expressions worn by a stranger. We asked what kinds of experience might mediate the development of infants' sensitivity to facial expression. Is mere exposure to maternal facial expressions critical? Or is more directive maternal experience the key, as when mothers encourage their infants to attend to the mothers' facial expressions? To address this question, we evaluated how infants' sensitivities to facial expression related to their experiences at home.

We studied the same infants both in the laboratory and at home; 30

3-month-olds and their mothers participated. In the home, we observed and recorded two infant activities, including smile at mother and look at mother, as well as five maternal activities, including smile at infant, look at infant, vocalize to infant, encourage the infant to attend to properties, objects, or events in the environment, and encourage the infant to attend to the mother herself (by positioning, touching, or directing the baby verbally or physically). In addition, a composite variable was constructed to document the co-occurrence of infant looking at mother and mother smiling at infant.

In the laboratory, we independently assessed infants' abilities to detect variations of smiling in a single face. During the laboratory procedure, the infant was seated alone in a test room while pairs of stimuli were projected for view. For this study, we developed two series of six chromatic slides of two women's faces. Each series included a neutral expression and five smiles ranging in approximately equal steps from a weak smile with slightly upturned corners of the mouth to a broad, toothy expression. Each infant saw 11 preference trials with one face series; on each preference trial, the infant saw the neutral expression paired with itself or with one of the five smiling poses of the same face. In these preference trials, the neutral–neutral pair was presented once, and each of the five neutral–smile pairs was presented twice with the left–right locations of the neutral and smiling expressions balanced.

We first analyzed the 3-month-olds' preferences and sensitivity to smiling expressions and then evaluated the association between infants' expressed perceptual sensitivities and their mothers' activities at home. As a group, 3-month-olds preferred poses of increasing intensity of smiling; however, individual infants showed different patterns of sensitivity to variation in the smiling series. Specifically, infants demonstrated differentially steep growth functions for preference; that is, some showed greater increases in looking earlier in the stimulus series, others only later in the stimulus series. Presumably, babies with steeper preference functions need fewer facial cues (e.g., smaller bow to the mouth, no teeth visible, less narrowing of the eyes) to distinguish among smiling expressions. To characterize growth rates of individual infants' sensitivity functions, we determined where in the stimulus series each infant reached a constant increment in looking over his or her looking at the neutral pose. In this formulation, greater increments earlier in the stimulus series indicate greater sensitivity. Infants showed considerable variation in their sensitivity; each infant's sensitivity index then served as a correlate for that infant's home experiences.

We then asked how infants' sensitivity to expressions of smiling related to their mothers' activities at home. We found that infants' sensitivity to facial expression was uniquely associated with their mothers' encouraging attention to themselves, $r = -.36$, $p < .05$. Mothers who actively encouraged their infants to attend to them more had infants who detected facial expressions of smiling more readily.

In order to compare the relative strengths of association of mere exposure to amount of maternal smiling on the one hand versus the role of maternal directiveness on the other, with infant sensitivity as a criterion variable, we conducted a series of multiple regression analyses in two steps. We let maternal smiling while infant looks at mother stand for a mere exposure hypothesis and maternal encouraging attention to self stand for a maternal directiveness hypothesis. We first compared these possible sources of variance for infants' perceptions in a simultaneous multiple regression analysis. This model accounted for 13% of the variance in infant performance. We reasoned, however, that infants experience their mothers' smiling in many contexts, including directive exchanges, and that the association between directiveness and infant performance may vary at different levels of exposure and vice versa. Therefore, in a second step of the analysis we used hierarchical multiple regression to evaluate the contribution of the interaction between these two variables with the pure effect of each partialed first (Cohen & Cohen, 1983). This model, including the interaction term, accounted for a significant 27% of the variance in infants' sensitivity. The increment in R^2 owing to the addition of an interaction term was a significant 14%.

In order to probe the nature of the interaction between mere exposure and maternal directiveness, we conducted a further analysis of slopes (beta weights) from the hierarchical regression equations (Cohen & Cohen, 1983). For this analysis, we tridivided the range for each variable into low, middle, and high values and inserted the midpoint for each range of one independent variable into the regression equation, thus allowing determination of the slope, or degree of relatedness, between the other independent variable and the dependent measure. Strong relations existed between maternal directiveness and infant sensitivity when the infant was exposed to low or to middle levels of maternal smiling, but as the infant experienced increasing amounts of maternal smiling, the association between maternal directiveness and infant sensitivity decreased. Corresponding examination of the relation between maternal smiling and infant sensitivity at varying levels of maternal directiveness yielded no statistically significant findings.

Infants are well known to discriminate smiling from other facial expressions, and so distinguish among categories of facial expression that signal different affects. The findings of our first study indicate that young infants also distinguish within a category of facial expression that signals a single affect. More pertinently, the study further indicates that mothers' encouraging attention to themselves, especially in the context of low to moderate levels of smiling while their infants are watching, is strongly associated with individual differences in infants' competence at distinguishing among such facial expressions. It is plausible therefore that mothers are promoting sensitivity in their infants.

Alternative interpretations are possible; however, they can be ruled out. If, for example, infants' precocious sensitivity engendered more maternal directiveness, we might expect that precocious infants would smile more at home as a way of cueing their mothers' behavior. No meaningful relations emerged between infants' smiling at home and infant sensitivity to smiling or maternal directiveness. Nor was mothers' smiling a correlate of infant perceptual acumen; this fact also substantiates the specialty and specificity of maternal directiveness. The association could also have been mediated by maternal demographic status, but when we evaluated the role of maternal education and social class in the correlation of infant sensitivity and maternal directiveness, we found that these factors played no part. Further, the interaction analysis demonstrated that mothers' drawing their infants' attention to themselves was most strongly associated with infants' sensitivity to smiles when the mothers' own smiling was tempered. Young babies seemed to learn about a phenomenon best when their attention was clearly directed by their mothers to less frequent but highly salient examples of the phenomenon.

3.2. Caretaking and Exploratory Competence

The first study indicates that infants only 3 months of age may be influenced in the expression of their perceptual sensitivity by specific maternal activities. In the second study series, we asked whether maternal style with somewhat younger and somewhat older babies could influence babies' visually and tactually exploring the environment. More specifically, in the first 6 months of the baby's life, some mothers tend to engage more in social forms of interaction, relatively speaking, whereas other mothers tend to engage more in didactic forms of interaction (Bornstein & Tamis-LeMonda, 1987a). We asked whether babies' tendencies in exploring the environment coordinated with their mothers' predominant organization of the babies' attention (Bornstein & Tamis-LeMonda, 1987b). In this main study of the second series, 29 primiparous mothers and their infants participated in two home observations, the first when the infants were 2 months of age and the second when 5 months of age.

We asked whether basic activities of mothers and basic activities of their infants interrelated at 2 and at 5 months. Approximately one-third of maternal and infant activities coordinated at each age, and in broad strokes patterns of intercorrelation between mothers and their 2-month-olds paralleled analogous patterns between mothers and their 5-month-olds. Consider, for example, patterns of conceptually corresponding relations between maternal stimulation of infant attention and infant attention itself and, relatedly, between maternal stimulation of infants and infants' tactual exploration. At 2 and at 5 months, respectively, mothers who stimulate their infants more have infants who attend more, $rs = .61$ and $.47$, $ps < .01$. Moreover, mothers and infants of both ages give evidence of a high degree of mutual specificity in these types of interaction: More maternal social encouragement is met with more infant social orientation at both ages, $rs = .55$ and $.30$, $ps < .001$ and $.05$, respectively, and more maternal didactic encouragement is met with more infant didactic orientation at both ages, $rs = .42$ and $.64$, $ps < .01$ and $.001$, respectively.

This relation is perhaps best summarized in the intercorrelation of how much mothers encouraged their infants to attend didactically vis-à-vis their total amount of stimulation and how much infants attended didactically vis-à-vis their total amount of attending: More maternal emphasis on didactic vis-à-vis social foci of interaction was met with more infant emphasis on didactic vis-à-vis social foci of attention at 2 months, $r = .53$, $p < .001$, as well as at 5 months, $r = .35$, $p < .02$. Relatedly, maternal stimulation of infant attention, especially didactic, is associated with infants' tactual exploration at the two ages, $r = .47$, $p < .01$, at 2 months and $r = .29$, $p < .05$, at 5 months.

Patterns of cross-relations between maternal speech and infant attention and exploration mostly followed the same course. At 2 months, maternal speech and infant attending were unrelated, whereas at 5 months maternal speech and infant attending were strongly coordinated activities, $r = .50$, $p < .01$. This general relation held, too, for mothers' use of the infant register as opposed to adult conversational tones. Maternal speech in total and especially in the infant register was positively associated with infants' tactual exploration, mean $r = .32$, $ps < .05$, whereas maternal speech to infants in adult conversational tones was negatively associated with infants' tactual exploration.

The specificity of maternal encouraging attention is also evident in an analysis of the difference in the correlations obtained in the first study series. The relation between infants' perceptual-cognitive sensitivity to smiling and mothers' social encouraging attention to themselves ($r = -.36$) tended to be stronger ($p < .07$) than it was to mothers' didactic encouraging of infants' attention to properties, objects, or events in the environment ($r = .01$).

Further, the specificity of maternal caretaking is maintained over time, as is shown in a comparison of lagged relations between maternal social versus didactic attention orientation at 2 months and infants' social versus didactic attention allocation at 5 months. For example, we found that mothers who tended more often to orient their infants didactically at 2 months not only had 2-month-olds who oriented didactically, but had 5-month-olds who favored a didactic orientation, $r = .38$, $p < .01$.

Significantly, the specificity of maternal orientation of infants' allocation of attention is not limited to American mothers and babies. In a parallel study of 31 Japanese mothers and their 5-month-old infants, we found analogous patterns of relations. Japanese mothers who more often encourage their infants to attend have infants who pay more attention, $r = .44$, $p < .01$; those who encourage more socially have infants who attend more socially, $r = .55$, $p < .001$; and those who encourage more didactically have infants who attend more didactically, $r = .65$, $p < .001$. Thus, mothers and babies in different cultures give evidence of comparably high degrees of specificity of interactions and their effects.

3.3. Caretaking and Verbal and Play Competence

The first two study series concerned the role of maternal social and didactic activities in young infants' developing perceptual–cognitive and exploratory competences. Infants were still in the first six months of life. In this third study series, we investigated the roles of these same maternal activities in older infants' developing verbal and play competences (Vibbert & Bornstein, 1987). Infants who participated were at the beginning of their second year.

The onset of the second year of life is harbinger to rapid language acquisition and the first referential uses of speech (e.g., Huttenlocher, Smiley, & Ratner, 1983; Snyder, Bates, & Bretherton, 1980). At this time, infants exhibit considerable variation in both comprehending and producing words. Extant research suggests that maternal social and didactic activities may relate positively to developing verbal competences among 1-year-olds. For example, Clarke-Stewart (1973) reported that mothers who stimulated their 1-year-olds to play with them in the context of objects had infants who performed higher on measures of cognitive competence at 1½ years of age. Likewise, Bradley et al. (1979) found a positive influence of maternal involvement (defined as, for example, "talking," "encouraging developmental advance," and "providing challenging toys") on Bayley Scale scores between 1 and 2 years.

Other studies have focused more specifically on children's verbal expressiveness. For example, Newport, Gleitman, and Gleitman (1977) found that mothers' use of yes/no questions and pointing related positively to growth in auxiliary verb use and noun inflections among 1-year-olds. Schwartz and Terrell (1983) found that 1-year-olds' acquisition of contrived lexical concepts (pairings of nonsense words with an object or action) linked directly to the frequency and distribution of examplars they heard during language intervention sessions. Furrow and Nelson (1984) found that mothers' use of references to people versus objects contributed to stylistic differences in language acquisition of 1- to 2-year-olds. Finally, Low (1985) reported that mothers who used shorter and simpler sentences had infants who were accelerated in acquiring their first words at 1 year.

In the same vein, researchers have attempted to map the development of play across the first 2 years (Belsky & Most, 1981; Nicolich, 1977; Wolf & Gardner, 1981) and to relate infants' play performance to their mothers' activities. For example, Belsky, Garduque, and Hrncir (1984) found that infants' early experiences (as evaluated on the HOME) exerted a positive influence on play motivation in samples of 1- to 1½-year-olds. Also, DeLoache and Plaetzer (1985) found that 1½-year-olds achieved higher levels of symbolic play when they played with their mothers than when they played alone. In overview, recent data support the general conclusion that parental input may influence development of infants' verbal and play competences.

In our study, 34 pairs of mothers and infants participated in two home visits, one designed to assess mother–infant interaction and the second to assess infant language and play. Home observations on the first visit were of two kinds: time sampling (already described) and global rating. One experimenter conducted time-sample observations. In order to aggregate observation data into more powerful and conceptually sophisticated variables for hypothesis testing, one global social and one global didactic composite score were created. A second experimenter periodically rated the degree to which mother or infant was responsible for initiating didactic and social interactions. The didactic control score from global ratings, which represents the degree of mother- versus infant-perceived control over didactic interactions, showed a positive correlation with the didactic composite, suggesting a consistent association between the frequency of various maternal didactics and perceived maternal control.

On the second home visit, a trained experimenter blind to the observational data administered the Reynell Developmental Language Scales (Reynell, 1981) and conducted play assessments based on a procedure reported by Belsky (Belsky & Most, 1981; Belsky, Garduque et al., 1984). The first part of the session consisted of a "free-play" period during which infants were rated for spontaneous play acts according to a 14-point scale. During a second "semistructured" part of the session, the experimenter offered infants a systematic series of demonstrations designed to elicit play acts at more advanced developmental levels than those attained during the free-play period. Each infant received a single elicited play score corresponding to the highest level of play attained during either the spontaneous or semistructured parts of the session. While the infant was occupied with the Reynell and play assessments, another experimenter interviewed the mother for detailed accounts of her infant's abilities to understand and to produce over 100 words and phrases (Bates, 1979; Bates, Bretherton, & Snyder, 1982).

We found that infants' language comprehension and production from the maternal interview correlated positively, $r = .40, p < .02$, as did their comprehension and production scores from the Reynell Scales, $r = .36, p < .04$. In order to fully represent infant language skills based on data from both the maternal interview and the independent assessment, a composite language score was created by transforming the maternal interview and the Reynell into z scores and adding them. In play, infants' elicited scores were significantly higher than their spontaneous scores, and the two were positively correlated, $r = .65, p < .01$. Play scores were also transformed and added together to create a composite variable that more fully represented infant play behavior.

We also looked at the relation between the didactic composite and the social composite, which we found to be independent, $r = .22$. When, finally, we evaluated the relation between mother and baby we found that maternal didactic activity in the home correlated significantly with both infant language and play, $rs = .38$ and $.37, ps < .05$, respectively, and that maternal social activity in the home was significantly associated with infant play, $r = .52, p < .01$. This pattern of results supports the conclusion that maternal didactic and social activities are independently associated with the development of infant language and play skills.

In order to examine the simultaneous contribution of maternal activities to infant language and play and to explore different paths of associations among these activities and abilities, we generated structural equation (path) models. Our initial model represented a unique, theory-based (*a priori*) hypothesis about the potential direction of effects among relevant activities. Maternal didactic and social activities were given equal weight in these models. Our model specified direct causal paths from maternal activities to infant skills; we also acknowledged the obvious endogenous contribution of maturation on infant language and play by an equivalent path from infant age to infant skill. When we tested this model with the language and play composite variables as criteria, the resulting solutions offered quite reasonable fits to the data. For example, the model provided an excellent overall fit to the language score, and the parameter estimate associated with the path from maternal didactics to infant language was uniquely significant. The model provided an excellent overall fit to the play score as well, and this time the parameter estimate associated with maternal social input was uniquely significant.

Further examination of infant language and play outcomes suggested the following conclusions. Maternal didactic input at this age appears to be a positive factor in developing infant skills, but maternal social input achieves this status only in conjunction with high levels of maternal didactic input and/or high maternal control (initiating) over didactics. For example, in the case of language, maternal social input was negatively associated with infant skill when maternal didactic control was low and infants were more active in controlling didactic exchanges. However, maternal social input seems to hold especial significance for the level infants attain in play performance.

3.4. Caretaking and Intellectual Competence

Whereas the first three study series mostly concerned concurrent associations between maternal social and didactic activities and diverse infant competences at points across the first year of life, the fourth study set investigated the short- and long-term predictive validity of maternal activities with infants for the same children's developing intellectual competence. This study set comprised several separate longitudinal observations: One focused on a group of singletons, a second on twins, and a third on singleton children from a different culture, Japan (Bornstein, 1985; Bornstein, Miyake, & Tamis-LeMonda, 1985–1986; Bornstein & Ruddy, 1984).

In the first study, we observed singleton children with their mothers at three points in development, initially when the babies were 4 months old, again when they celebrated their first birthday, and finally when they turned 4 years of age and were about to enter preschool. At 4 months and at 1 year, we coded mother–infant interactions at home specifically for mothers' didactically encouraging their infants to attend to properties, objects, and events in the environment. At 1 year we assessed productive vocabulary size in the toddlers, and at 4 years we assessed children's intelligence by the Wechsler series. Pertinently, we found that the 4-month-olds whose mothers didactically prompted them more often possessed larger expressive vocabularies at 1 year, $r = .61$, $p < .05$, and scored higher on a standardized intelligence test at 4 years, $r = .51$, $p < .05$.

We cross-validated the influences of didactic caretaking by capitalizing on the greater naturally occurring variability in maternal activity that arises among different populations of children. Specifically, we compared singletons with twins, for in this contrast the economics of maternal didactics (among other things) is taxed through mothers' necessary time sharing with two babies instead of one. At 4 months and at 1 year, mothers of twins interacted with their infants didactically at less than half the rate of mothers of comparable singletons ($p < .05$); presumably in consequence, at 1 year the twins possessed less than half the productive vocabulary of singletons ($p < .10$), and at 4 years the twins scored significantly lower on the Wechsler intelligence test ($p < .05$). Twins are widely acknowledged to perform consistently, if marginally, less well than singletons on psychometric assessments of language development, verbal reasoning, and intelligence (Mittler, 1970; Myrianthropoulos, Nichols, Broman, & Anderson, 1972), except perhaps when they are reared as singletons (Record, McKeown, & Edwards, 1970). Amidst the plethora of biological and experiential factors that could contribute to this established twin disadvantage, these data suggest that twins' relative deprivation in didactic experiences may play a contributing role (see, too, Lytton, 1980; Tomasello, Mannle, & Kruger, 1986).

Finally, we asked whether these maternal activities at 5 months possess a more general predictive relevance for developing intellectual competence by assaying their parallel role in children's cognitive growth in a culture outside America. A total of 26 Japanese infants who were observed in interaction with their mothers at 5 months were tested on the Japanese version of the Peabody Picture Vocabulary Test when they reached 2½ years of age. Two kinds of maternal didactic activities with infants predicted children's PPVT performance. Infants whose mothers verbally stimulated more or stimulated more often by introducing new things to their attention later scored higher on the PPVT, $rs = .35$ and $.36$, $ps < .05$, respectively. Our research in the United States has shown long-term predictive value of maternal interaction style in infancy for cognitive competence in childhood. This longitudinal study reveals similar patterns among Japanese mothers and their infants. The fact that interactive mechanisms that have been found to have predictive value in one culture function analogously in a considerably different culture argues for their potential universal worth.

3.5. Summary

The four study sets reviewed above demonstrate consistent concurrent and predictive relations between two forms of maternal caretaking and a variety of cognitive competences in infancy and early childhood. Moreover, each of these studies specifies associations between particular caretaking and particular developmental competences. This specificity may be the rule, rather than the exception. Many antecedent-consequent relations in the cognitive domain exhibit like specificity. This means that to understand the nature of caretaking effects it is necessary to differentiate inputs, patterns of association, and outcome variables. For example, general intelligence psychometrically measured is the childhood cognitive consequence most often evaluated in studies of mother–infant interaction, but intelligence is not a monolithic construct: There are many dimensions of intelligence (Gardner, 1984), and even many subabilities of psychometrically assessed intelligence (Guilford, 1967, 1979; Hunt, 1983). The same is true of language, which is perhaps the next most often assessed competence related to caretaking (e.g., Hoff-Ginsberg & Shatz, 1982). As we have found, specific interaction experiences can be expected to relate to specific outcomes.

It is clear from our data as well that associations between caretaking and competence are often direct. Sometimes, however, they may be indirect: Many studies of caretaking consequences are designed on the assumption that interactions exert independent and linear effects in development; yet, this assumption precludes consideration of significant complex or conditional effects that categories of caretaking may exert in concert. For example, Olson et al. (1984) found that mothers' social interactions with their 6-month-olds predicted a composite measure of children's cognitive competence at 2 years. However, path analysis of the investigators' longitudinal panel revealed that maternal social interactions at 6 months affected child outcome only indirectly through the influence of social interactions on maternal didactics at 1 year, which directly predicted children's cognitive competences at 2 years.

Likewise, in two of our studies we uncovered influential conditional effects among social and didactic forms of caretaking. In one, babies whose mothers at home more often encouraged them didactically to attend to the mothers' own faces distinguished expressions of smiling in the laboratory more acutely, but only when their mothers had not been overly social; high degrees of maternal social interaction in conjunction with didactics actually attenuated the otherwise direct relation between didactics and infant perceptual sensitivity. In the second study, infants whose mothers more often prompted them didactically scored higher on a standardized measure of language comprehension, whereas maternal social caretaking did not contribute to this infant competence. The language of infants whose mothers exerted high control over didactic object-centered exchanges profitted most from frequent social input. When infants were more controlling of didactic exchange, maternal social input was negligibly, even negatively, associated with language competence.

Categories of caretaking might therefore exchange during development to maintain their efficacy; similarly, to take advantage of input infants must be able to distinguish the signal of one category from noise of another. Human infants experience a complex mélange of caretaking interactions in their everyday life. Beyond the univariate effects of caretaking, developmentally changing and conditional relations among classes of caretaking constitute important factors in an emerging multivariate model of experiential determinants of development.

To effect their concurrent or predictive, and univariate or conditional consequences, caretaking interactions must function in specifiable and, perhaps, time-delimited ways. I take up these two considerations in the next section.

4. MECHANISMS OF ACTION AND TEMPORAL MODELS OF CARETAKING EFFECTS

Once categories of caretaking are defined and their effects on children's developing cognitive competences are identified, it is next of interest to attempt to specify the mechanisms of action as well as the temporal models by which such caretaking effects function. By mechanisms of action, I mean the exact means and conditions in which "transfer" of learning between caretaker and child—however that transfer is instantiated—is effected. By temporal models, I mean that these caretaking modes surely vary over the course of development in their concurrent and predictive validity for developmental outcome, and it is valuable to assess which are effective when.

4.1. Mechanisms of Action

How do social exchanges influence the child's cognitive performance? *How* do didactic experiences affect the child's intellectual accomplishments? In answering these questions several separate issues must be raised: first, direct versus indirect paths of influence must be distinguished; second, specific versus common mechanisms of action must be dissociated; third, short- versus long-term effects must be clarified;

and fourth, the functional relation between level of caretaking and developmental outcome must be specified.

Researchers and theoreticians who have linked social and didactic modes of caretaking to mental growth have postulated both direct and indirect pathways of influence. As defined by Parke (1978), direct influences encompass processes by which a social agent or physical event affects the child with no intervening stage, whereas indirect influences encompass processes by which a social agent or physical event affects the child through the mediation of some other agent or event. Many of the associations described above might be direct, but certainly indirect influences are common. It may be, for example, that toys and books in the home are positively associated with a child's developmental progress, but the extent to which such material aspects of the child's life actually influence development outside of interpersonal mediation has been questioned (e.g., Clarke-Stewart, 1973).

Beyond the issue of direct versus indirect paths of influence, some researchers and theoreticians have hypothesized that mechanisms of action must be specific to the nature of an interaction, whereas others have opined that influential interactions may reflect much more common processes. Consider some possible mechanisms of action that are specific to the domains of social and didactic caretaking, respectively. It could be that caretakers' social involvement with children promotes security in them, that secure children explore the environment more efficaciously, and that exploration translates into mental growth through information acquisition (Ainsworth & Bell, 1974). Matas, Arend, and Sroufe (1978) found that securely attached 1½-year-olds were more enthusiastic, persistent, cooperative, and in general more effective problem solvers at 2 years. Similarly, it could be that caretakers' didactic interactions cumulate to shape and texture the child's mental life (Bornstein, 1987a). Miner and Bornstein (1987) used moment-to-moment microanalytic techniques to explore those didactic interactions that possess long-term predictive validity for children's cognitive development. They found that mothers' prompting regularly anticipated their 3-month-olds' attending and vocalizing.

Explanations that could be common to more than one class of caretaking are of the following sorts. Social and didactic caretaking alike could stimulate brain growth that in turn underpins higher mental functioning. Responsiveness could inculcate feelings of self-efficacy and control and thereby contribute to children's competences, and responsiveness could be instantiated in caretaker social activities (e.g., Bell & Ainsworth, 1972; Bradley et al., 1979; Coates & Lewis, 1984; Lewis & Goldberg, 1969) or didactic ones (e.g., Bornstein & Tamis-LeMonda,

1987c; Riksen-Walraven, 1978). Indeed, attentive caretaking *per se* could promote self-regulation in children that facilitates attention and learning; it could strengthen children's motivation to acquire information or to succeed at solving problems; or it could simply provide caretakers and children with shared opportunities to learn about one another and thereby assist learning—in adults to structure experiences to enhance their informativeness and in infants to learn that their actions are correct and matter.

However direct or indirect the paths of influence, however specific or common the mechanisms of action, effective caretaking must exert an influence either in the short- or in the long-term. Consider two common models of the time course of caretaking effects. One possibility is that a given interaction experienced at a particular time affects the child at that time and that the consequent change in the child endures. This model is consonant with a dramatic "sensitive period" interpretation of experience effects (e.g., Bornstein, 1987b; Colombo, 1982). For example, Bornstein (1985) found that maternal didactic interactions at 4 months contributed more strongly to child IQ test performance at 4 years than did the same maternal didactic interactions at 12 months, even though mothers remained relatively stable in their didactic activities between 4 and 12 months.

An alternative possibility is that caretaking exerts an influence over development through its consistency. That is, that any caretaking experience at any one time does not necessarily exceed threshold in affecting the child, but longitudinal relations are structured by similar interactions continually repeating and aggregating over shorter time periods. Temporal stability in the child's social or didactic caretaking thereby underwrites the cumulation of experiences that eventually exceed a threshold of change (Bornstein, 1987a; Bornstein & Sigman, 1986; Stern, 1985). For example, Olson et al. (1984) found that the continuity of maternal interactions they measured over the first 2 years predicted children's 2-year cognitive competence, above the unique contribution of early or later maternal interactions they measured. Similarly, a number of studies have resulted in an attenuation of early caretaking effects when the contributions of later ones are partialed (e.g., Bradley & Caldwell, 1980; Gottfried & Gottfried, 1984). Thus, both the sensitive period and cumulative impact interpretations find empirical support in the extant developmental literature. Of course, there is nothing to prevent each from operating in separate spheres.

Finally, consider four simple models of possible functional relations between caretaking level and developmental outcome. The first is a straightforward linear relation: the more caretaking, the higher the developmental outcome. The second is a threshold relation: increasing caretaking has minimal effect on the asymptote of the outcome up to a certain point, above which its effect is constant. The third is an inverted-U curvilinear relation: the more caretaking, the higher the developmental outcome to a certain level, above which caretaking is increasingly deleterious to developmental outcome. The fourth is a U-shaped curvilinear relation: little caretaking is associated with a high developmental outcome, more with a low outcome, and still more with a high outcome again.

These are some of the basic models of possible functional associations of caretaking with developmental outcome. Of course, these associations have several variations. For example, the first relation described need not be strictly linear, but at some point the growth curve could inflect to reach an asymptote above which increments in caretaking do not affect developmental outcome. Further, these are simple models in the sense that they do not take into consideration variations in child sensitivity ascribable to general developmental changes or to individual differences among children. It may be that species-general characteristics dictate sensitivity to particular types of caretaking only above a certain level. Caretaking below that level is not effective. Alternatively, individual differences could dictate that different forms of the caretaking-outcome function apply to different people. For a temperamentally "passive" infant a linear relation might function, but for a temperamentally "active" infant a curvilinear relation might suit.

In overview, caretaking interactions may affect development by direct paths of influence or by indirect ones. Some mechanisms of action may be specific, others could be common. Some caretaking effects may obtain immediately, others only over long periods. Finally, caretaking may exert its influences according to linear, threshold, or more complex curvilinear functions. A signal future course of developmental study will be to identify and further elucidate the precise processes by which specific forms of caretaking affect specific developmental outcomes in children.

4.2. Temporal Models

Development is too subtle, dynamic, and intricate to admit that immediate availability or even the simple aggregation of social and didactic caretaking determine the course of ontogeny. Even if all types of caretaking were available to the child at different developmental periods, which they are not (at least in equal proportions), caretaking modes wax and wane in effectiveness, modulated at least in part by the developmental status of the child.

For example, one category of interaction may have telling consequences at an early developmental period but not at a later one, whereas a second category may have inconsequential impact at the first time period, but considerable effect at the second. Bee et al. (1982) found that mothers' instructional techniques predicted their children's language skills at 3 years and IQ at 4 years with increasing power between 4 months and 4 years, whereas maternal attentiveness, mood, and the like during feeding reciprocally lost predictive force over the same time period. In the extreme case, an interaction beneficial at one developmental period may adversely affect growth at another, again depending on the developmental status of the child. Goldberg (1977) found that kinesthetic stimulation of infants in the first 6 months positively predicted their concurrent and future test performance over the first year, whereas kinesthetic stimulation in the second 6 months impacted negatively on infant performance. Proximal contact could constitute a kind of primary stimulation in the newborn period or most effectively engage and organize newborn attention and thereby promote performance, whereas the same kind of contact later in infancy might inhibit infants' developing exploratory skills. Doubtlessly, motor, mental, and social status in the child help to determine whether and modify how different caretaking experiences will affect growth.

Research shows that even subtypes of caretaking vary in effectiveness depending on children's developmental status. Belsky and his coworkers (Belsky et al., 1980) and Bornstein and his coworkers (Bornstein, 1985; Bornstein & Ruddy, 1984; Bornstein & Tamis-LeMonda, 1987b) found that mothers' physical strategies of encouraging attention were more effective in influencing young infants' competences than were their verbal strategies dating from the same period. Prompting as opposed to independence and physical strategies rather than verbal ones seem to possess more immediacy, meaningfulness, and efficacy for the young, motorically incompetent, nonverbal infant. Presumably, the changing nature of the active and more independent child underlies the changing predictive significance of different subtypes of caretaking modes (see Carew, 1980).

The developmental perspective defines a kind of dynamic that integrates the evolving nature of the child with the changing effectiveness of different categories of caretaking vis-à-vis different developmental outcomes. This dynamic reflects both prior experiences and intrinsic maturational forces in the child. These two combine to render organism and new experience at any given time optimally or nonoptimally matched. The two trajectories—effective caretaker change and change in effective caretaking—together support Hunt's (1981) dictum: "For any experience to have maximal effect, it is essential that it match the existing achievements of the infant" (p. 23). This dynamic association between caretaking experience and developmental level also confirms the aptness of a "sensitive period" orientation to experience and development (Bornstein, 1987b).

5. CONCLUSIONS

A central fact of developmental advance in childhood is transaction in the caretaker–child dyad, and a central concern of developmental study is evaluation of forces bound up in developmental advances (Bornstein & Lerner, 1987). The studies I have recounted were designed to evaluate the roles of two important modes of caretaking in developmental advances in infancy. Several brief caveats are warranted in advance of reaching any general conclusions about the foregoing data and theory.

First, in discussing these studies I have referred uniformly and neutrally to "caretakers," but in practice mothers were the subjects of study. There is no intention here to place the onus of child-rearing solely on mothers (whether or not in the Western family mothers are traditionally principal caretakers for infants). Rather, typicality and convenience dictated this choice. Whether or not the mechanisms of interaction uncovered in studying mothers generalize to fathers, grandparents, extrafamilial caretakers, and others remains open to study. Parallel observations designed to explore these alternatives are currently underway in my laboratory.

Second, our studies focused on caretaker effects in the development of competence, leaving aside complementary "child effects." Child effects that are direct or indirect are highly relevant, however. It could be that infants simply carry inborn competences to childhood that are independent of their caretakers, or it could be that infant competences (or other aspects of infants) differentially affect caretakers in ways that subsequently redound to the infants-as-children (see Bornstein, Gaughran, & Homel, 1986; Sameroff & Chandler, 1975). It will be the work of future research to integrate caretaker and child effects together into a comprehensive model of transactional forces influencing development.

Third, a threat to the psychological independence—and, hence, meaningfulness—of caretaking effects derives from genetic variance shared between caretaker and child. Perhaps children's didactic experiences predict their language proficiency, not on account of any direct relation between caretaking and cognition, but because more educated and affluent caretakers, who would tend to interact didactically with their children more often, themselves tend to be smarter and to bear smarter children. Genetic endowment undeniably contributes to individual differences in cognitive development. However, several arguments weaken the force of this genetic critique of caretaking effects. The most significant is that caretaking appears to influence development even in situations where caretakers and their children are unrelated genetically. Adoption studies consistently show positive effects of caretaking interactions on cognitive and communicative functioning between unrelated mother–child pairs (e.g., Beckwith, 1971; Hardy-Brown, Plomin, & DeFries, 1981; Plomin & DeFries, 1985). Moreover, different categories of caretaking that are individually effective are not themselves perfectly correlated; that is, it is not necessarily the case that social caretakers are didactic and vice versa. Lastly, even among biologically related dyads different categories of caretaking retain unique predictive effects in development.

Fourth, modes of caretaking seem naturally to array themselves hierarchically in the everyday ecology of the child. In terms of the "economics of caretaking," nurturant interactions place the first and perhaps greatest demand on allocation of resources of infant caretakers; and, however life sustaining it may be, solicitousness seems to contribute least to the mental life of babies. Certainly, social interactions are next most engaging for parents—perhaps their popularity reflects their inherent ease and happy aspect. Unfortunately, didactic interactions, especially with infants, are the most taxing and, perhaps, stilted and are usually relegated to a last position of leftover time. Thus, caretakers typically make toys available to their young children and play together with them, but engage in instruction with considerably diminished consistency. Moreover, in life these categories of caretaking do not sort themselves out neatly, but may be confounded. Straightforward and intuitive as a connection between the child's social experiences and the child's developmental progress appears, the extent to which social caretaking influences development outside of didactic mediation may be questioned. These possibilities to the contrary notwithstanding, the research I have reviewed indicates that nurturant, social, and didactic caretaking are theoretically and conceptually distinct psychological categories, and each is a meaningful mode of interaction in itself.

Fifth, our studies demonstrate that different caretaking strategies deployed at different periods in different combinations affect the development of different child competences. Whether and how caretaking bears on the growth of the child depends on many factors, and no theoretically meaningful or potentially relevant interaction experience can be ruled out on the basis of a single-instance failure of investigators to uncover its effects. In this domain of research, highly specific associations as well as "sleeper effects" are to be expected, and both these sorts of phenomena can obscure potentially significant findings. By the same token, specifying means of promoting development in cognitive competence does not constitute an exhortation or even a recommendation to lift the common and right-minded injunction against "hothousing" children. Nevertheless, the identification of caretaking experiences especially efficacious in promoting development (of the mental sort or any other) has manifest epistemological implications that accrue undeniable additional practical significance when we consider that they may be taught and that they may play a useful role in intervention and compensation with normal as well as with at-risk populations of children.

The child's life is populated with many experiences that no doubt have identifiable implications in the course of development. Significant among these is caretaking, of which there are at least three main kinds, the nurturant, social, and didactic. Conceptual theoreticians and research investigators alike ask, not *whether* caretaking affects development, but *which* caretaking experiences affect *what* aspects of development *when* and *how*. Most have tended to promulgate the view that it is principally aggregate-level variables, like social class (e.g., Kagan, 1979; McCall, 1981) or cultural practice (Rogoff, Gauvain, & Ellis, 1984), that influence development of children generally and cognitive growth specifically. Logically, however, individual modes of *caretaking* must mediate between global influences on the one hand and individual differences in growth on the other. Indeed, two major perspectives within developmental study, those of Piaget (e.g., 1926) and of Vygotsky (e.g., 1934/1962, 1978), hold that mental advance in childhood develops out of classes of interpersonal experience such as these. Modern developmental psychology has come to see that however much children may accomplish alone in developing more can be achieved through their interactions.

That caretaking experiences influence development by no means implies that they monistically predestine or fix the child's eventual stature. Many factors contribute to human growth, and experiences of later life are widely acknowledged to account for large proportions of variance in every domain of mature human competence. Thus, throughout the life course, individuals are open to change, and they may be motivated to change on account of new or old experiences. Nonetheless, infancy seems to be an especially susceptible phase of the life cycle with regard to caretaking: Not only is caretaking at its most intensive in this period, but infants are thought to be particularly plastic to such external experiences because of the still fluid state of the nervous system, because of primacy effects in learning, and because of the lack of established competing responses. This perspective helps to explain why many life-long characteristics might assume their basic form in infancy and why infants' caretaking experiences might be so influential later in life.

Acknowledgments

Supported by research grants (HD20559 and HD20807) and by a Research Career Development Award (HD00521) from the National Institute of Child Health and Human Development. I thank H. Bornstein, A. Kuchuk, C. Miner, K. Miyake, M. Ruddy, C. Tamis-LeMonda, and M. Vibbert for collaborative assistance.

6. REFERENCES

Ainsworth, M. D. S., & Bell, S. M. (1974). Mother–infant interaction and the development of competence. In K. S. Connolly & J. S. Bruner (Eds.), *The growth of competence.* London: Academic Press.

Allen, M. J., & Yen, W. M. (1979). *Introduction to measurement theory.* Monterey, CA: Brooks/Cole.

Barrera, M. E., & Maurer, D. (1981a). The perception of facial expressions by the three-month-old. *Child Development, 52,* 203–206.

Barrera, M. E., & Maurer, D. (1981b). Recognition of mother's photographed face by the three-month-old infant. *Child Development, 52,* 714–716.

Bates, E. (1979). *The emergence of symbols: Cognition and communication in infancy.* New York: Academic Press.

Bates, E., Bretherton, I., & Snyder, L. (1982). *Language comprehension and production interview.* Unpublished manuscript, University of California at San Diego.

Bates, J. E., Olson, S. L., Petit, G. S., & Bayles, K. (1982). Dimensions of individuality in the mother–infant relationship at 6 months of age. *Child Development, 53,* 446–461.

Beckwith, L. (1971). Relationships between attributes of mothers and their infants' IQ scores. *Child Development, 42,* 1083–1097.

Beckwith, L., & Cohen, S. E. (1983). *Continuity of caregiving with preterm infants.* Paper presented to Society for Research in Child Development, Boston.

Beckwith, L., Cohen, S. E., Kopp, C. B., Parmelee, A. H., & Marcy, T. G. (1976). Caregiver–infant interaction and early cognitive development in preterm infants. *Child Development, 47,* 579–587.

Bee, H. L., Barnard, K. E., Eyres, S. J., Gray, C. A., Hammond, M. A., Spietz, A. L., Snyder, C., & Clark, B. (1982). Prediction of IQ and language skill from perinatal status, child performance, family characteristics, and mother–infant interaction. *Child Development, 53,* 1134–1156.

Bell, S. M., & Ainsworth, M. D. S. (1972). Infant crying and maternal responsiveness. *Child Development, 43,* 1171–1190.

Belsky, J., Garduque, L., & Hrncir, E. (1984). Assessing performance, competence, and executive capacity in infant play: Relations to home environment and security of attachment. *Developmental Psychology, 20,* 406–417.

Belsky, J., Gilstrap, B., & Rovine, M. (1984). The Pennsylvania infant and family development project I: Stability and change in mother–infant and father–infant interaction in a family setting—1- to 3- to 9-months. *Child Development, 55,* 692–705.

Belsky, J., Goode, M. K., & Most, R. K. (1980). Maternal stimulation and infant exploratory competence: Cross-sectional, correlational, and experimental analyses. *Child Development, 51,* 1163–1178.

Belsky, J., & Most, R. (1981). From exploration to play: A cross-sectional study of infant free play behavior. *Developmental Psychology, 17,* 630–639.

Bornstein, M. H. (1985). How infant and mother jointly contribute to developing cognitive competence in the child. *Proceedings of the National Academy of Sciences, 82,* 7470–7473.

Bornstein, M. H. (1987a). *The multivariate model of interaction effects in human development: Categories of caretaking.* Unpublished manuscript, New York University.

Bornstein, M. H. (Ed.). (1987b). *Sensitive periods in development: Interdisciplinary perspectives.* Hillsdale, NJ: Erlbaum.

Bornstein, M. H., Gaughran, J., & Homel, P. (1986). Infant temperament: Theory, tradition, critique, and new assessments. In C. E. Izard & P. B. Read (Eds.), *Measuring emotions in infants and children* (Vol. 2). New York: Cambridge University Press.

Bornstein, M. H., & Lerner, R. M. (1987). The development of human behaviour. *Encyclopaedia Britannica,* 708–723.

Bornstein, M. H., Miyake, K., & Tamis-LeMonda, C. (1985–1986). A cross-national study of mother and infant activities and interactions: Some preliminary comparisons between Japan and the United States. *Research and Clinical Center for Child·Development Annual Report,* 1–12.

Bornstein, M. H., & Ruddy, M. (1984). Infant attention and maternal stimulation: Prediction of cognitive and linguistic development in singletons and twins. In D. Bouma & D. G. Bouwhuis (Eds.), *Attention and performance X.* London, England: Erlbaum.

Bornstein, M. H., & Sigman, M. D. (1986). Continuity in mental development from infancy. *Child Development, 57,* 251–274.

Bornstein, M. H., & Tamis-LeMonda, C. S. (1987a). *Stability and continuity in maternal activities towards firstborn infants still in the first six months of life.* Unpublished manuscript, New York University.

Bornstein, M. H., & Tamis-LeMonda, C. (1987b). *Mother-infant interaction: Specificity of mutual relations in the infant's first half-year.* Unpublished manuscript, New York University.

Bornstein, M. H., & Tamis-LeMonda, C. (1987c). *Short-term effects of two kinds of maternal responsivity for infant exploration and information processing.* Unpublished manuscript, New York University.

Bowlby, J. (1969). *Attachment and Loss: Vol. 1. Attachment.* New York: Basic Books.

Bradley, R. H., & Caldwell, B. M. (1980). Competence and IQ among males and females. *Child Development, 51,* 1140–1148.

Bradley, R. H., Caldwell, B. M., & Elardo, R. (1979). Home environment and cognitive development in the first 2 years: A cross-lagged panel analysis. *Developmental Psychology, 15,* 246–250.

Carew, J. V. (1980). Experience and the development of intelligence in young children at home and in day care. *Monographs of the Society for Research in Child Development, 45* (Serial No. 187).

Clarke-Stewart, K. A. (1973). Interactions between mothers and their young children: Characteristics and consequences. *Monographs of the Society for Research in Child Development, 38* (6–7, Serial No. 153).

Clarke-Stewart, K. A., & Apfel, N. (1979). Evaluating parental effects on child development. In L. S. Shulman (Ed.), *Review of research in education* (Vol. 6). Itasca, IL: Peacock.

Coates, D. L., & Lewis, M. (1984). Early mother–infant interaction and infant cognitive status as predictors of school performance and cognitive behavior in six-year-olds. *Child Development, 55,* 1219–1230.

Cohen, J., & Cohen, P. (1983). *Applied multiple regression/correlation analysis for the behavioral sciences.* Hillsdale, NJ: Erlbaum.

Colombo, J. (1982). The critical period hypothesis: Research, methodology, and theoretical issues. *Psychological Bulletin, 91,* 260–275.

Consortium for Longitudinal Studies, The. (1983). *As the twig is bent: Lasting effects of preschool programs.* Hillsdale, NJ: Erlbaum.

DeLoache, J. S., & Plaetzer, B. (1985). Tea for two: Joint mother–child symbolic play. In J. S. DeLoache & B. Rogoff (Chairs), *Collaborative cognition: Parents as guides in cognitive development.* Symposium conducted at the meeting of the Society for Research in Child Development, Toronto, Canada.

Dunn, J. F., Plomin, R., & Nettles, M. (1988). Consistency of mothers' behavior toward infant siblings. *Developmental Psychology.*

Ekman, P. (1972). Universals and cultural differences in facial expressions of emotion. In J. Cole (Ed.), *Nebraska symposium on motivation.* Lincoln: University of Nebraska Press.

Field, T., Woodson, R., Greenberg, R., & Cohen, D. (1982). Discrimination and imitation of facial expressions by neonates. *Science, 218,* 179–181.

Furrow, D., & Nelson, K. (1984). Environmental correlates of individual differences in language acquisition. *Journal of Child Language, 11,* 523–534.

Gardner, H. (1984). *Frames of mind: The theory of multiple intelligences.* New York: Basic Books.

Goldberg, S. (1977). Social competence in infancy: A model of parent–infant interaction. *Merrill-Palmer Quarterly, 23,* 163–177.

Gottfried, A. W. (Ed.). (1984). *Home environment and early cognitive development.* Orlando, FL: Academic Press.

Gottfried, A. W., & Gottfried, A. (1984). Home environment and cognitive development in young children of middle socioeconomic status families. In A. Gottfried (Ed.), *Home environment and early cognitive development.* New York: Academic Press.

Guilford, J. P. (1967). *The nature of human intelligence.* New York: McGraw-Hill.

Guilford, J. P. (1979). Intelligence isn't what it used to be: What to do about it. *Journal of Research and Development in Education, 12,* 33–44.

Hardy-Brown, K., Plomin, R., & DeFries, J. C. (1981). Genetic and environmental influences on the rate of communicative development in the first year of life. *Developmental Psychology, 17,* 704–717.

Harlow, H. F., & Harlow, M. K. (1966). Learning to love. *American Scientist, 54,* 244–272.

Hoff-Ginsberg, E., & Shatz, M. (1982). Linguistic input and the child's acquisition of language. *Psychological Bulletin, 92,* 3–26.

Hunt, E. B. (1983). On the nature of intelligence. *Science, 219,* 141–146.

Hunt, J. McV. (1981). Comments on "The modification of intelligence through early experience" by Ramey and Haskins. *Intelligence, 5,* 21–27.

Huttenlocher, J., Smiley, P., & Ratner, H. (1983). What do word meanings reveal about conceptual development? In T. R. Wannenmacher & W. Seeler (Eds.), *The development of word meanings and concepts.* Berlin: Springer-Verlag.

Izard, C. E. (1971). *The face of emotion.* New York: Appleton-Century-Crofts.

Kagan, J. (1979). Structure and process in the human infant: The ontogeny of mental representation. In M. H. Bornstein & W. Kessen (Eds.), *Psychological development from infancy: Image to intention.* Hillsdale, NJ: Erlbaum.

Kuchuk, A., Vibbert, M., & Bornstein, M. H. (1986). The perception of smiling and its experiential correlates in 3-month-old infants. *Child Development, 57,* 1054–1061.

LaBarbera, J. D., Izard, C. E., Vietze, P., & Parisi, S. A. (1976). Four- and six-month-old infants' visual responses to joy, anger, and neutral expressions. *Child Development, 47,* 535–538.

Lamb, M. E., & Bornstein, M. H. (1987). *Development in infancy: An introduction.* New York: Random House.

Lewis, M., & Goldberg, S. (1969). Perceptual–cognitive development in infancy: A generalized expectancy model as a function of mother–infant interaction. *Merrill-Palmer Quarterly of Behavior and Development, 15,* 81–100.

Low, J. M. (1985). *The relationships between measures of mothers' speech and indices of first word acquisition.* Paper presented at the meeting of the Society for Research in Child Development, Toronto, Canada.

Lytton, H. (1980). *Parent–child interaction: The socialization process observed in twin and singleton families.* New York: Plenum Press.

Maccoby, E. (1980). *Social development—Psychological growth and the parent–child relationship.* New York: Harcourt Brace Jovanovich.

Matas, L., Arend, R., & Sroufe, L. A. (1978). Continuity of adaptation in the second year: The relationship between quality of attachment and later competence. *Child Development, 49,* 547–556.

McCall, R. B. (1981). Early predictors of later I.Q.: The search continues. *Intelligence, 5,* 141–147.

Mill, J. S. (1873/1924). *Autobiography of John Stuart Mill.* New York: Columbia University Press.

Miner, C. R., & Bornstein, M. H. (1987). *Maternal stimulation of infant vocalization and infant visual attention at 4 months: A time-series analysis of dyadic transactions.* Unpublished manuscript, New York University.

Mittler, P. (1970). Biological and social aspects of language development in twins. *Developmental Medicine and Child Neurology, 12,* 741–757.

Myrianthropoulos, N. C., Nichols, P. L., Broman, S. H., & Anderson, V. E. (1972). Intellectual development of a prospectively studied population of twins in comparison with singletons. In J. de Grouchy, F. J. G. Ebling, & I. W. Henderson (Eds.), *Human genetics: Proceedings of the Fourth International Congress of Human Genetics.* Amsterdam: Excerpta Medica.

Newport, E. L., Gleitman, H., & Gleitman, L. R. (1977). Mother, I'd rather do it myself: Some effects and non-effects of maternal speech style. In C. Snow & C. A. Ferguson (Eds.), *Talking to children: Language input and acquisition.* Cambridge: Cambridge University Press.

Nicolich, L. M. (1977). Beyond sensorimotor intelligence: Assessment of symbolic maturity through analysis of pretend play. *Merrill-Palmer Quarterly, 23,* 89–100.

Nunnally, J. (1978). *Psychometric theory.* New York: McGraw-Hill.

Olson, S. L., Bates, J. E., & Bayles, K. (1984). Mother–infant interaction and the development of individual differences in children's cognitive competence. *Developmental Psychology, 20,* 166–179.

Parke, R. D. (1978). Children's home environments: Social and cognitive effects. In I. Altman & J. F. Wohlwill (Eds.), *Human behavior and environment* (Vol. 3). New York: Plenum Press.

Pettit, G. S., & Bates, J. E. (1984). Continuity of individual differences in the mother–infant relationship from 6 to 13 months. *Child Development, 55,* 729–739.

Piaget, J. (1926). *The language and thought of the child.* London: Routledge & Kegan Paul.

Plato. (ca. 355 B.C./1970). *[The laws]* (T. J. Saunders, Trans.). Harmondsworth, Middlesex, England: Penguin.

Plomin, R., & DeFries, J. C. (1985). *The origins of individual differences in infancy: The Colorado Adoption Project.* Orlando, FL: Academic Press.

Ramey, C. T., Farran, D. C., & Campbell, F. A. (1979). Predicting IQ from mother–infant interactions. *Child Development, 50,* 804–814.

Record, R. G., McKeown, T., & Edwards, J. H. (1970). An investigation of the differences in measured intelligence between twins and single births. *Annals of Human Genetics, 34,* 11–20.

Reynell, J. (1981). *Reynell developmental language scales* (revised). Windsor, England: NFERNUSON.

Riksen-Walraven, J. (1978). Effects of caregiver behavior on habituation rate and self-efficacy in infants. *International Journal of Behavioral Development, 1,* 105–130.

Rogoff, B., Gauvain, M., & Ellis, S. (1984). Development viewed in its cultural context. In M. H. Bornstein & M. E. Lamb (Eds.), *Developmental psychology: An advanced textbook.* Hillsdale, NJ: Erlbaum.

Ruddy, M., & Bornstein, M. H. (1982). Cognitive correlates of infant attention and maternal stimulation over the first year of life. *Child Development, 53,* 183–188.

Russell, A. (1983). Stability of mother–infant interaction from 6 to 12 months. *Infant Behavior and Development, 6,* 27–37.

Rutter, M. (1979). Maternal deprivation, 1972–1978. New findings, new concepts, new approaches. *Child Development, 50,* 283–305.

Sameroff, A. J., & Chandler, M. J. (1975). Reproductive risk and the continuum of caretaking casuality. In F. D. Horowitz, E. M. Hetherington, S. Scarr-Salapatek, & G. Siegel (Eds.), *Review of child development research* (Vol. 4). Chicago: Chicago University Press.

Schwartz, R. G., & Terrell, B. Y. (1983). The role of input frequency in lexical acquisition. *Journal of Child Language, 10,* 57–64.

Sears, R. R., Maccoby, E. E., & Levin, H. (1957). *Patterns of child rearing.* Stanford: Stanford University Press.

Seitz, V. (1988). Methodology. In M. H. Bornstein and M. E. Lamb (Eds.), *Developmental psychology: An advanced textbook.* Hillsdale, NJ: Erlbaum.

Snyder, L. S., Bates, E., & Bretherton, I. (1980). Content and context in early lexical development. *Journal of Child Language, 8,* 565–582.

Solkoff, N., & Matusak, D. (1975). Tactile stimulation and behavioral development among low birthweight infants. *Child Psychiatry and Human Development, 6,* 33–37.

Solkoff, N., Sumner, Y., Weintraub, D., & Blase, B. (1969). Effects of handling on the subsequent development of premature infants. *Developmental Psychology, 1,* 765–768.

Spitz, R. A., & Wolf, K. (1946). The smiling response: A contribution to the ontogenesis of social relations. *Genetic Psychology Monographs, 34,* 57–125.

Stern, D. N. (1974). Mother and infant at play: The dyadic interaction involving facial, vocal, and gaze behaviors. In M. Lewis & L. Rosenblum (Eds.), *The effect of the infant on its caregiver.* New York: Wiley.

Stern, D. (1985). *The interpersonal world of the infant.* New York: Basic Books.

Tomasello, M., Mannle, S., & Kruger, A. C. (1986). Linguistic environment of 1–2-year-old twins. *Developmental Psychology, 22,* 169–176.

Vibbert, M., & Bornstein, M. H. (1987). *Mothers interacting with their 13-month-olds: Effects on language and play.* Unpublished manuscript, New York University.

Vygotsky, L. S. (1934/1962). [*Thought and language*] (E. Hanfmann & G. Vakar, Trans.). Cambridge, MA: The M.I.T. Press.

Vygotsky, L. S. (1934/1978). *Mind in society: The development of higher psychological processes.* Cambridge, MA: Harvard University Press.

Wachs, T. D., & Gruen, G. E. (1982). *Early experience and human development.* New York: Plenum Press.

Wolf, D., & Gardner, H. (1981). On the structure of early symbolization. In R. Schiefelbusch & D. Bricker (Eds.), *Early language intervention.* Baltimore, MD: University Park Press.

Yarrow, L. J., Rubenstein, J. L., & Pedersen, F. A. (1975). *Infant and environment: Early cognitive and motivational development.* New York: Wiley.

Young-Browne, G., Rosenfeld, H. J., & Horowitz, F. D. (1977). Infant discrimination of facial expressions. *Child Development, 48,* 555–562.

## 3

The Maternal Self-Report Inventory

A Research and Clinical Instrument for Assessing Maternal Self-Esteem

E. SHEA AND EDWARD Z. TRONICK

1. INTRODUCTION

Maternal self-esteem can be viewed as a psychological final common pathway mediating the effects of the biosocial factors that influence a woman's adaptation to motherhood. Such factors include variations in the infant's and the mother's health, the sex of the infant, demographics, separation at birth, delivery route, social support, and other circumstances. By modifying the mother's self-esteem these factors modify the quality of the mother's behavior with her infant. For example, a mother with low self-esteem is expected to be less facilitative and more disruptive of the infant's goals for maintaining homeostatic regulation and engagement with the external environment. This quality of her behavior is thus more likely to compromise her infant's development.

Unfortunately, there exists no standard or comprehensive instrument for assessing maternal self-esteem and there are only a few, mostly clinical, studies that have evaluated the factors that affect it. Our pur-

---

E. Shea and Edward Z. Tronick • Department of Psychology, University of Massachusetts, Amherst, Massachusetts 01003.

pose was to develop and validate such an instrument, the Maternal Self-Report Inventory (MSI), and to assess some of the factors that affect it.

2. FACTORS IMPLICATED AS AFFECTING MATERNAL SELF-ESTEEM

Many diverse factors have been implicated as affecting a woman's adaptation to motherhood. Seashore, Leifer, Barnett, and Leiderman (1973), in one of the few systematic investigations of maternal self-esteem, found that mothers who were denied early contact with their infants had less self-confidence than mothers who had early contact. But self-confidence, at least for the Seashore study, was not simply a function of separation. Primiparous mothers had less self-confidence than multiparous mothers regardless of contact experience. This effect of parenthood is reported in several other studies (e.g., Westbrook, 1978). Researchers have also reported that following a Caesarean section delivery—a variable confounded by the factors of maternal health, infant health, and separation—mothers generally experience significantly more feelings of depression, anxiety, and negative feelings toward pregnancy and motherhood than do mothers who delivered vaginally (Pederson, Zaslow, Cain, & Anderson, 1980; Grossman, 1980; Field & Widmayer, 1980). Similar findings on separation and parity have been reported in many other studies, although the effects are often attributed to bonding (Kennell, Trause, & Klaus, 1975) rather than disruption of maternal self-esteem.

Infant medical status affects maternal self-esteem. Rose, Boggs, and Alderstein (1960) and Kennell and Rolnick (1960) found that even mild and temporary illnesses that separated the mother and infant produced feelings of anger, anxiety, and postpartum "blues." These minor problems had long-lasting effects on the mother–infant interaction as well. More significant infant health problems more seriously disrupt mother–infant interactions and lead to stronger maternal feelings of guilt, anxiety, and incompetence (Prugh, 1953; Mason, 1963; Caplan, Mason, & Kaplan, 1965; Kaplan & Mason, 1969; Klaus & Kennell, 1976).

Dramatic and intense feelings of inadequacy and failure are reported when an infant is born with a congenital anomaly or a chronic disease (Greenberg, 1979). Mothers perceive the infant as a "defective or bad part of the self." Mothers find that they are helpless to care for the infant, heightening feelings of failure and causing them to withdraw even more from their infants.

The birth of a premature infant, a more typical problem, produces maternal feelings of failure along with feelings of anxiety and guilt. To quote Klaus and Kennell (1976), "The birth of a premature infant is a severe blow to the mother's self-esteem, mothering capabilities, and feminine role. It is conceived of as a loss of a body part, an insult of her bodily integrity, and a sign of inner inferiority."

A review of these studies suggests that despite the initial narcissistic injury to self-esteem, the continued development of maternal self-esteem largely depends on the mother's success in interacting and caring for her infant. This suggests the hypothesis that more competent infants facilitate caretaking, an outcome which then enhances a mother's self-esteem. The hypothesis finds much support with respect to the infant's impact on caretaking. Variations in an infant's alertness, habituation, cuddliness, irritability, activity levels, and responsiveness to stimulation affect an infant's interaction with his or her mother (Scanlon, Scanlon, & Tronick, 1983). However, again, there are few studies relating infant behavior directly to maternal self-esteem. Moreover, confounding the evaluation of this relationship are the findings demonstrating that many of the factors that affect infant behavior (e.g., birth weight, gestational age, obstetric medication, Caesarean section, jaundice, neurological syndromes, size for gestational age, pH, P_{O_2}, as well as demographic variables such as sex, age, birth order, parental age, education, occupation (Scanlon et al., 1983; Brazelton, 1974; Coopersmith, 1967), are variables that also seem to affect maternal self-esteem directly.

Research has demonstrated (Cohen, 1966; Barnard & Gortner, 1977; Feiring & Taylor, 1977) the importance of family support and family acceptance in predicting positive maternal attitudes as well as high ratings of maternal involvement immediately after delivery. A lack of this familial support and acceptance causes a mother to worry more about the health of the baby or herself and portends later attachment problems. Another variable that has been found to affect maternal adaptation and the mother–infant interaction is the mother's perception of her infant (Broussard & Hartner, 1971). Mothers who saw their infants as "better than average" had better interactions with their infants and better attitudes toward themselves.

There are several problems related to these studies. First, with few exceptions most studies have been retrospective. Second, the discussion of self-esteem has been based on clinical impressions. No objective or validated method was used to assess maternal self-esteem. Third, the factors investigated were often confounded with one another and little or no attempt was made either analytically or conceptually to separate out their effect. And fourth, many of the confounded factors directly impact on each other, adding even greater complexity to the picture. Nevertheless, despite all these findings, maternal self-esteem is repeatedly given a central role as a factor affecting maternal adaptation.

Given these findings and these methodological problems, our goal was to develop and validate a questionnaire for assessing self-esteem and to avoid some of these methodological problems by using a prospective study to establish validity of the questionnaire. Our first task was to establish the dimensions or characteristics of maternal self-esteem.

3. DIMENSIONS COMPRISING FEELINGS OF SELF-ESTEEM

Self-esteem is thought to have general as well as specific components. General self-esteem has been found to be a relatively stable and enduring characteristic of a person. It is more at the core of one's personality. It does not show much change with changes in circumstance, though it will change slowly over time with changes in the person's life. More specific components of self-esteem relate to the person's evaluation of himself or herself in a particular domain of functioning. These self-evaluations are often more transitory and related to specific situations and conditions.

"Self-esteem may vary across different areas of experience and role-defining conditions" (Coopersmith, 1967). As Epstein (1979) has stated, "The overall findings indicate that self-esteem is both unified and differentiated, and has wide ramifications for general functioning." As for maternal self-esteem, one might expect that a woman's feelings about her capacity to be a mother would be at the core of her personality whereas her feelings about her ability to engage in routine caretaking tasks maybe much more based on her evaluation of her performance.

Epstein (1979) found that situations that frequently preceded increases in self-esteem included difficult undertakings, the development of love relationships, new social roles, and situations forcing individuals to assume greater autonomy and responsibility, whereas events that frequently preceded decreases in self-esteem included exposure to a new environment, demonstration of inadequacy, immoral behavior, being negatively evaluated, being rejected by a loved one, death of a loved one, disturbed love relationship, loss of group affiliation, and introspective negative self-assessment. Clearly, the experience of becoming a mother and caring for a newborn contains many of these elements and as such is likely to have an effect on one's specific self-esteem as a mother in either a negative or a positive direction. Moreover, to the extent that maternal self-esteem is central to women's identity the adaptation to motherhood has the potential to modify a woman's general self-esteem.

What are the dimensions that make up maternal self-esteem? Leifer (1977); Shereshefsky and Yarrow (1973); Greenberg and Hurley (1971); Blau et al. (1963); Shaefer and Bell (1958); and Cohler, Weiss, and Grunebaum (1970) have provided in-depth accounts of the feelings and attitudes of mothers toward pregnancy and motherhood. Their descriptions are based on years of observation, clinical interviews with mothers, and data from questionnaires designed to identify and assess the critical factors comprising maternal adjustment toward motherhood.

Referring to this literature, we identified a number of factors we thought were dimensions of maternal self-esteem; i.e., a mother's feelings of self-confidence in her mothering ability. These dimensions are (1) maternal caretaking ability, (2) general ability as a mother, (3) acceptance of the baby, (4) expected relationship with the baby, (5) complications during labor and delivery, (6) parental influence, and (7) body image and maternal health. Besides having good face validity, these dimensions have been found by many researchers to be related to successful adaptation to motherhood. They will now be explored in more depth.

3.1. Caretaking Ability

Leifer (1977) found that a mother's beliefs about her adequacy were tied to such events as ability to nurse successfully and calm her baby. During pregnancy and immediately following delivery, a mother typically must make a decision as to whether or not to breast feed her baby. In making this decision, a mother must consider her own needs, fears, and ability to meet the demands of her baby. For some the choice is a very easy one, particularly when the mother receives spousal and/or familial support for her decision. However, for other mothers who choose to breast feed but fail to be able to continue or for mothers who feel pressured to breast feed against their own desire, this experience can lead to feelings of failure and inadequacy in the mothering role (Coopersmith, 1967; Cohen, 1966).

Seashore et al. (1973) devised a paired comparison questionnaire to assess maternal self-confidence. Mothers were asked to compare themselves with five other possible caretakers (father, grandmother, experienced mother, pediatric nurse, and doctor). Comparisons were made on six caretaking tasks, three of which were classified as instrumental and three as social. The three instrumental tasks were feeding the baby, bathing the baby, and diapering the baby. The three social caretaking tasks were showing affection to the baby, holding and calming the baby, and understanding what the baby needs. Seashore et al. (1973) found that these two measures, social and instrumental caretaking tasks, correlated very highly ($r = .80$). In addition, Schaefer and Bell (1958) have suggested that mothers who were more irritable with their infants were less confident in their caretaking ability. Greenberg (1979) found that mothers of handicapped infants who had very low self-esteem also felt as though they might be potentially dangerous or harmful to their infant. They reported not trusting their own caretaking ability.

3.2. General Ability as a Mother

Schaefer and Bell (1958) have data suggesting that a mother's enjoyment and pleasure in caregiving is related to how confident she is in her overall ability to care for her child. A mother's overall ability to care for her child differs from caretaking ability in that it comprises feelings concerning more general competence in assuming and fulfilling the responsibilities of being a mother, such as being there when needed, teaching one's child all that he or she will need to learn, and being a loving and caring parent. In addition, they found that a mother's acceptance or rejection of her role as a mother and her feelings about sacrificing personal time and activities were strongly related to maternal expectations of her abilities. Blau et al. (1963) suggested that a mother's perception of her ability to provide unique contributions to her infant's development and to teach her infant important new tasks is related to her feelings of competence.

Mothers normally experience some anxiety and apprehension concerning all the responsibility they must assume as mothers of newborn infants. But as Bibring (1959) and Brazelton (1976) have suggested, the mother's ability to cope with these feelings and adjust to this new developmental crisis is strongly related to how she feels about her ability to care for her infant. Thus, maternal feelings of anxiety, depression, and emotional preparedness for mothering appear to be factors related to maternal self-esteem. It is expected that these self-appraisals are basic to a mother's beliefs about her general ability as a mother.

3.3. Acceptance of Baby

During pregnancy, an expectant mother evaluates her capacities to be a mother. This generally includes visualizing what the baby will look like, what the sex of the infant will be, and whether or not the baby will develop normally. Brazelton (1976) has suggested that the mother's ability to adjust her expectations and fantasies of the baby she expected to the infant she "gets" is important if the mother is to adapt positively to her new role and to her infant. It is expected that the mother's acceptance of and happiness with the characteristics of her infant will influence her feelings of competence as a mother. Greenberg and Hurley (1971) found that mothers whose expectations of the "wished-for" infant were not realized had very low self-esteem. Mothers who viewed their infant as a negative extension of themselves also had low self-esteem. Berger (1952) found that expressed acceptance of self is positively correlated with expressed acceptance of others. It may be that mothers who have negative feelings toward themselves will also express negative feelings toward their infant.

3.4. Expected Relationship with Baby

Benedek (1949) suggests that "the capacity of the mother to receive from the child, her ability to be consciously gratified by the exchange and to use this gratification unconsciously in her emotional maturation is the specific quality and function of motherliness." Benedek goes on to suggest that a mother who finds fulfillment and gratification in interacting with her infant and developing a close and mutual relationship with her infant will then develop more confidence in her mothering ability and fulfillment in her role as a mother. Using clinical interviews, Greenberg and Hurley (1971) found that parental self-esteem was not only related to the mental image of the "wished-for-infant," referred to above, but was also closely tied to the parental "wished-for" relationship with the infant. In addition, Greenberg found that mothers who devalued themselves or their infants also had very low self-esteem.

3.5. Feelings during Pregnancy, Labor, and Delivery

Research that has assessed the influence of a mother's initial desire to have an infant on her later ability to adapt to her mothering role has reported conflicting results. A study mentioned earlier by Bibring (1959) and a later study by Davids (1968) indicate that mothers who initially did not want to get pregnant later frequently had disturbed relationships with their infants. However, Seashore et al. (1973) tested the relationship between self-confidence and mothers' initial desire to have an infant and reported no significant relationship. The subjects in the Seashore et al. study were all from middle-class, intact families, so that social and economic problems concerning unplanned pregnancies of a single mother were not encountered.

It has been reported that mothers who have experienced very difficult labor or who required large amounts of anesthesia and sedation often experience a lag in the development of "mothering" attitudes (Grossman, 1980). Benedek (1949) found that many mothers reacted to very long and difficult labor with depressive symptoms that produced withdrawal from the child. Others became rejecting toward the baby and perceived the child as the person responsible for the unacceptable feelings within them.

More recently, Grunebaum, Weiss, Cohler, Harman, and Gallant (1975) found that complications during delivery such as breech presentation, the need for high forceps, and anoxia produce maternal feelings of guilt and inadequacy. In the past few years, researchers have also begun investigating the ramifications of Caesarean section delivery on both infant development and maternal adaptation. Although various methods have been used to assess maternal adaptation following a Caesarean section delivery, the findings indicate that there is a high incidence of maternal depression, anxiety, and negative feelings toward pregnancy following a Caesarean section, particularly when it is unexpected (Pederson et al., 1980; Grossman, 1980; Field & Widmayer, 1980).

Deutsch (1945) and Brody (1956) have discussed at length the process whereby the mother's "instinctive forces" and maternal feelings in response to her infant pull her out of this "blue" period and allow her to develop a positive relationship with her infant. However, as the above research indicates, the mother does not always succeed and the mechanisms that the mother uses to overcome this depression are still not clearly understood.

3.6. Parental Acceptance

Benedek (1949) emphasized the effect of childhood events and experiences such as the mother's own mother–child relationship, her identification with her own mother, and her feelings of parental acceptance and love (Rosenberg, 1979) on her mothering. Davids (1969) found that mothers who had not yet resolved their negative attitudes toward childrearing later had frequent problems in their relationships with their own children. Ricks (1981) found that mothers of securely attached infants evaluated their relationship with their parents as significantly more accepting and supportive than mothers of infants not considered securely attached. Mothers of securely attached infants also had significantly higher self-esteem than mothers of infants who were not securely attached. However, no correlation between parental acceptance and self-esteem was mentioned in this study.

Psychoanalytically oriented research (Blau et al., 1963; Deutsch, 1945) indicates that in preparing for the experience of motherhood, women frequently reflect back on their experiences with their mothers and evaluate their ability as mothers in relation to their own parents. Given this heightened awareness of a mother's relationship with her mother, it is quite possible that there is an influence on her perception of her own ability to be a good mother.

3.7. Body Image and Health after Delivery

Body image has been found to be closely linked to one's feelings of self-esteem (Rosenberg, 1979). In a factor analysis of his Self-Report Inventory, Epstein (Epstein & O'Brien, 1976) found that satisfaction with physical appearance correlated very strongly with general self-esteem. Satisfaction with body functioning as defined by resistance to illness or by physical ability was not strongly related to general self-esteem in the college student population of the Epstein study. However, as women go through such dramatic changes in physical appearance as well as bodily functioning, during and after their pregnancy, it is quite likely that their self-concept will be affected. Blau et al. (1963) found that two factors that were related to maternal adaptation were a feeling of looking well before and after pregnancy and a lack of concern about one's postnatal figure.

In summary, we see these seven dimensions as the major components of maternal self-esteem. The first four of these (caretaking ability, general ability as a mother, acceptance of the baby, and expected relationship with the baby) are very closely related to each other and expected to correlate highly with each other. However, it is expected that they each measure a distinct component of maternal self-esteem.

4. DEVELOPMENT OF THE MATERNAL SELF-REPORT INVENTORY

With these seven primary conceptual dimensions identified, a large number of self-report items were written for each dimension aimed at revealing how a mother rated her own feelings concerning each of the dimensions. All items are written in the first person and mothers were requested to indicate on a Likert scale how accurately each statement described how they felt by circling the answer that best expressed the degree to which the statement was true for her. Some of the items on the scale were modified versions of items from questionnaires concerning child rearing attitudes (Schaefer & Bell, 1958), maternal attitudes toward pregnancy (Blau et al., 1963), *The Maternal Personality Inventory* (Greenberg & Hurley, 1971), and a structured interview designed to assess maternal adaptation (Barnard & Gortner, 1977).

To start, a large number of questions were written for each of the dimensions. On the caretaking ability dimension questions were designed to assess the possible conflicts concerning the decision to breast feed, ability in various caretaking tasks such as bathing and diapering, ability to show affection to the baby and to hold and to calm the baby. Questions were also included concerning how irritable a mother expected she would feel in response to a crying baby. For the dimension of general ability as a mother, questions were devised that measure more global feelings of maternal competence. For the dimension of acceptance of baby, questions were designed to measure the mother's pleasure with the sex and appearance of her infant and her confidence that her infant will grow and develop normally. In order to measure the dimension of expected relationship with baby, questions were devised regarding the mother's ability to develop a loving relationship with her baby and her expectations about the baby loving her. Questions were also devised concerning the dimensions of feelings during pregnancy, labor, and delivery and parental acceptance. Finally, to assess the dimension of body image and health after delivery, questions were written to measure feelings about postnatal appearance, health, and energy.

To choose among the large number of questions generated, ten mothers and five psychologists were given each question on a separate index card and asked to sort them into categories that seemed psychologically homogeneous. They were also asked to label each category. The majority of raters sorted the questions into six or seven categories and their category labels closely matched those we had assigned. Items that were not consistently placed in the same category by different raters were said not to match up with their categories or just "didn't seem correct" and were dropped. This process indicated the face validity of the items and resulted in a total of 100 self-report items, about 15 questions for each dimension. These questions were compiled in a self-report questionnaire—the Maternal Self-Report Inventory. Items from the seven dimensions were randomly mixed in the inventory and an equal number of positive and negative items were written for each dimension to avoid response sets. Appendix A presents the full instrument organized in terms of the seven dimensions.

Once the MSI was developed to measure maternal self-esteem, the purpose of the present study was to validate the instrument by assessing its relationship to a standard measure of self-esteem and to a set of nine factors—demographic variables, delivery route, maternal health, infant health, separation, parity, feeding problems, family support, maternal perception and mother–infant interaction—that we had found in the literature review for the first postpartum month among a group of normal and relatively healthy infants and mothers. It was hypothesized that even within the context of normal infants and mother, differences exist in maternal self-esteem that are related to differences in maternal experiences and newborn characteristics.

4.1. Method

4.1.1. Selection of Sample

Thirty mother–infant pairs were randomly selected from the normal newborn nursery of the Baystate Medical Center in Springfield, Massachusetts. The only criteria for inclusion in the study was that the mother and infant had to be discharged home from the hospital together. This made for a relatively healthy full-term sample of mothers and infants.

4.1.2. Measures

The Parmelee Obstetrical Complications Scale (Littman & Parmelee, 1978) was used to assess the mother's prenatal delivery and postnatal course and includes 36 possible risk factors such as maternal age, parity, hypertension, type of delivery, placenta previa, and premature rupture of membranes. This information was obtained from each mother's medical record during the perinatal period and data on complications occurring post discharge were obtained from maternal report. The total number of medical complications was used as the index of maternal health, with high scores reflecting increased risk to the mother's health.

The Parmelee Postnatal Complications Scale (Littman & Parmelee, 1978) was used to assess the infant's postnatal course and includes 17 possible risk factors such as respiratory distress, hyperbilirubinemia, metabolic and temperature disturbances, and feeding problems. This information was obtained from each infant's medical record during the perinatal period and from maternal report during the postnatal period.

The total number of medical complications was used as the index of infant health, with high scores reflecting increased risk.

The Neonatal Behavioral Assessment Scale (Brazelton, 1973) was used to screen the newborn's neurological status on 20 reflexes and to assess the newborn's behavior on 26 behavioral items. These behaviors are summarized by four *a priori* scoring dimensions labeled Interactive Processes, Motoric Processes, State Organization Processes, and Physiological Response to Stress (Als, Tronick, Adamson, & Brazelton, 1976). These scoring dimensions were summed to produce a total score, with lower scores indicating more optimal performance. All examinations were conducted by a trained and certified examiner who was blind to the mother's response to the questionnaires. Interrater reliability scores with another trained certified examiner were obtained twice during the study and were greater than 90% absolute agreement each time.

A 16-item Family Support Questionnaire was used to determine the degree of family, especially paternal, support that the mother felt she was receiving. Included were questions concerning the father's or secondary caretaker's involvement in caretaking activities and participation in decision making and the mother's satisfaction with her relationship with the baby's father or secondary caretaker.

Broussard's Neonatal Perception Inventory (Broussard & Hartner, 1970) was used to assess the mother's perception of her infant as compared with "the average baby." This inventory consists of two derived scores, the first being the discrepancy score and the second the bothersome score. To derive the discrepancy score, the inventory asks the mother to first rate the "average baby" on six measures or behaviors on a 1 to 5 scale, and then these ratings are summed. The mother is asked to rate her baby on the same six measures. The discrepancy between the "average baby score" and "your baby score" constitutes the NPI Discrepancy Score. A mother is considered to have a positive perception of her baby if she perceives her baby to be better than the average baby and thus has a positive score. A mother who perceives her own baby to be the same as or worse than the average baby is considered to have a negative perception of the infant. The second score, the bothersome score, is derived by summing the number of bothersome behaviors the mother perceives her infant to have and the degree of difficulty the mother perceives with the problem of behavior. A high bothersome score reflects a more "bothersome" infant and a more difficult mother–infant relationship.

A teaching task designed by Spietz and Eyres (1977) was used to assess maternal and infant behavior in an interactive situation. In this assessment the mother is asked to teach her infant two tasks, an easy and a hard task. The easy task for the 1-month-old infants is adapted from the Bayley Scales of Infant Development and involves teaching the infant to turn to look at a small shielded flashlight and follow the light as it is moved through several excursions from left to right. The "hard" task, also adapted from the Bayley Scales of Infant Development, involves teaching the infant to follow a red ring for at least 30 degrees to each side and to reach for the ring. Mothers were not given any instructions as to how to engage their infant in the tasks and if they asked, they were told to do what they felt would work best for their baby. The two tasks were presented in succession but the length of time spent on each task was determined by the mother and recorded by the investigator. A summary score referred to as the "Disbrow Interactive Score" was used to reflect the mother's overall quality of interaction. A high Disbrow Interactive Score is indicative of more positive maternal behavior.

Fifty items from the Epstein-O'Brien Self-Report Inventory (Epstein & O'Brien, 1976), which measures a person's general self-esteem, were used as a concurrent validity measure.

As an additional measure of self-esteem, maternal statements during the home visit were rated as indicative of the mother being high or low on self-esteem. Interrater reliability on this measure was over .90.

4.1.3. Dependent Measure

The Maternal Self-Report Inventory was used as the dependent measure.

4.1.4. Procedure

A research assistant who was blind to the purpose of the study performed the screening and subject selection and reported the names of potential subjects for the study to a second investigator. This investigator then contacted each infant's mother one day after delivery and discussed with her the general nature and purpose of the study. If the mother wished to participate in the study, written informed consent was obtained from her.

4.1.4a. Time 1. Two days after delivery, all mothers completed the MSI and the Family Support Questionnaire. In addition, at this time each infant was assessed with the Brazelton Neonatal Behavior Assessment Scale. The mother was not present and only minimal feedback was given to the mothers concerning their infant's performance on the exam so as not to bias the mothers' perceptions of their infants. The Parmelee

Postnatal Complications Scale and the Obstetrical Complications Scale were completed to assess infant and maternal health.

4.1.4b. Time 2. One month after discharge from the hospital, a home visit was conducted during which mothers again completed the MSI and the Family Support Questionnaire. During this home visit, infant behavior and health were again assessed using the Brazelton Neonatal Behavior Assessment Scale and the Parmelee Postnatal Complications Scale. Mother–infant interaction was assessed using the teaching task designed by Spietz and Eyres (1977). Mothers also completed the Broussard Neonatal Perception Inventory.

Throughout the course of the study, all mothers were assured of complete confidentiality concerning all the information obtained.

4.2. Results

4.2.1. Descriptive Data on Independent Variables

4.2.1a. Demographic Data. Maternal demographic data is presented in Table 1. Of particular interest is the limitation of race and religion, with a majority of mothers identifying themselves as white and Catholic, the generally high education level, and the large majority of mothers in this study who were married and living with the father of their baby.

4.2.1b. Maternal Obstetric History. Obstetrical information for these mothers is presented in Table 2. The majority of mothers had generally good obstetric histories. The most typical problems included increased blood pressure, hyperemesis, premature rupture of membranes, nuchal cord, meconium staining, and anemia. A few of the mothers had more serious complications including one mother with a seizure disorder, one mother with mild toxemia, one mother with a history of a drug overdose during pregnancy, and a few mothers with either positive or suspicious stress tests. The data from the obstetric complications scale indicates that on average these mothers had few complications.

4.2.1c. Infant Health. As indicated by the infant health complications scale, the infants were generally quite healthy in the immediate perinatal period and experienced few health complications during their first month of life. The mean score was 1.3 (S.D. 1.5) at Time 1 and .77 (S.D. .04) at Time 2. In the perinatal period the typical problems included hypotonia, feeding problems, postmaturity, transient tachypnea, suspected infections, and medical interventions such as phototherapy for elevated bilirubin levels. Other problems were small-for-gestational-age infants, three infants with heart murmurs, and two infants with

TABLE 1. Maternal Demographic Information

	Mean	S.D.	Range	
Maternal age	24.2	4.65	17–33 years	
			N	%
Religious affiliation				
Catholic			21	70.0
Protestant			9	30.0
Jewish			0	0.0
Race				
White			25	83.3
Black			3	10.0
Puerto Rican			2	6.7
Occupation				
Housewife			11	36.7
Clerical			6	20.0
Semiskilled, unskilled, or student			7	23.3
Skilled			2	6.7
Sales, managerial, or professional			4	13.3
Education				
12 years or less			19	63.3
1 year of college or more			11	36.7
Marital status				
Married			25	83.3
Separated			1	3.3
Single, living with baby's father			1	3.3
Single, not living with baby's father			3	10.0
Family income				
0–$5,000			3	10.0
5–$10,000			8	26.7
10–$15,000			3	10.0
15–$20,000			7	23.3
20–$25,000			4	13.3
Paternal education				
12 years or less			15	50.0
1 year of college or more			15	50.0

TABLE 2. Maternal Obstetrical History

	N	%
Parity		
Primiparous	18	60.0
Multiparous	12	40.0
Type of delivery		
Vaginal	20	66.7
Repeat Caesarean section	2	6.7
Emergency Caesarean section	8	26.7

Obstetrical complications		
Mean	S.D.	Range
4.5	2.9	1–10

congenital anomalies, one involving a cleft palate and the other post-eromedial deviation of a leg. At and during the first month, the majority of health complications included minor colds (10 infants), diaper rash (2 infants), colic (2 infants), feeding problems (5 infants), infections (2 infants), and weight loss (2 infants). As for feeding, 46% of the infants were breast fed, 43% bottle fed, and 10% were both breast and bottle fed.

It is important to emphasize that there is an extremely limited range of infant and maternal health problems in this sample. Such truncation of the range of a variable works against the finding of relationships between the truncated variable and other variables. In this study strong relations were found despite truncation.

4.2.2. Maternal Self-Report Inventory Scores

Descriptive statistics are presented for the self-report inventory in Tables 3 and 4. Several aspects of these data are important in this context. For each of the subscales as well as the total score, the scores are relatively high and the range of scores observed is relatively narrow. Furthermore, the scores on each of the scales increased from the newborn period to one month, although these increases were not significant. The correlations between subscales at both time points were significant, indicating a great deal of stability in maternal self-esteem. Such stability

TABLE 3. Summary Data from MSI at Time 1

MSI—Time 1	Raw score means	Standard deviations	Range	Number of items
Caretaking Ability	110.83	9.30	90–127	26
General Ability as a Mother	111.40	9.93	77–125	25
Acceptance of Baby	41.97	5.07	28–50	10
Relationship with Baby	38.87	3.18	31–45	9
Body Image and Health after Delivery	35.83	6.39	21–45	9
Parental Influence	27.67	2.89	19–30	6
Pregnancy, Labor, and Delivery	60.63	9.51	36–73	15
Total MSI Score	427.20	36.91	322–481	100

may well indicate that maternal self-esteem is more at the core of the mother's personality than at the periphery and is relatively unaffected by immediate circumstance.

4.2.2a. Face Validity. Face validity was demonstrated in the initial evaluation of the questions by the mothers and psychologists.

4.2.2b. Concurrent Validity. A new test can be said to have concurrent validity to the extent that it correlates with another concurrently obtained criterion. For the purposes of assessing the concurrent validity of the MSI, one of the criterion used was a shortened version of the Self-Report Inventory (SRI) developed by Epstein and O'Brien (1976). High

TABLE 4. Summary Data from MSI at Time 2

MSI—Time 2	Raw score means	Standard deviations	Range	Number of items
Caretaking Ability	113.23	8.61	93–128	26
General Ability as a Mother	112.83	10.92	80–124	25
Acceptance of Baby	43.27	4.86	28–50	10
Relationship with Baby	39.30	3.39	31–45	9
Body Image and Health after Delivery	36.40	5.76	22–45	9
Parental Influence	27.67	2.83	16–30	6
Pregnancy, Labor, and Delivery	62.03	9.84	34–75	15
Total MSI Score	434.73	37.44	346–481	100

correlations between the MSI and the SRI were found at the first and second administrations of the questionnaires. At Time 1, a correlation of .74 ($p < .001$) was found between the MSI total score and the SRI total score. Furthermore, all of the MSI subscales significantly correlated with the SRI total score. The correlations ranged from .44 ($p < .007$) for Parental Influence to .75 (p $< .001$) for General Ability as a Mother. At Time 2, a correlation of 0.76 ($p < .001$) was found between the MSI total score and the SRI total score. At Time 2, all subscale correlations were significant at $p \leq .02$ and ranged from 0.37 ($p < .02$) for Parental Influence to .70 ($p < .001$) for General Ability as a Mother.

However, although all of the subscales of the MSI significantly correlated with the total score of the SRI at Times 1 and 2, these correlation are not high enough to suggest that the two scales are indeed measuring identical factors. Given the fact that both scales were combined when administered to mothers and thus share the same measurement technique, time and setting of administration, it is likely that some of the variance in the MSI not explained by the SRI maybe due to the unique aspects of maternal self-esteem that are not assessed by a measure of adult self-esteem.

The other method for assessing the concurrent validity of the MSI was to assess the correlation between the MSI and clinical ratings of maternal self-esteem, in order to demonstrate the relationship between different methods purporting to measure the same construct. The correlation between the clinical ratings of maternal self-esteem and MSI scores was .35 with $p < .02$. This correlation lends support to the validity of the MSI as a measure for assessing maternal self-esteem.

4.2.2c. Construct Validity. In order to further demonstrate the validity of the MSI scale, data pertaining to the construct validity of the test must be presented. The construct validity of the scale can be demonstrated by examining each of the following: (1) the internal validity of the scale; (2) the homogeneity of the construct being measured; and (3) the correlations between MSI scores and those independent variables that are logically and/or theoretically expected to correlate with maternal self-esteem, as well as the correlations between MSI scores and those independent variables that logically and/or theoretically are not expected to correlate with maternal self-esteem. Number 3 is most important to the clinician so the results of the analyses on numbers 1 and 2 will be presented briefly.

4.2.2d. Internal Validity. The first process in the validity analyses involved assessing the internal validity of the scale in order to ascertain what variables, other than the construct in question, may be determining the observed response. This process involved assessing the degree of defensiveness associated with responses to the questionnaires. In order to determine the degree of defensiveness/social desirability that may have been influencing scores from the MSI and the SRI, 10 of the defensiveness items from the Epstein-O'Brien Self-Report Inventory were intermixed with items from both questionnaires. An equal number of positive and negative items were included. For the purposes of this study, defensiveness was defined as "a stereotypical response which reflects what is socially acceptable or valued, rather than individual differences on the construct" (Wells & Marwell, 1976).

At Time 1 the correlations between MSI and the defensiveness items were generally low and ranged from $r = -.05$ ($p < .39$) for Body Image and Health after Delivery to .57 ($p < .001$) for the Parental Influence subscale. Thus most of the subscales on the MSI were not highly influenced by defensiveness/social desirability factors and the one subscale that did appear to be highly influenced by social desirability was the Parental Influence subscale, which might be expected to be most influenced.

At Time 2, the correlations between both self-esteem measures increased but were still generally low. The correlations between the individual subscales of the MSI and defensiveness measure ranged from $r = .18$ ($p < .17$) for Body Image and Health after Delivery to .55 ($p < .001$) for Feelings Concerning Pregnancy, Labor, and Delivery. Of interest is the finding that body image was consistently the factor least affected by defensiveness. Overall, it does not seem that the scales were strongly influenced by social desirability or defensiveness.

4.2.2e. Homogeneity of the Scale. As concerns the construct validity analysis, the MSI subscale score-to-total score correlations were all significant at the $p < .001$ level, and ranged from $r = .64$ for Body Image and Health after Delivery to $r = .89$ for General Ability as a Mother at Time 1, and $r = .60$ for Body Image and Health after Delivery to .92 for General Ability as a Mother at Time 2.

Because of the high correlation between subscale scores and total score at both the time points and because of the central concern of validating the MSI, it was decided that the rest of the analyses would utilize only the total score as the dependent measure. But note that the results of those analyses were found to conform closely to the analyses using the total score.

4.2.2f. External Validity: Correlations between the Maternal Self-Report Inventory and Other Independent Measures. The external validity of the inventory is critical if the scale is to have any research or clinical utility.

Demographic Variables. Table 5 indicates that there were no significant correlations between the MSI and demographic variables. However, note that many of these variables had restricted ranges and nonnormal distributions. Two of the variables, family income and father's

**TABLE 5. Pearson Product-Moment
Correlations between Demographic
Variables and the MSI Times 1 and 2**

Demographic variables	Time 1[a]	Time 2
Mother's age	.23	.02
Mother's religion	−.01	.08
Mother's race	−.20	−.10
Mother's occupation	−.21	−.14
Mother's education	−.10	−.23
Family income	.27*	.02
Marital status	−.23	−.07
Father's age	.27*	.08
Father's race	−.08	.02
Father's occupation	.01	.03
Father's education	.03	−.09

[a]Significance levels are indicated as follows:
  *$p < .10$.

age, despite these limitations had correlations that approached significance and were in the expected direction at Time 1. Yet, as will be shown
below, more proximal variables had much stronger relationships to maternal self-esteem. This result argues that maternal self-esteem is not a
demographic or population variable but rather is a characteristic of the
individual and the individual's unique situation (see below).

Infant Health Status. Infant health status at Time 1, despite its limited
range, had a large and significant correlation, $r = -.52$ ($p < .01$) with
MSI at Time 1 and at Time 2, $r = -.41$ ($p < .01$) (see Tables 6 and 7).
Mothers of healthier infants, even in this relatively very healthy population of infants, had higher self-esteem. This relationship held up even at
one month when mothers' self-esteem was more related to their infant's
newborn health status. Maternal self-esteem was unrelated to infant
health status at one month but then it had almost no variability.

Maternal Health Status, Time of Delivery, and Parity. Maternal health at
Time 1 had a large and significant correlation, $r = -.38$ ($p < .01$), with
maternal self-esteem at Time 1 but not at Time 2, $r = -.15$ ($p < .10$) (see
Table 6 and 7). The lack of a significant effect at Time 2 is probably the
result of the finding that almost all the mothers at that time were essentially recovered from any insult they may have experienced at Time 1.
However, neither type of delivery nor parity were significantly related to
maternal self-esteem as evaluated by correlations or Student t tests, al-

TABLE 6. Pearson Product-Moment Correlations and Student's t Test for Independent Variables and the MSI at Time 1

Independent variables	MSI-1[b]
Infant Health Status	$-.52$***
Mother's Health	$-.38$**
Type of Delivery	$t = 1.07$
Parity	$t = 1.21$
Family Support	$.69$***
Maternal Separation[a]	$-.43$***
Brazelton Total Score	$.04$
Infant Sex	$t = 2.19$**

[a] There are only three cases of separation.
[b] Significance levels are indicated as follows:
  *$p < .10$.
  **$p < .05$.
  ***$p < .01$

TABLE 7. Pearson Product-Moment Correlations and Student's t Test for Independent Variables and the MSI at Time 2

Independent variables	MSI-2[a]
Infant Health Status—Time 1	$-.41$***
Infant Health Status—Time 2	$-.19$
Maternal Health—Time 1	$-.35$
Maternal Health—Time 2	$-.15$
Parity	-1.01
Type of Delivery	$.72$
Separation	$-.38$**
Family Support	$.79$***
Brazelton Total Score—Time 2	$-.08$
Maternal Perception—Discrepancy Score	$.36$**
Maternal Perception—Bothersome Score	$-.36$**
Disbrow Interactive Score	$.33$**
Feeding Problems	$-.35$**

[a] Significance levels are indicated as follows:
  *$p < .10$.
  **$p < .05$.
  ***$p < .01$.

though in all cases the relationships were found to be in the expected direction.

Family Support. The relationship between family support and maternal self-esteem was very strong and in the expected direction at both points in time (see Tables 6 and 7). Mothers who received more emotional and physical support from the baby's father and the mother's immediate family had significantly higher self-esteem, $r = .69$ ($p < .01$) at Time 1 and $r = .79$ ($p < .01$) at Time 2.

Newborn Behavior. The one variable that was predicted to significantly correlate with maternal self-esteem but did not was the infant's behavioral responsiveness and competence (see Tables 6 and 7). Virtually no correlation was found between Brazelton examination total scores (or dimension scores not shown) and mother's MSI score at either points in time. One reason for this was a restricted range and a distribution of scores skewed toward the more optimal range of performance.

Maternal Perception of Infant (Time 2 only). As measured by Broussard's questionnaire, mothers who saw their infants as better than average and the mothers who saw their infants as less bothersome had significantly higher maternal self-esteem, $r = .36$ ($p < .01$) and $r = -.36$ ($p < .01$) respectively (see Tables 6 and 7). Thus, how mothers experience their infants may have more effect on their self-esteem than does behavior objectively assessed, especially when the range of the latter is so limited.

Mother–Infant Interaction (Time 2 Only). Maternal interactive competence as assessed by the Disbrow Interactive Score and by the maternal sensitivity measure was positively related to maternal self-esteem (see Table 7). The Disbrow Interactive Score's correlation with self-esteem was $r = .33$ ($p < .05$). Mothers with higher self-esteem are more sensitive to their infants.

Infant Sex. A significant difference in maternal self-esteem ($t = 2.19$, $p < .05$) was found between mothers of male or female infants with mothers of male infants having a higher index of self-esteem (see Table 6).

A *post hoc* analysis of sex of infant was examined. Mothers of male infants were found to have significantly higher self-esteem than mothers of female infants at both Time 1 and Time 2 (Time 1 mean male = 442.23 vs. mean female 415.17 ($p < .04$) and Time 2 mean male = 453.31 vs. mean female 420.53 ($p < .01$). However, this difference was not independent of either infant health or family support. Additional covariate analyses indicated that mothers of male infants received more familial support, resulting in greater self-esteem. Thus the relation between sex and self-esteem appears to be mediated by the familial support.

Feeding Problems. A negative relationship was found between feeding problems and maternal self-esteem, $r = -.35$ ($p < .05$). Mothers who had infants who did not feed well, even though there were quite minor problems, had significantly lower self-esteem than mothers who reported having no feeding problems.

Relations among the Independent Variables. It is obvious that the different independent variables are not independent of one another. Table 8 presents the intercorrelations among the 16 independent variables. There are many significant correlations. Of particular interest are the ones involving Brazelton scores, family support, maternal perception, and maternal interaction. Given these relations, it would be useful to be able to carry out some form of multiple regression analysis to evaluate the independent relations of these variables to maternal self-esteem. However, such an analysis is precluded by statistical considerations.

In sum, these results indicate that the MSI has a great degree of external validity. It is related to infant and maternal health, maternal perceptions, and maternal behavior with infant.

4.2.2g. Test-Retest Reliability or Individual Stability. The construct measured by the MSI appears to have very good stability over time, as indicated by the four-week test-retest Pearson product moment reliability coefficient of .85. Examination of mean scores from Time 1 and Time 2 indicates that on the average, maternal self-esteem increased by approximately seven points over this period of time. Further analysis of the correlation between MSI scores at Time 1 and Time 2 via a scatter diagram revealed a normal distribution of scores around the regression line.

4.3. Short Form of the MSI

Given the results on the validity of the scale and our goal for developing a research instrument as well as a clinically useful instrument, we developed a shortened version of the MSI. Our approach was first to apply reliability analysis, Cronbach's (1955) alpha, to the seven dimensions in order to reduce the number of items making up each of the dimensions. Then the external validity of the reduced dimensions was assessed as a criterion for keeping an item or a dimension in the MSI-Short Form.

Five reiterations of the Cronbach analysis were carried out, the first with the full set of items and the last with 33 items. There was little change

TABLE 8. Intercorrelations between 16 Independent Variables[a]

	Infant health 1	Infant health 2	C-section	Parity	Mother's health 1	Mother's health 2	Separation	Family support 1	Family support 2	Braz 1	Braz 2	Maternal perception	Mother–infant interaction	Infant sex	Feeding problems	SES
Infant health 1	—															
Infant health 2	.18	—														
C-section	.06	-.11	—													
Parity	-.27	-.13	-.09	—												
Mother's health 1	.29	.17	.65*	-.31*	—											
Mother's health 2	.11	.57*	-.18	.28	-.08	—										
Separation	.37*	-.30*	.30*	.14	.16	-.09	—									
Family support 1	-.21	-.33*	-.33*	.05	-.27	-.20	-.33*	—								
Family support 2	-.26	-.24	-.21	.06	-.14	-.34*	-.34*	.85*	—							
Brazelton 1	.34*	-.19	.23	.31	.04	.02	.21	-.41*	.24	—						
Brazelton 2	-.05	.06	.19	.24	-.05	.05	.33*	-.35*	-.23	.10	—					
Maternal perception	-.01	-.36*	.08	-.13	-.26	-.12	.59*	-.25	-.38*	-.26	.01	—				
Mother–infant interaction	-.06	-.26	-.13	.02	-.26	-.12	-.17	.49*	.34*	-.13	-.26	-.44*	—			
Infant sex	.14	.08	.11	-.20	.26	.13	.05	-.35*	-.52*	-.40*	.13	.09	-.05	—		
Feeding problems	.16	.24	-.08	-.09	-.07	.53*	-.12	-.42*	-.49*	-.15	.25	.03	-.003	.40*	—	
SES	.01	-.37*	.03	-.01	-.17	.16	-.05	.44*	.15	.14	-.21	-.01	.31*	.12	18	—

[a] Asterisks indicate $p < .05$.

in the alpha values over the iterations. Three dimensions—Expected Relationship with Baby, Parental Acceptance, and Body Image and Health after Delivery—had relatively low alphas in the last reiteration, .66, .71, and .68 respectively. The other dimensions had alphas above .80. This suggested that these three dimensions should be dropped. However, before the dimensions with low alphas were dropped the external validity of each of the dimensions was evaluated using the variables of family support, infant health, maternal health, Brazelton score, and teaching task. In this analysis we found that despite its low alpha the shortened dimension of Expected Relationship with Baby still had four out of five significant relationships the longer version had. It was decided that this dimension would be kept. The dimensions of Parental Acceptance and Body Image were dropped. Two dimensions with a relatively large number of items, Caretaking Ability with 8 items and General Ability as a Mother with 13, were reduced to 6 and 8 items by applying further reiterations of the Cronbach analysis.

The final version of the MSI-Short Form consisted of five dimensions with 26 items: Caretaking Ability (alpha = .83) with 6 items, General Ability as a Mother (alpha = .88) with 8 items, Acceptance of Baby (alpha = .81) with 3 items, Expected Relationship with Infant (alpha = .66) with 3 items, and Feelings during Pregnancy, Labor, and Delivery (alpha = .89) with 4 items. The MSI-Short Form is presented in Appendix A.

4.4. Discussion

These results demonstrate the face, concurrent, internal, and external validity of the Maternal Self-Esteem Inventory. It now becomes, especially in its short form, a useful instrument for clinically evaluating maternal self-esteem and in its long and short forms a valuable research instrument on maternal self-esteem *per se* and on how maternal self-esteem is related to other factors. Since this study was primarily designed to evaluate this instrument, its results with regard to clinical and research implications must be taken as preliminary. Nonetheless, they are intriguing.

The configuration of results confirms the two-sided nature of maternal adaptation, "bio" in the driving force of infant health and other health factors, and "social" in the importance of family support and other social factors, as well as in the linkage between these biosocial factors. It is our view that maternal self-esteem can be seen as the psychological final common pathway for these biosocial factors as they affect a woman's adaptation to motherhood.

It is most striking that even mild and very temporary illnesses impact so significantly on maternal self-esteem. To the extent that infant
health outweighs the impact of the other factors examined, it emphasizes that the delivery of a healthy infant is the primary concern to the
mother, just as it is to the physician. As can be seen, not even maternal
health or other aspects of the delivery experience weighed as much on
the mother's feelings of competence.

Of particular interest was the finding that infant health problems
during the first few days following delivery still were having a strong
effect upon maternal self-esteem one month later. This is in agreement
with Minde, Brown, and Whitelaw's (1981) findings that it was not until
three months after discharge that parents of healthy prematures had
recovered emotionally enough to engage in appropriate parent–infant
social interactions and had begun to develop a healthy attachment to
their infants. This delay occurred despite the fact that the infants had
recovered from their earlier illnesses and were doing very well. Apparently, and not surprisingly, the health of the infant at birth has a salient
and long-lasting effect on the mother's (and likely the father's) self-
perception and adaptation to the infant. This period of time may be one
of vulnerability to insults, as would be expected by Brazelton's (1976)
and Bibring's (1959) characterization of maternal psychological disor-
ganization at this time.

Family support directly and strongly relates to maternal self-esteem.
This relationship was expected. Positive attitudes toward mothering,
and the quality of the mother–infant interaction, are largely influenced
by a positive family support system. Given the insignificant relationships
between demographic variables and maternal self-esteem, it is evident
that the basis of self-esteem is more influenced by proximal personal
relationships than by more psychologically distant demographic factors.
This effect of proximal variables is noted in the literature on depression
(Grunebaum, Weiss, Cohler, Harman, & Gallant, 1975) but there is a
lack of examples in the literature on postpartum depression. It is also
consistent with findings by Epstein (1979) in the general adult self-esteem literature that one of the major factors associated with low self-
esteem is disturbed love relationships.

Yet, despite the power of these two variables, other factors are still
of interest for it is only out of their mutual interaction that an understanding of maternal adaptation can be achieved. This interaction is well
illustrated by the relationship of maternal health with other variables
and self-esteem.

Mothers in this study who encountered even mild health problems received less family support, resulting in a lowering in their self-esteem. This conditional type of family support has been noted before in the literature (Blake, 1954). As have others, we have observed a tendency of the hospital staff to withdraw support from mothers who complain of aches, pains, or headaches. There appears to be little sympathy for a mother who does not feel able to care for her infant, unless she is extremely ill. Certainly, it is of clinical import and somewhat poignant that despite problems of her own, a mother is expected to shift her attention to her infant if she is to receive more family support. Further-more, it is insidious that mother's health is related to infant health, C-section, separation, feeding problems, mother–infant interactions, and income in such a fashion that all act synergistically to *lower* family sup-port for a mother with health problems. Such configurations of variables characterize much of this data and are extremely important for identify-ing mothers who are in need of extra support. Of course, there are other configurations that can be considered optimal.

Infant behavior did not show a direct relation to maternal self-esteem. However, mothers who perceived their infants as "better than average" or "less bothersome" had higher self-esteem. And infants whose mothers received more support initially after delivery had better Brazelton scores at Time 2 than did infants whose mothers received less family support. In addition, the more family support a mother receives, the more likely it is that her baby is more responsive and alert and that she then receives more family support and more maternal self-esteem. It is also part of this configuration that mothers with higher self-esteem were more sensitive to their infant's cues and they received more family support.

This configuration of relations suggests that there may be an "op-timal" group of mothers whose infants are born without complications and are healthy, perform well on the Brazelton, and who receive a high degree of family support. This "optimal" group of mothers are likely to have high self-esteem. One would be hard put to find causality in this configuration. Yet when all these conditions are "in place," these women are buffered from a singular event that might lower their self-esteem and their general functioning. Of course, there is also a less optimal group of mothers and infants. In this group complications during labor, minor health problems in the infant, and lowered family support are associated. These mothers have lower self-esteem. These mothers are at risk for interactive problems with their infants. Single events can have a powerful effect on the self-esteem and functioning of these mothers.

This perspective has important implications for the concept of bonding (Klaus & Kennell, 1976). The conceptualization of bonding, a characteristic of many mammalian species, makes much of the relationship between the quality of bonding and many of the variables in this study, in particular separation, Caesarean section, and infant health and behavior. While these variables have for the most part been confounded in bonding studies, it has generally been interpreted that the occurrence of them may exceed the limits of maternal adaptability and disturb the bonding process. An alternative is presented in this study—maternal self-esteem is seen as the psychological final common pathway mediating the effect of factors that disturb a woman's adaptation. Mothers whose self-esteem is lowered by any of a host of biosocial factors become less available emotionally to their infants and less effective with them, disturbing not only their initial adaptation and relationship but their subsequent adaptation as well.

This interpretation explains the finding in the literature on bonding, but unexplained by it is the fact that the "bonding" of multiparous mothers is often equal to or exceeds the bonding even of those primiparous mothers given extra contact with their infants. From the perspective of maternal self-esteem multiparous mothers come to the delivery experience with a more stable sense of maternal self-confidence. Relatedly, the encouragement of contact and caretaking by mothers and fathers of their ill newborns can be seen as providing them with a way of increasing their self-esteem rather than bonding them to their infant. The self-esteem view also suggests that if such initial contact with their ill infant exceeds their emotional capacities or caretaking abilities their self-esteem will be lowered and their adaptation compromised; that is, not all contact may be useful or effective. More generally, thinking about the process in terms of maternal (and paternal) self-esteem allows for a consideration of a broad range of variables—income and education levels to minor infant illnesses that often occur long after the birth—as affecting maternal adaptation rather than considering only mother–infant contact over a very limited time period as having the major structuring effect on a woman's adaptation.

The mothers in this study were drawn for the most part from an optimal group and maternal self-esteem was stable and high. With a more heterogenous sample that included more at-risk mothers and infants, less stability and even more powerful affects of the variables studied would be expected. A clinical case from one of the most stressed mother–infant pairs illustrates this expectation. In this case, the infant was born with a minor cleft palate but no facial abnormalities, after a normal full-term pregnancy. Her mother suffered from migraine headaches following delivery and was very depressed and tired. During her hospital stay she encountered many feeding problems with her infant and expressed much anxiety about her ability to properly feed her baby. The nursing staff was very impatient with the mother's fears and anxieties, which the mother said made her feel guilty about these feedings. Following delivery, the mother's husband retreated from helping with caretaking chores and began working an extra shift. At the same time, her other two young children began requiring more attention from her. After being home for one month, the infant had not gained weight, had encountered more feeding problems, had developed a rash, and required two doctor's visits. Although this mother's maternal self-esteem was relatively low following delivery, by Time 2, her maternal self-esteem had significantly decreased. By Time 2, this mother was requesting psychological services as she no longer felt competent to care for her two children or the baby.

4.5. Clinical Implications

A woman's adaptation to motherhood is affected by a host of interacting biosocial factors of which the most important, but not the only, were infant health and family support. Such a configuration of factors can appear confusing and to some extent overwhelming to the practitioner; everything seems to affect everything else. This need not be the case. When maternal self-esteem is viewed as a psychological final common pathway mediating the effects of these factors, the central question becomes: How does this factor and its interaction with other factors affect maternal self-esteem and what can be done to mitigate its effects and to scaffold maternal self-esteem? With this view in mind many interventions, direct and indirect, are available, indeed.

Minor and transitory health problems impact strongly on maternal self-esteem. These problems are of only minor and transitory concern to the practitioner, but the practitioner must appreciate their impact on the mother and work to alleviate their negative effects. Such interventions can be direct by taking the mother's concerns seriously, allowing for their expression and then providing her with a picture of their course and how she as the child's mother can have a role in their resolution. Interventions can also be indirect by supporting family members as they support the mother. And, as emphasized by Brazelton (1974), the practitioner must not forget the infant as a partner to the intervention; for the infant, in almost all cases, can be relied on to improve behaviorally and the practitioner by helping mother and her family to recognize their role in that improvement can then bank on its positive transactional effects on maternal adaptation. Most important, the support services themselves must guard against communicating to the mother that she is not doing an adequate job. This will not occur if intervention is directed toward supporting maternal self-esteem rather than showing or telling a mother what she should be doing or feeling.

5. SUMMARY

This study has demonstrated the validity of the Maternal Self-Report Inventory and argued that maternal self-esteem can be viewed as a psychological final common pathway mediating the effects of the biosocial factors that affect a woman's adaptation to motherhood. Such factors are truly biological and social. Small variations in infant health, even in this population of healthy infants, and small variations in family support, even in this population of stable and intact families, strongly affects maternal adaptation. Other factors—maternal health, sex of infant, demographics, separation, delivery route—affect the adaptation process primarily through maternal self-esteem. These results emphasize that practitioners must pay special attention to maternal and familial concerns about even minor infant health problems. The interaction of factors indicates that mothers who are ill may receive a very conditional form of support from their families that may compromise their adaptation. The results suggest that interactions aimed at fostering maternal adaptation should be geared to support maternal self-esteem by intervening directly with the mother around her concerns and her effectiveness or indirectly through the family or infant since their effects on the mother are so powerful.

Finally, one may raise the question of the limitations of measuring only maternal self-esteem during the one-month postpartum period given the uniqueness of the experience during this time period. And relatedly one may ask if an intervention strategy based on this perspective would be adequate. Since our work was not focused on an intervention strategy, further study is required to answer these questions. However, given the findings on the stability of maternal self-esteem over this time period, one might expect that measuring it during even this unique period permits one to generalize beyond this time period. Furthermore, the relations to the independent variables not only are strong and consistent but they are also sensible, strengthening our claim that maternal self-esteem can indeed be viewed as a final psychological common pathway reflective of the factors affecting the mother.

6. APPENDIX A

Maternal Self-Report Inventory
E. Shea
Edward Z. Tronick

Instructions for use of the appendix:

The 100 questions of the MSI are presented in the appendix. They are grouped by dimension but they are numbered according to the order that they are to be presented to a mother in the questionnaire. Thus to create a questionnaire the items must be retyped in proper order. They should be administered in the sequence of item numbers, not dimension by dimension. Twenty-six of the questions are additionally labeled *Short (#)*. These are the 26 items that make up the Short Form of the MSI.

Coding instructions:

Change all scales to have scores run into positive scores indicating higher self-esteem. Then add scores within each dimension or all scores for total score.

INSTRUCTIONS FOR MATERNAL SELF-REPORT INVENTORY

Please note how accurately the following statements describe how you feel. Read each item carefully and when you are sure you understand it, indicate your answer by drawing a circle around the answer which best expressed the degree to which the statement is true for you.

Rate each statement as follows:

CF	MF	Un	MT	CT
Completely False	Mainly False	Uncertain or Neither True	Mainly True	Completely True

For example, circle CR if you feel that statement is completely false, circle MR if the statement is mainly false, circle MT if the statement is mainly true, and circle CT if the statement is completely True. If you are uncertain or feel that the statement is neither true nor false, circle Un.

Please answer each item as honestly as you can, and work rapidly as first impressions are as good as any. Try to answer every question, and if in doubt, circle the answer which comes closest to expressing your feelings. Although some of the statements seem to be similar, they are not identical, and should be answered separately. All of your answers will be treated with complete confidentiality. There are no right or wrong answers, so please feel free to note them at the end of the questionnaire. Your comments are very much appreciated.

Thank you very much.

******

CARETAKING ABILITY

Total Number of Items = 26

# of Item	Items
2.	Feeding my baby is fun.
5.	I feel confident at being able to satisfy my baby's physical needs.
7.	I feel confident at being able to know what my baby wants.
9.	I feel unable to give my baby the love and care which he/she needs.
16.	If it is true that breast feeding is important, it is because it brings the mother and baby closer together.
17.	I sometimes feel very angry when a baby won't stop crying.
25.	I worry that feeding my baby will be a burden for me.
27.	Having to bathe my baby makes me very nervous as he/she is so hard to handle.
30.	I am worried that I will have difficulty changing my baby's diapers.
33.	I doubt that I will be able to satisfy my baby's emotional needs.
38.	& Short (#8). I often worry that I may be forgetful and cause something bad to happen to my baby.
46.	I will not mind getting up in the middle of the night to feed my baby.
47.	& Short (#10). I am concerned that I will have trouble figuring out what my baby needs.
54.	I feel competent at being able to feed my baby.
62.	I am not very good at calming my baby.
64.	I never feel like spanking a crying baby.
69.	& Short (#17). I worry that I will not know what to do if my baby gets sick.
70.	& Short (#18). It is difficult for me to know what my baby wants.

# of Item	Items
71.	I feel that I am too good a mother to ever lose my temper with my baby.
74.	& Short (#20). I am afraid I will be awkward and clumsy when handling my baby.
75.	I looked forward to breast feeding my baby.
76.	I feel like I have lots of love to give my baby.
85.	I am worried about being able to feed my baby properly.
89.	I am afraid that someday I will hurt my baby.
91.	As long as I love my baby, it doesn't matter if I breast feed or bottle feed.
98.	& Short (#25). I worry about being able to fulfill my baby's emotional needs.

GENERAL ABILITY AND PREPAREDNESS FOR MOTHERING ROLE

Total Number of Items = 25

# of Item	Items
1.	I feel that being a mother will be a very rewarding experience.
10.	I do not mind having to sacrifice my present personal activities in order to stay at home with my baby.
11.	& Short (#2). I think that I will be a good mother.
14.	This is a very happy time in my life.
15.	& Short (#4). I don't have much confidence in my ability to help my baby learn new things.
24.	I feel reasonably competent in taking care of my new baby.
31.	I look forward to taking my baby home.
39.	I feel like I am (or will be) a very good mother.
40.	I have no anxieties about all there is to do as a mother.
41.	I feel emotionally prepared to take good care of my baby.
44.	I have some unique contributions which I alone can make to my baby's life.
45.	& Short (#9). I am confident that I will be able to work out any normal problems I might have with my baby.
53.	I feel guilty about bringing a baby into this troubled world.

# of Item	Items
56.	& Short (#12). I expect that I won't mind staying home to care for my baby.
59.	I feel like I am (or will be) a failure as a mother.
66.	& Short (#16). It really makes me feel depressed to think about all there is to do as a mother.
68.	I am enthusiastic about taking responsibility for caring for my baby.
77.	& Short (#21). I feel confident about being able to teach my baby new things.
80.	I am frightened about all the day-to-day responsibilities of having to care for my baby.
90.	I do not find being a mother to be as fulfilling an experience as I thought it would be.
93.	I feel somewhat anxious about all the things a mother must do.
94.	& Short (#23). I feel that I will do a good job taking care of my baby.
95.	I do not feel emotionally secure enough to care for my baby by myself.
96.	& Short (#24). I know enough to be able to teach my baby many things which he/she will have to learn.
100.	I have mixed feelings about being a mother.

ACCEPTANCE OF BABY

Total Number of Items = 10

# of Item	Items
3.	My baby is very fragile and I worry that I will be too rough with him/her.
4.	I am disappointed with the sex of my baby.
18.	I was overjoyed when I first saw my baby.
23.	I think my baby is very beautiful.
22.	& Short (#6). I have real doubts about whether my baby will develop normally.
42.	When I first saw my baby I was disappointed.
61.	& Short (#14). I am concerned about whether my baby will develop normally.

# of Item	Items

79. & Short (#22). I am confident that my baby will be strong and healthy.
82. I am concerned about whether my baby will develop normally.
84. I have great expectations for what my baby will be like.

EXPECTED RELATIONSHIP WITH BABY

Total Number of Items = 9

# of Item	Items

13. & Short (#3). I am confident that I will have a close and warm relationship with my baby.
19. & Short (#5). Looking forward to having a baby gave me more pleasure than actually having one.
35. The thought of holding and cuddling my baby is very appealing to me.
49. I feel I don't relate very well to little babies.
52. & Short (#11). I worry about whether my baby will like me.
60. I need more time to adjust to my baby.
65. & Short (#15). I doubt that my baby could love me the way I am.
73. I think I will enjoy my baby more when he/she is older and has a personality of his/her own.
99. & Short (#26). I am confident that my baby will love me very much.

PARENTAL ACCEPTANCE

Total Number of Items = 6

# of Item	Items

8. I expect I will be at least as good a mother as my mother was.
29. My mother was rarely affectionate to me and I worry that I will not be able to be affectionate with my baby.

# of Item	Items
55.	My mother was a very caring and loving person and I expect I also will be a very loving mother.
67.	My father made me feel very loved, and I feel I too can give my baby love and affection.
78.	I feel that my parents did a very bad job raising me and I am sure that I will not make the same mistakes with my baby.
92.	I did not like my mother and I worry that my baby will not like me.

BODY IMAGE AND HEALTH

Total Number of Items = 9

# of Item	Items
20.	I am concerned about losing my figure after having had a baby.
28.	In general, I don't worry about my own health interfering with my ability to care for my baby.
32.	I think I am at least as good looking now as I was before I had a baby.
36.	I worry whether I am healthy enough to take care of my baby.
50.	I feel as though I have plenty of energy to take care of my baby.
57.	I do not like the way I look after having had my baby.
83.	It will take me a long time to get back my energy so I can properly take care of my baby.
88.	I doubt that my figure will ever look as good after having had a baby.
97.	I felt I looked very good during my pregnancy.

FEELINGS CONCERNING PREGNANCY, LABOR, AND DELIVERY

Total Number of Items = 15

# of Item	Items
6.	& Short (#1). I found the experience of labor and delivery to be one of the most unpleasant experiences I've ever had.

# of Item	Items
12.	I felt emotionally "empty" after delivering my baby.
21.	I felt slightly depressed and "blue" soon after delivery.
26.	I was extremely pleased when I found out I was pregnant.
34.	& Short (#7). I found the delivery experience frightening and very unpleasant.
37.	When I found out I was pregnant, I had mixed feelings about having a baby.
43.	I feel that something I did during my pregnancy may have caused (or will cause) problems for my baby.
48.	I missed the feeling of being pregnant after delivering my baby.
51.	When I was pregnant I eagerly awaited the birth of my baby.
58.	& Short (#13). I found the delivery experience to be very exciting.
63.	I took good care of myself during my pregnancy.
72.	& Short (#19). I found the whole experience of labor and delivery to be one of the best experiences of my life.
81.	I found labor to be very frightening.
86.	When I was pregnant I often had frightening fantasies that I would deliver an abnormal baby.
87.	I felt emotionally prepared for my baby's birth.

7. REFERENCES

Als, H., Tronick, E., Adamson, L., & Brazelton, B. (1976). The behavior of the full-term yet underweight newborn infant. *Developmental Medicine and Child Neurology, 18*, 590–602.

Barnard, K. E., & Gortner, S. R. (1977, May). *Nursing Child Project*. Division of Nursing, Bureau of Health Resources and Development, Department of Health, Education, and Welfare.

Benedek, T. (1949). The psychosomatic implications of the primary unit, mother-child. *American Journal of Orthopsychiatry, 4*, 63–72.

Berger, E. (1952). The relationship between expressed acceptance of self and acceptance of others. *Journal of Abnormal and Social Psychology, 47*, 778–782.

Bibring, E. M. (1959). Some considerations of the psychological processes in pregnancy. *Psychoanalytical Study of the Child, 14*, 113–121.

Bibring, E. M., Dwyer, T. F., Huntington, D. S., & Valenstein, A. F. (1961). A study of the psychological processes in pregnancy and the earliest mother-child relationship. *Psychoanalytic Study of the Child, 16*, 9–27.

Blake, F. G. (1954). *The child, his parents, and the nurse*. Philadelphia: J. B. Lippincott.

Blau, A., Slaff, B., Easton, R., Welkowitz, J., Spingain, J., & Cohen, J. (1963). The psycho-genic etiology of premature births, a preliminary report. *Psychosomatic Medicine, 25,* 210–211.

Brazelton, T. B. (1973). *Neonatal behavioral assessment scale.* London: Spastic International Medical Publications.

Brazelton, T. B. (1974). Does the neonate shape his environment? In *The Infant at risk, birth defects, Original Article Series, The National Foundation, 10*(32), 131–140.

Brazelton, T. B. (1976). The parent–infant attachment. *Clinical Obstetrics and Gynecology, 19,* 373–389.

Brody, S. (1956). *Patterns of mothering.* New York: International Universities Press.

Broussard, E. R., & Hartner, M. S. (1970). Maternal perception of the neonate as related to development. *Child Psychiatry and Human Development, 1,* 16–25.

Broussard, E. R., & Hartner, M. S. (1971). Further considerations regarding maternal perception and the first born. In J. Hellmuth (Ed.), *Exceptional Infant: Vol. 2. Studies in abnormalities.* New York: Brunner/Mazel.

Caplan, G., Mason, E., & Kaplan, D. M. (1965). Four studies of crisis in parents of pre-matures. *Community Mental Health Journal, 1,* 149–161.

Cohen, R. L. (1966). Some maladaptive syndromes of pregnancy and the puerperium. *Obstetrics and Gynecology, 27,* 562–570.

Cohler, B., Weiss, J., & Grunebaum, H. (1970). Child care attitudes and emotional distur-bance among mothers of young children. *Genetic Psychological Monographs, 82,* 3–47.

Coopersmith, S. (1967). *The antecedents of self-esteem.* San Francisco: Freeman.

Cronbach, L., & Meehl, P. (1955). Construct validity in psychological tests. *Psychological Bulletin, 52,* 281–302.

Davids, A. (1968). A research design for studying maternal emotionality before childbirth and after social interaction with the child. *Merrill-Palmer Quarterly, 14,* 345–354.

Deutsch, H. (1945). *The psychology of women: A psychoanalytic interpretation: Vol. 11. Moth-erhood.* New York: Grune & Stratton.

Disbrow, M. A., Doers, H. O., & Caulfield, C. (1977, March) *Measures to predict child abuse.* Report submitted to Maternal and Child Health Division, U.S. Department of Health, Education and Welfare.

Epstein, S. (1979). The ecological study of emotions in humans. In D. Plinar, K. R. Blank-stein, & I. M. Spigel (Eds.), *Advances in the study of communication and affect: Vol. 5. Perception of self and other.* New York: Plenum Press.

Epstein, S., & O'Brien, E. (1976). *Self-report inventory.* Unpublished manuscript, University of Massachusetts.

Feiring, C., & Taylor, J. (1977). Further considerations regarding maternal perception and the first born. In J. Hellmuth (Ed.), *Exceptional Infant: Vol. 2. Studies in abnormalities.* New York: Brunner/Mazel.

Field, T., & Widmayer, S. (1980, April). *Eight-month follow-up of infants delivered by Caesarean section.* Paper presented at the International Conference of Infant Studies, New Haven, Connecticut.

Greenberg, D. M. (1979). *Parental reactions to an infant with a birth defect: A study of five families.* Paper presented at the biennial meeting of the Society for Research in Child Development, San Francisco.

Greenberg, N. H., & Hurley, J. (1971). The maternal personality inventory. In J. Hellmuth (Ed.), *Exceptional Infant: Vol. 2. Studies in abnormalities.* New York: Brunner/Mazel.

Grossman, F. K. (1980, April). *Psychological sequelae of Caesarean delivery.* Paper presented at the International Conference on Infant Studies, New Haven, Connecticut.

Grunebaum, H., Weiss, J., Cohler, B., Harman, C., & Gallant, D. (1975). *Mentally ill mothers and their children.* Chicago: University of Chicago Press.

Kaplan, D. N., & Mason, E. A. (1969). Maternal reactions to premature birth viewed as an acute emotional disorder. *American Journal of Orthopsychiatry, 30,* 539–552.

Kennell, J. H., & Rolnick, A. (1960). Discussing problems in newborn babies with their parents. *Pediatrics, 26,* 832–838.

Kennell, J. H., Trause, M. A., & Klaus, M. H. (1975). Evidence for a sensitive period in the human mother. In *Parent–infant interaction,* Ciba Foundation Symposium 33, Amsterdam: Elsevier.

Klaus, M. H., & Kennell, J. (1976). *Maternal infant bonding.* St. Louis: C. V. Mosby.

Leifer, M. (1977). Psychological changes accompanying pregnancy and motherhood. *Genetic Psychology Monographs, 55*–96.

Littman, B., & Parmelee, A. (1978). Medical correlates of infant development. *Pediatrics, 61,* 470–474.

Mason, E. A. (1963). A method of predicting crisis outcome for mothers of premature babies. *Public Health Report, 78,* 1031–1035.

Minde, K., Brown, J., & Whitelaw, A. (1981). *The effect of severe physical illness on the behavior of very small premature infants.* Paper presented at the Society for Research in Child Development, Boston, Massachusetts.

Pederson, R., Zaslow, M., Cain, R., & Anderson, B. (1980, April). *Caesaren childbirth: The importance of a family perspective.* Paper presented at the International Conference on Infant Studies, New Haven, Connecticut.

Prugh, D. (1953). Emotional problems of the premature infant's parents. *Nursing Outlook, 1,* 461–464.

Ricks, M. (1981). *Relationships between the quality of infant attachment and maternal personality: Secure babies have secure mothers.* Unpublished manuscript, University of Massachusetts.

Rose, J., Boggs, T., & Alderstein, A. (1960). The evidence for a syndrome of "mothering disability" consequent to threats to the survival of neonates: A design for the hypothesis testing including prevention in prospective study. *American Journal of Disabilities in Childhood, 100,* 776–777.

Rosenberg, M. (1979). *Conceiving the self.* New York: Basic Books.

Scanlon, J., Scanlon, K., & Tronick, E. Z. (1983). *Physiological variables and the behavior of extremely small infants.* Unpublished manuscript, University of Massachusetts.

Schaefer, E. S., & Bell, R. Q. (1958). Development of a parental attitude research instrument. *Child Development, 29,* 339–361.

Seashore, M. H., Leifer, A. D., Barnett, C. R., & Leiderman, P. H. (1973). The effects of denial of early mother–infant interaction on maternal self-confidence. *Journal of Personality and Social Psychology, 26,* 369–378.

Shereshefsky, P. M., & Yarrow, L. J. (1973). *Psychological aspects of a first pregnancy and early postnatal adaptation.* New York: Raven Press.

Spietz, A. L., & Eyres, S. J. (1977, May). Instrumentation and findings: The environment. In K. E. Barnard & S. R. Rartner (Eds.), *Nursing child assessment project,* Division of Health, Education, and Welfare.

Wells, L., & Marwell, G. (1976). *Self-Esteem: Its conceptualization and measurement.* Beverly Hills, Sage.

Westbrook, M. T. (1978). The effect of the order of birth on women's experience of childbearing. *Journal of Marriage and Family,* 165–172.

## 4

Social Support and Parenting

SUSAN CROCKENBERG

1. INTRODUCTION

Social support refers to the emotional, instrumental, or informational help that other people provide an individual. With respect to families, *emotional support* refers to expressions of empathy and encouragement that convey to parents that they are understood and capable of working through difficulties in order to do a good job in that role. *Instrumental* support refers to concrete help that reduces the number of tasks or responsibilities a parent must perform, typically household and child-care tasks. *Informational support* refers to advice or information concerning child care or parenting. As practitioners and researchers, our interest in social support derives in part from the belief that having adequate support can affect parenting and facilitate the child's development. One purpose of this chapter is to review the theory and research that is the basis for this belief.

Social support is just one of many possible influences on parents—other factors include characteristics of the child, the parent, and the marital or partner relationship (Belsky, 1984; Crockenberg, 1981). Unlike these other influences, however, social support is assumed to be relatively changeable. If families do not have enough social support, it may be possible to increase that support in order to improve parenting. It is this possibility for change, along with the potential impact of that

Susan Crockenberg • Department of Applied Behavioral Sciences, University of California, Davis, California 95616.

change on parents and children, that has focused the attention of service providers on social support. Whether the assumption of changeability is warranted and what role health professionals might have in facilitating a change in social support are central questions in this chapter.

Consideration of health professionals as providers of social support is both a sign of the times and a manifestation of long-established historical roots. In recent years there has been a tendency for professionals to take over tasks that were once the responsibility of kin. This tendency is nowhere more apparent than in the partial replacement of the extended family by professionals in the transmission of culturally valued parenting skills (Rossi, 1968).

The reasons for this shift are many. There has been a decrease in the size of families and with it reduced opportunities for children of both sexes to learn about parenting as they grow up. The emphasis on mothering as the sole or primary role available to females has diminished and a focus on females learning other skills than those related to house and child care has emerged. At the same time, it is now more common for men to take on greater responsibility for early nurturing. Further, with the greater mobility of families, relatives are less likely to be readily available as sources of parenting wisdom. Even when family members are ready and willing to provide advice and assistance, new parents may prefer professional advice for its presumed scientific validity and its appropriateness to the life style they have adopted. Mothers who stayed at home with their children are sometimes ill-prepared to advise their daughters on combining mothering with working, and daughters, for their part, may be reluctant to ask for advice when they anticipate it might be accompanied by disapproval. Similarly, fathers, who typically engaged in little caregiving with their young children, may be unable to assist their sons in their new nurturing role.

Whatever the causes there is evidence that parents, and mothers in particular, look to professionals for advice on baby and child care. In a sample of mothers seeking care in private pediatric offices, only 30% were most worried about their child's physical health. The remaining 70% were most concerned about problems related to parenting and child development (Hickson, Altemeier, & O'Connor, 1983). Similarly, 76% of a sample of adolescent mothers said they wanted more information about child care from professionals (Crockenberg, 1986). Although professionals are often identified as advice givers, advice is not the only type of support professionals can provide. Another focus of this chapter is to consider different types of professional support and to explore ways professionals can help families obtain the social support they need.

2. HOW SOCIAL SUPPORT WORKS

The main assumption underlying this chapter is that the receipt of social support by families affects parents positively and translates into benefits to their children. We will begin by examining the theoretical basis of this assumption. How might social support influence parents and children? What is the process or processes by which the expected benefits are conveyed to families?

2.1. Support as a Reducer of Stressful Events

The simplest and most direct impact of social support may be to reduce the sheer number of stressful events and their cumulative impact on parents. A family may be able to draw on its own resources and cope effectively with one stress—a new baby, a sick child, an accident. But stresses often multiply, and it may be the accumulation of stress upon stress that is most disrupting to families. To illustrate: a family with a child in the hospital experiences a stressful event—a child with an illness or injury who typically is separated from the rest of the family. The stressful event is a given. All parents worry about a sick or injured child. Will he recover? Will there be long-term effects? Will she be affected by the hospitalization?

The stressful experience of having a hospitalized child derives not just from these worries, but from a series of associated and potentially preventable stresses. The parents may have difficulty making contact with their child's physician; hospital policies might prevent parents from staying with their child; the need to care for other children at home may separate parents from each other, limit the amount of contact between the sick child and the parent or lead to exhaustion as parents try to attend to the children in both places and to maintain their other responsibilities. These conditions make demands on the parents' physical and emotional energy and may deplete their internal resources to the point that they are unable to respond appropriately to their children's needs, needs that are also intensified under stress.

Social support in the form of a responsive and understanding physician and hospital staff who facilitate contact between families and children and instrumental assistance from family, friends, or community members in caring for the children at home should reduce the amount of stress these parents experience. By reducing stress, social support should facilitate responsive and nurturant parenting.

2.2. Support as a Buffer or Mediator of Stress

Another view is that social support serves as a buffer between a stressful event and the individual's response to that event (Cobb, 1976; Dean & Lin, 1977). According to this view, stressful life events tend to be associated with physical and psychiatric illness and behaviorally with patterns of parenting considered maladaptive for the child's development. If, however, the person touched by the experience receives adequate and appropriate social support, he or she will remain physically or emotionally healthy and will continue to parent in a manner that allows the child's needs to be met. This is an interesting description of the role social support might play with respect to parenting behavior, but it does not explain how the support works. What is it about the provision of support that accounts for its apparent buffering effect?

2.3. Social Support as a Generator or Activator of Active Coping

We know that individuals respond differently to the same external stressors. Some people experience loss of a job, multiple roles, or city life as anxiety producing and debilitating, while others experience them as challenging and stimulating. Often these different psychological experiences are accompanied by different repertoires of resources available for coping. People who experience the potentially or initially stressful event as challenging feel they can deal with what life has served up to them. They believe they are competent and that somehow they will manage in the face of adversity. In contrast, people who experience the event as anxiety producing and severely distressing feel they have no control over what has happened to them or what will happen to them as a result of the initial event (Seligman, 1975; Abramson, Seligman, & Teasdale, 1978). They may feel, as some adolescent mothers do, that they are incompetent, simply not up to the task of caring for an infant. As a consequence, they may become frustrated more quickly than mothers who feel more competent in their new role. For example, a mother who feels she has no influence on her baby might allow him to cry after the first attempt to soothe doesn't work, or she might withdraw altogether by failing to respond to any of the baby's cues, or eventually by relinquishing the baby to the care of someone else.

The difference between these two coping styles is typically presented as a difference internal to individuals, the result of past experiences with success and failure. It is likely, however, that ongoing experiences outside the individual also influence how she responds to a potentially stressful event. Noninstrumental social support may intervene between the experience of a stressful event and behavior by helping the individual develop effective and appropriate strategies for dealing with the event. To the extent that a woman receives confirmation that she is doing a good job with her baby, her view of herself may change. Instead of telling herself that she is not competent, she may begin to believe that she is capable of caring for her baby. Moreover, if these messages are coupled with suggestions for soothing a crying baby, for amusing an active baby during diapering, or for interesting a bored baby, she may continue to develop a repertoire of skills that will increase her competence as a mother and allow her to generate from within the message that she is competent.

2.4. Social Support as the Presence of an Intimate Relationship

It has been suggested that the love and caring characteristic of intimate relationships is an essential aspect of social support (Cobb, 1976; Lowenthal & Haven, 1968). This conceptualization comes primarily from the clinical insights of psychologists, such as Bowlby (1958) and Erickson (1959), who identify intimacy and trust as basic needs and the establishment of relationships characterized by these qualities as the crux of subsequent development.

In the parlance of developmental psychologists, through their experiences with their parents, children develop "working models" of relationships they carry forward with them into new relationships (Main, Kaplan, & Cassidy, 1985). According to this view, children who have experienced rejection and hostility will view themselves as unworthy of love and unlikely to elicit nurturance from others. This expectation will in turn interfere with their ability to give love and nurturance to others, including their children. They may fear the love will not be reciprocated, they may focus on meeting their own unmet needs, or, because they have repressed the affective experiences associated with these early painful events, they may be unable to empathize with the pain and fear in their own children (Frailberg, 1980). In contrast, if their experience has been one of acceptance and nurturance, the child, and subsequently the adult, views himself or herself as worthy of love and likely to elicit nurturance from others. In this way, a loving relationship with parents is thought to support adaptive development in children.

How might this developmental process be useful to understanding the impact of emotional support on parenting behavior? Although a working model of relationships begins to form in infancy, it is likely that its maintenance depends on experiences the individual has throughout childhood and into adulthood. Thus, if a baby expects to be loved and nurtured, this expectation may lead the baby both to engage in behaviors designed to elicit love and nurturance, and it may allow the baby to withstand a certain amount of subsequent rejection. Nonetheless, because a working model is not impervious to ongoing experience, an extended period of rejection, or even the absence of love and nurturance during a time when the individual is called on to provide nurturance to another, may eventually undermine the individual's sense of herself or himself as a person deserving of love and care and capable of caring for someone else. Ongoing emotional support or nurturance may affirm this sense and in doing so encourage the individual's inclination to be nurturant to others.

If a parent failed to form a positive working model of relationships as a young child, the receipt of emotional support as an adult should be even more important in facilitating the parent's ability to nurture a child. There is considerable evidence that parents who abuse their children were themselves abused in childhood, either physically or emotionally (Herrenkohl, Herrenkohl, & Toedter, 1983; Main & Goldwyn, 1984). This finding does not imply that childhood experiences have a determining effect on adult behavior, but they may have such an effect *if no other nurturing experience intervenes*—if no other person in the child's life loves and nurtures the child (Epstein, 1986; Epstein & Erskine, 1983). At the same time, it may be more difficult to nurture such a person because she or he does not expect to be nurtured and may fail either to seek it out or to recognize the nurturance for what it is (Crittenden, 1985).

One goal of emotional support and nurturance in this context is no less than that of reshaping the adult's working model of relationships. In view of the enormity of this task and the resistance the nurturing person may encounter, the amount of support needed under these circumstances could be extensive. Fraiberg (1980) suggests that when the adult with this background is a parent with a baby, nothing short of infant–parent psychotherapy will be sufficient to undo the painful effects of the past. Other studies indicate, however, that a supportive partner may mediate the impact of the mother's developmental history on her parenting behavior: mothers with histories of separation and rejection exhibited appropriate behavior with their young children when they had supportive spouses (Quinton & Rutter, 1985; Crockenberg, 1987). The implications of these differing perspectives for intervention will be discussed in the final section of the chapter.

2.5. Social Support as a Direct Impact on the Child

In discussing the process by which social support works, the implicit assumption has been that the impact of social support on the child is indirect: social support encourages appropriate parental behavior, which in turn benefits the child. It is likely, however, that social support affects children directly as well (Bryant, 1985). The relationships grandparents develop with their children and grandchildren are a case in point. While grandparents may provide parents with advice, general emotional support, and eager babysitters, at the same time they can provide their grandchildren with loving caregiving (Crockenberg, 1981; Tinsley & Parke, 1983). This kind of loving care is undoubtedly valuable to all children, but it may be essential to children whose parents are undergoing some kind of stress and who for that reason are unable to provide the kind of responsive, involved caregiving on which children thrive.

Evidence from Werner and Smith's (1982) study of the "vulnerable" children is consistent with this prediction: one of the events that distinguished the vulnerable children who developed normally from those who did not was the opportunity to establish a close bond with at least one caregiver during the first year of life. Often this nurturing came from substitute caregivers within the family—siblings, aunts and uncles, and grandparents. Similarly, studies of adolescent mothers indicate that grandmothers, primarily the mother's mother, are a major source of social support, both emotional and instrumental, especially when the babies are very young (Crockenberg, 1987b, 1987, in press). Although no attempts have been made to assess whether the impact these grandmothers have on their grandchildren's development is direct or indirect, it seems likely that some of the benefit that accrues to the child must come from direct contact with the grandmother. Often she lives in the same home with the child and is the person who cares for the child during the day while the mother works or attends school. She may also be the person most likely to get up with the baby when he or she cries at night.

2.6. Summary

The theories advanced to explain the means by which social support affects parental behavior and child development are not mutually exclusive. It is quite probable that support works in all these ways, sometimes simultaneously. Thus, by being supportive a partner may reduce the stress a mother experiences by taking on greater than usual household responsibilities, and he may buffer the stress associated with having a sick or irritable baby by telling his partner that he thinks she's a capable parent. Moreover, his love and nurturance may affirm the mother's sense of being cared for herself. Together these experiences will support her ability to be responsive and nurturant toward her baby. Developmental theory and research indicate that the baby benefits from responsive and nurturant maternal caregiving, and he or she may benefit further from direct contact with a second adult—in this instance his or her father (Lamb, 1981).

The complexity of the association between social support, parenting, and child behavior is illustrated in Figure 1.

3. REVIEW OF RESEARCH ON SOCIAL SUPPORT

Theory predicts that social support will have an ameliorative or facilitating impact on parenting and on the child's development. This would seem a straightforward hypothesis to test, but as is typically the case in scientific investigation, the adequacy of that testing depends on the adequacy of the methodology employed. In research on the impact of social support on parenting, a number of conceptually based methodological issues have surfaced. (1) Several sources and dimensions of social support have been identified. Are certain types of support more or less important with respect to parenting? Does it matter who provides the support? (2) Is it the objective amount of support available to a family that is important to parenting, or is it the perception that whatever support is available is enought? If it is the latter rather than the former, what are the factors that influence that perception? (3) Is social support equally important for all families, or are there certain families for whom social support is particularly important and for whom it will be most related to differences in parenting? (4) Is it social support that has

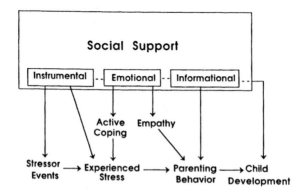

FIGURE 1. Ways in which social support may affect parenting behavior and child development.

an impact on parenting, or is it some other uncontrolled variable that accounts for the effect? For example, if a history of rejection during childhood decreases the likelihood that a mother will have or seek to obtain social support as an adult, developmental history and social support may be intercorrelated, and the former variable may account for any association between social support and parenting behavior.

In response to these issues, our review will be organized in the following way. Studies will be presented concerning whether the families can be considered at high or low risk for maladaptive parenting by virtue of the child's characteristics, the parents' characteristics, or the particular stresses in the social environment. If the source or type of social support is identified, findings will be presented in relation to those specific sources or types, e.g., family/partner, peer; intimate, child-care, or household support. Professional support will be treated in a separate section. Studies that have taken particular care to establish a causal relation between social support and parenting behavior will be identified and any association between social support and the child's development will be noted. Each section will begin with a brief statement of the major finding with respect to social support and parenting, present the specific studies that confirm the association, and end with a summary and interpretation of the findings and a discussion of contradictory results.

Theories linking social support with parenting behavior emphasize the special importance of that support when family members are experiencing a great deal of stress in their lives. For that reason, the review will begin with studies that have examined the association between social support and parenting in "high-risk" families—those considered to be under particular stress.

3.1. Social Support in High-Risk Families

The classification of high-risk has been applied to a diverse collection of families—families with premature or highly irritable babies and with handicapped children, families in which the mother is an adolescent or has been identified as abusing a child, families that live in poverty, families that are experiencing a divorce. These diverse families have in common a potentially high level of stress associated either with the specific characteristics of their babies, the characteristics of the parents as defined by their age or background, or the external conditions of their lives. Because of their exposure to potential stressors, these families are considered to be at high social risk to have difficulty parenting.

Parents of premature infants and handicapped children may worry more than other parents about their children's very survival, about their immediate health or development, and about their future. In addition, their children may require more care than other children by virtue of their special characteristics. Even children without special needs require considerable time and energy from their parents, and parents who have many other pressing concerns may have difficulty responding to the ordinary needs of their children.

Thus, adolescent mothers engaged in developmental transitions around issues of identity and intimacy may have other concerns that compete with the baby for time and attention. Similarly, mothers who are going through a separation and divorce may be concerned about where they will live and how they will support themselves, while low-income mothers may be struggling just to keep themselves and their families fed, housed, clothed, and safe. There may be little energy left to respond effectively to their children's needs. To the extent, then, that parents experience these circumstances, it can be anticipated, for all the reasons outlined above, that social support could facilitate sensitive and responsive parenting.

Even within a high-risk classification, however, not all parents will experience the high levels of stress thought to impede parenting. Not only do the specific experiences of individual families vary, but some individuals have effective internal resources for coping with stressful life events (Gottlieb, 1983). It follows that although social support is an important predictor of parenting behavior, other aspects of the individual's character and circumstances must be considered in evaluating the independent impact of social support on parenting.

3.1.1. Studies of Babies with Special Needs

Studies of families with babies with special needs report that better social support is associated with better maternal adjustment and more optimal parenting practices. Three studies investigated the association between social support and maternal adjustment or behavior in families with a premature infant (Affleck, Tennen, Allen, & Gershman, 1986; Boukydis, Lester, & Hoffman, 1987; Crnic, Greenberg, & Slough, 1986); an additional study investigated the association in families with a retarded, handicapped, or developmentally at-risk child (Dunst & Trivette, 1986); a fourth project considered the association between support and maternal behavior for a group of irritable babies (Crockenberg & McCluskey, 1986); and another study looked at social support in families with twins (Glaser, 1987).

In the Affleck et al. (1986) study, the sample consisted of mothers of infants who had been treated for severe perinatal medical problems. Two months following hospital discharge, measures of the mother's emotional, informational, and tangible support were obtained, as well as measures of the need for and satisfaction with that support and questionnaire data on maternal adaptation. Social support was not associated with maternal adaptation in the whole sample, but was associated with maternal adaptation for infants whose conditions were more severe. Mothers of infants with more worrisome conditions exhibited more positive adaptation when they were more satisfied with the emotional, informational, and tangible support they received.

Crnic et al. (1986) reported similar findings in a sample of 52 mothers and their preterm infants. A composite measure of nonprofessional social support, collected one month after hospital discharge, was associated with more positive affect and dyadic synchrony during interaction at 8 months and with better language development, less noncompliance, and more secure attachment in the infants at 12 months. When social support was considered separately by source, intimate support from family members correlated most highly with maternal measures, social support from friends the least.

This latter finding, while consistent with the results of other studies, may underestimate the value of support from friends to parents of preterm babies. In Boukydis, Lester, and Hoffman's (1987) study of term and preterm infants and their families, parents of preterm infants reported receiving significantly more emotional support from friends during the first month postdischarge of their baby from the hospital. Moreover, parents who had contact with other parents of preterm babies made fewer calls to health professionals during that first month. From these findings we may infer that support from friends can be quite important to parents of premature infants, particularly during the first few weeks the baby is home from the hospital.

Although frequently parents of disabled and handicapped children display interactive styles characterized by intrusiveness and coercion (see Dunst, 1985, for a review), social support is associated with more positive patterns of interaction in this population. Dunst and Trivette (1986) studied 102 mothers of retarded, handicapped, and developmentally at-risk infants and preschoolers. Mothers were interviewed to obtain a measure of social support (the number of members of mothers' personal network who provided six types of support) and a measure of the absence of support or role accumulation (the number of roles the mothers performed without assistance). They were also observed interacting with their children. Mothers with good social support employed a more engaging maternal style, while mothers with more task assistance showed greater involvement of various types with their children. The authors interpret these findings as evidence that mothers with exclusive responsibility for a larger number of household and childcare chores were less able to either initiate interaction with or respond to their child's bids for attention. Social support, in the form of household and childcare assistance, gives the mother time to attend to her child.

While social support may affect maternal behavior simply by freeing mothers to interact with their children, research on mothers with irritable infants suggests that social support may affect the quality of interaction even under circumstances when mothers have the same opportunity to interact. Mothers of babies identified as irritable during the neonatal period were more or less sensitive to their 1-year-old babies in the laboratory "strange situation" depending on the amount of social support they had received (Crockenberg & McCluskey, 1986a). Mothers with greater social support were more sensitive than mothers with less social support, and more sensitive mothers were more likely to have securely attached babies (Crockenberg & McCluskey, 1986b). It is possible, of course, that over time mothers with less support have less time for their babies and develop a pattern of insensitivity and unresponsiveness that carries over into other situations. On the other hand, social support may affect a mother not just by reducing the number of competing tasks she must perform, but in other ways as well, possibly by giving her confidence in her ability to parent an irritable baby. Evidence that social support predicts parenting self-efficacy (the expectation that one will cope well as a parent) is consistent with this view (Cutrona & Troutman, 1986).

Glaser's (1987) study of mothers of twins confirms the fact that both instrumental and emotional support are associated with differences in maternal adjustment. Questionnaire data on support and maternal adjustment to having twins was obtained from 250 mothers with infant twins. For women who needed help, instrumental, informational, and emotional support all correlated significantly with the adjustment indicators. Moreover, the combination of adequate physical help, information about twins, and emotional reassurance about their maternal role predicted adjustment more strongly than any single type of support.

In sum, the research to date suggests that social support is associated with sensitive, involved interaction between parents and their infants with special needs. Studies differ, however, in the type of social support they identify as most predictive of differences in parenting. Several studies indicate that child-care and household help account for differences in parenting, while others suggest that intimate support is more important. The idiosyncratic nature of the circumstances faced by families in different samples makes it difficult to generalize about what type of support is more important. Depending on the demands of a particular event and on the developmental status of the infant and the parent–infant relationship, different informational and instrumental support may be needed.

Moreover, in statistical terms, the type of support that will predict differences in parenting will depend in part on which dimensions of support vary in a given sample. If most families have good intimate support but vary widely with respect to child care support, only child care support would show any correlation with measures of parenting. We would not wish to conclude, however, that other types of social support were unimportant to the family. They may have been consistent and adequate in all families in a given sample. For this reason, we will proceed cautiously with respect to the inferences drawn from the *absence* of association between specific types of support and parenting behavior.

It is also unclear from these studies whether differences in social support account for the observed differences in parent–child interaction. In all the reviewed studies, characteristics and circumstances other than social support likely distinguished the more and less sensitive and involved mothers, yet only one study used a statistical model designed to control for the possible confounding effect of other variables (Crockenberg & McCluskey, 1986a). It is possible, therefore, that some of the observed associations between social support and parenting behavior are a function of some other, unmeasured, variable, such as the mother's beliefs about childrearing and her developmental history. We will continue to question whether the studies reviewed were designed to adequately test a possible causal link between social support and parenting.

3.1.2. Studies of Low-Income Families

Evidence that social support is positively associated with parenting in low-income families comes from several independent research projects. Feiring and Taylor (1982) found that in their low-income, primarily black inner-city sample, mothers who were rated as involved and responsive also perceived a high amount of positive support from the secondary parent, typically the mother's mother or the baby's father. Ryan et al. (1985) reported similar findings in a two-year follow-up of 38 low socioeconomic status, primarily Caucasian mothers and babies. Current maternal social support correlated positively with home stimulation and accounted for the largest portion of the variance, in comparison with the family's race and income. Moreover, mothers who reported high stress and low support provided significantly lower amounts of home stimulation than families characterized by any other combination of support/stress factors. With high support, highly stressed mothers were able to provide the same level of home stimulation as less stressed mothers.

Longfellow, Zelkowitz, Saunders, and Belle (1979) confirm these findings with a sample of 40 low-income women with young children and specify both the sources and the nature of the social support that shows the strongest association with parenting outcomes. Mothers who received more child care help of all kinds were less dominant and more affectionate in their interaction with their children and more responsive to their children's dependency needs. Although women with partners reported having more help of this type than did single women, the same association between child-care support and maternal behavior was observed within each group.

Most women in the sample of Longfellow et al. did not turn to their partners for help with personal problems. However, the women who did receive intimate emotional support from their partners were more responsive to their children's dependency requests and used fewer negative response styles. In addition, women who turned to their partners for emotional support had children who turned to him for nurturance as well (Zur-Szpiro & Longfellow, 1983). In contrast, neither the amount of neighborhood exchange, nor the extent of contact with friends was related to differences in parenting. There was evidence, however, that mothers who were engaged in greater neighborhood sociability and exchange reported more depressive symptoms and higher stress.

In sum, there is evidence that social support is associated with "desirable" parenting behavior in low-income samples and that within such samples the impact of support is strongest for those families experiencing higher levels of stress. Intimate support from partners appears particularly beneficial to mothers and children, but for single mothers help with child care is also associated with positive, responsive caregiving. In contrast, contact and exchange with friends and neighbors does not appear to facilitate caregiving of that type. Contact *per se* does not constitute support and it may be that the exchange of services, which requires reciprocity, may result in no overall benefit to the mother. It may also be that mothers who depend heavily on this type of support have less support from family members, and this lack rather than any deficit in exchange support may account for the greater stress and depression reported.

3.1.3. Studies of Adolescent Mothers

Of the studies that have explored the link between social support and adolescent maternal behavior and interaction, all but one suggest a positive impact of social support on parenting.

Lee and Colletta (1983) studied 40 adolescents under 19 years of age, most of whom had one child between 1 and 3 years of age. Mothers who were highly satisfied with their total support reported that they were more affectionate with their children, while mothers who were dissatisfied with their support reported more hostility, indifference, and rejection of their children. When type and source of social support were analyzed, emotional but not task support from family members was associated with less aggression and rejection, nagging, ridicule, and threats from mother to child. Mercer, Hackley, and Bostrom (1984) confirmed an association between social support and adolescents' self-reported feelings, but identified both emotional and instrumental support as important. At one-month postpartum, adolescent mothers with high instrumental support had stronger feelings of love toward their babies and a greater sense of competency in the maternal role. Emotional support was also associated with feelings of love and with the young woman's gratification in the mothering role.

Subsequent studies have confirmed the association between support and parenting in diverse samples of adolescent mothers, using independent behavioral assessments of mother–child interaction. Epstein (1980) reported that adolescent mothers who had part-time help from grandparents and/or the baby's father stimulated their babies appropriately, knew when and how to intervene to change behaviors, and evidenced clear enjoyment of their child. Levine, Garcia-Coll, and Oh (1985) studied 30 mothers, half of whom were 17 years of age or younger, eight months after the baby's birth. More child-care support was associated with higher quality of the face-to-face interactions between the mothers and babies. Similarly, Crockenberg (in press) reported that English adolescent mothers who received emotional and instrumental support from family members during the postnatal period reported more responsive attitudes and were independently observed to respond more quickly when their babies cried.

Other studies of adolescent mothers confirm the association between social support and parenting behavior, but suggest that the source of support most predictive of sensitive and responsive caregiving may change over time. Unger and Wandersman (1985) studied 35 adolescent mothers beginning during the prenatal period and continuing until the babies were 8 months old. Mothers were predominantly black, low-income, and single. Greater perceived support was related to fewer concerns about parenting and to better parenting skills. At one month after birth, family support and friend support were associated with lower parenting anxiety, but mothers provided better environments for their babies (had higher scores on the Home Observation for Measurement of the Environment (HOME) Scale) when the baby's father and relatives provided child care for the baby. By eight months, only support from the baby's father was associated with fewer concerns about parenting. In a second study of 87 adolescent mothers and their babies, family support measured prenatally predicted higher HOME scores at eight months, but again it was partner support at eight months that was positively associated with HOME scores.

Additional evidence that the nature of the social support most beneficial to adolescent mothers and their babies may change over time comes from a follow-up at two years of babies first studied at 3 months postpartum (Crockenberg, 1987). Mothers rejected by their mothers as children but with good current support from a partner were less angry and punitive with their toddlers than similarly rejected mothers with poor partner support. Table 3 from that paper illustrates this finding in the significant association between the interaction of maternal acceptance and partner support. Current support from family members, which at three months predicted several aspects of maternal behavior, showed no such buffering effect. Initially, it may be helpful to the young mother to have a number of people to facilitate the transition to parenthood. Continued reliance on a large number of family members may either reflect or contribute to a lack of competence on the mother's part.

TABLE 1. Predictors of Maternal Anger and Punitive Control[a]

	R^2 increase	df	F
Maternal acceptance	.081	1,38	3.28
Partner support	.000	1,37	<1
Time to calm	.008	1,36	<1
Acceptance × support	.108	1,35	4.55*
Time to calm × support	.006	1,35	1.23

[a]Variables were entered one at a time in the order listed. Significance levels are based on the increase in R^2 for each variable at entry.
*, $p < .05$.
From "Predictors and Correlates of Anger toward and Punitive Control of Toddlers by Adolescent Mothers" by Susan Crockenberg, 1987, *Child Development, 50,* 971.

If, for example, the adolescent's mother and sisters take over a substantial share of the childrearing, they may unintentionally deprive her of the role as primary caregiver and interfere thereby in the developing mother–child relationship.

These studies of adolescent mothers, like those of other high-risk families, establish an association between social support and the way mothers care for their infants, but typically fail to rule out the possible influence of other variables on the observed association. An exception is a study of 61 adolescent mothers and their 3-month-old infants (Crockenberg, 1987b). More family or more overall daily support were associated with greater rated sensitivity and accessibility and faster responsiveness to crying, even after differences associated with mothers' developmental history, childrearing attitudes, and current stress were taken into account. There was also evidence that for certain maternal behaviors the effect of social support depended on the amount of stress in the mother's life. Contrary to expectations, when the amount of stress reported was extremely high, social support had no beneficial impact. It may be that unusually high stress in a population already considered stressed by virtue of the mother's age and circumstances may increase the need for support beyond what family members can provide. Evidence in this study that additional stressors often had to do with conflict or tragedy involving the family suggests further that the families may have been unable to meet the supports needs of the young mother. Under such circumstances special professional services may be particularly necessary.

Only one study of adolescent parents failed to find an association between social support and maternal behavior (Lamb & Elster, 1985). The study's approach of observing the mother, father, and baby as a triad distinguishes it from all other studies in this section, which focused primarily or exclusively on the mother and infant, and likely accounts for the lack of association. Evidence that maternal behavior in dyadic, but not triadic, contexts predicts the security of infant–mother attachment suggests that a mother's behavior with her baby may be atypical when the father is present (Belsky, personal communication, 1983, cited in Lamb & Elster, 1985). It is noteworthy, however, that social support in this study was associated with differences in interaction between fathers and babies; fathers with more support engaged in more overall interaction.

In sum, there is considerable evidence that social support is associated, quite likely in a causal way, with adolescent maternal behavior that is sensitive and responsive during the first months after birth, stimulating and involved during the second half of the first year, and less angry and punitive at the end of the second year or life. Not all sources of support are equally valuable, however. Support from the adolescent's family or partner appears to be particularly advantageous with respect to parenting, but the source and nature of the support most beneficial to the adolescent mother may shift over time. What may be essential is that the support person, whoever it is, walks the fine line of helping the mother without intruding on her role as primary caregiver and without undermining her developing sense of herself as a competent mother.

3.1.4. Studies of Single-Parent Families

In light of the findings concerning social support and parenting among adolescent mothers, many of whom are also without partners, it is not surprising to find that social support is associated with more sensitive and responsive maternal behavior among single mothers as well.

Weinraub and Wolf (1983) studied social support and mother–child interaction in 28 mother–child pairs—14 single mothers and their preschool children were matched with 14 married women and children. Single mothers tended to be more socially isolated than married mothers, and they received less emotional and less parental support. At the same time they experienced more potentially stressful life changes. Although the single mothers reported more difficulty in the areas of household responsibilities than did married mothers, no significant difference between groups were found in mother–child interaction. However, within the single-parent sample, parenting supports and satisfaction with these supports were associated with more appropriate maternal control, better mother–child communication, and greater nurturance. In contrast, single mothers with a large number of social contacts were less nurturant and exercised less appropriate control.

Subsequent research confirms the negative association between frequent contact with friends and neighbors and parental behavior (Flesock, 1985). Flesock studied 135 white mothers of preschool children, 59 single and 76 married, from lower-class and middle-class backgrounds. Mothers described their social support and also their childrearing practices. Single and married mothers did not differ in the total amount of social support they reported, but increased contact with friends and number of neighbors known were related to an increased reported use of power assertion for single mothers only. In addition, mothers who expressed greater satisfaction with their support were less likely to use power-assertive discipline with their children.

While the few studies of single-parent families demonstrate the potentially positive impact of social support on parenting behavior, they illustrate again the problem of equating social contacts or size of social networks with social support. Contact that is stressful for the mother or that distracts her from the task of parenting may have a debilitating rather than a facilitating effect on her interaction with her child. If friends actually provide support for parenting, the effects can be quite different, as the Boukydis et al. (1987) study discussed earlier indicates.

Alternately, it may be that the causal explanation of the association between social contact and less optimal or appropriate parenting runs in the opposite direction. Those single mothers who work long hours and spend a considerable amount of their remaining time with friends may be less attuned to their children's needs and therefore less responsive to them (Weinraub & Wolf, 1983). In addition, children of mothers who both work and engage in frequent activities with friends may be more demanding of the mother's attention when she is at home, and possibly more resistant to her attempts to control their behavior, thereby eliciting more power-assertive discipline.

3.1.5. Studies of Abusing Parents

For some time social isolation and lack of support have been linked to child abuse and neglect (Young, 1964). Newberger, Reed, Daniel, Hyde, and Kotelchuck (1977) found a lack of social support to be correlated highly with abuse, controlling for social class, age, and ethnicity. Polansky, Chalmers, Buttenweiser, and Williams (1979) compared a sample of neglectful families with a matched sample of control families. The neglectful families reported significantly less formal and informal social participation and had lower scores on a scale measuring the adequacy of their core social network.

More recently, investigators have expanded their investigations to consider the possible mediating effect of social support on the association between stress and abuse and to test more precisely how powerful differences of support are for discriminating abusing and nonabusing mothers. Gaudin and Pollane (1983) studied 41 abusive mothers and 59 nonabusive mothers. Abusing mothers reported significantly weaker, less supportive informal social networks and more situational stress than the nonabusing mothers. Both the kinship networks and the neighbor/friend networks of the nonabusing mothers were stronger than those of the abusing mothers. The findings also support the mediating effect of strong social support on the relation between situational stress and abuse: mothers living in highly stressful life situations who reported strong social networks were less likely to be abusers than mothers living in high-stress situations who reported less social support.

Similar findings were reported by Turner and Avison (1985). In that study, 78 mothers either known or suspected to have abused or neglected a child physically or emotionally were compared with 293 nonabusing mothers on several variables, including social support. Using only the measures of social support as predictors, 90.8% of the abusing and nonabusing mothers were correctly classified. Matching for variables that might have spuriously inflated identification of the two groups of mothers (age, education, socioeconomic circumstance, and recency of childbirth) decreased the accuracy rate only slightly.

It appears from the studies reviewed above that poor social support is associated with child abuse and it is tempting to conclude, in light of the number of variables eliminated as sources of potential confounding, that the association is causal in nature.

Not considered in these studies, however, is the possibility that characteristics of the mothers account both for their low support and their abusive parenting. Mothers rejected as children may lack the usual sources of support because they may not elicit or make use of potential sources of support (Crittenden, 1985). Thus, their behavior with their children may be as much a function of their own developmental history as it is a result of current, but correlated, social support.

The results of two other studies suggest, however, that despite the impact of developmental history on current parenting, there is an independent, interactive effect of partner support on maternal behavior (Quinton & Rutter, 1985; Crockenberg, 1987). In both studies, mothers with histories of separation and rejection avoided negative patterns of parenting when they had good social support from their partners. It seems reasonable to conclude, therefore, that social support may reduce the possibility of abusive behavior in families who are at risk for developing such behavior by virtue of their own experience of being parented.

3.2. Social Support in Low-Risk Families

Fewer studies have investigated the link between social support and maternal behavior in low-risk samples, but those that have done so report findings similar to those with high-risk samples: social support is positively associated with mothers' emotional well-being and with sensitive and responsive maternal behavior.

Shea and Tronick (1982) investigated the predictors of maternal self-esteem—the mother's confidence in her ability to mother during the first few days after birth and at one-month postpartum in a sample of 30 healthy, nonstressed, mother–infant pairs. Family support accounted for 30% of the variance in mothers' self-esteem immediately after birth, after differences associated with infant health were taken into account. Mothers who reported receiving more family support also had significantly higher maternal self-esteem than mothers who did not receive family support. By one-month postpartum, family support alone accounted for 52% of the variance in maternal self-esteem. Mothers who reported higher self-esteem behaved more positively and confidently when interacting with their infants and also were more sensitive and responsive to their infants' cues.

Leung (1985) reported similar results with a sample of 35 new Chinese mothers. Women who received support from their families had an easier adjustment to motherhood. They were likely to be less anxious and depressed than women who did not receive such support. Husbands were the most important source of assistance and emotional empathic understanding, while lack of marital support was correlated with depressed maternal mood.

Levitt, Weber, and Clark's (1986) study of 43 mothers and their 13-month-old infants confirms the importance of support from the spouse for the mother's well-being in intact families and extends the impact of that support to differences in the infant–mother relationship. Emotional and childcare support from the spouse, but not from other family members, was associated with greater life satisfaction and more positive maternal affect. In contrast, emotional support from mothers' friends was associated with lower life satisfaction and more negative maternal affect. There was no direct association between support and infant–mother attachment. However, maternal affect was related to security of attachment, with mothers of secure babies expressing more positive affect than mothers of anxious or resistant babies. This latter finding suggests a possible indirect effect of support on infant emotional development mediated through the mother's behavior.

Two additional studies have linked social support to maternal behavior with older infants and children. Luster (1986) studied 65 mothers and their children who ranged in age between 9 and 23 months. Most of the mothers were white, married, and not employed outside the home. Level of social support was related to the quality of care the mothers provided the infants: mothers with more extensive support networks had higher scores on the HOME Scale. In this study, the number of non-kin mentioned in the social support interview was more strongly related to the HOME scores than the number of kin mentioned.

In contrast, Roberts (1986) found that kin social support appeared to buffer the effect of stress on parenting in a sample of 30 families with preschool-age children. Stress was associated with less warm and less responsive parenting only for families with no emotional support from maternal kin. Contrary findings emerged for support from friends, especially fathers' friends. When fathers reported more contact and support from friends, parents were less warm and responsive toward their children. In addition, social support was directly associated with children's competence in preschool; even after differences in parenting were taken into account, children who were babysat by kin, typically grandparents, were more competent than children without such care.

Whether kin or friend support has the greater positive influence on parenting has been discussed above and remains a difficult issue to resolve. As Luster (1986) points out, kin support may be very important to the mother, but if there is little variability within the sample on that dimension of support, it will not show up as a correlate of maternal behavior. Moreover, as we discussed earlier, the source of support that will have the greater impact likely depends on the nature of the support provided by each source. When kin are disapproving of the mother or make excessive demands on her time and energy, any help they provide may be help the mother could well do without. Under these circumstances, or if kin are geographically distant, friends may provide support and encouragement for parenting along with an active exchange of babysitting and other types of instrumental assistance. Their support may be related in turn to differences in the way parents care for their children.

This analysis illustrates the danger of assuming the availability of support from the mere presence of network members capable of providing support and indicates the importance of determining from the parent's perspective whether she or he feels supported. Often, perceived support has little to do with objective indices of support, such as the number of network members (Cutrona, 1986). Not only does this subjective approach identify members of a support network who provide support and those who do not, but it also incorporates the results of an internal balancing that goes on inside the mother when she says to herself, "Yes, my mother takes care of the kids for me, but she always has something to say about how they're dressed and she manages to let me know that she doesn't think I should be leaving them to work." This is essential information in the assessment of a mother's social support and it will be discussed further in the final section of the chapter.

In sum, while it is unclear what kind or source of support is more likely to affect the ways parents care for their children, it appears from available research that social support is associated with patterns of parenting generally considered more appropriate or beneficial for the child's development, even in so-called "low-risk" samples. Another finding is that social support is associated in beneficial ways with the child's development, in one instance mediated through the mother's behavior and in another through direct contact between the support person and the child.

Evidence of an association between the availability of social support and parenting behavior in low-risk families raises an interesting theoretical question. If social support has its impact by reducing stress or by buffering the impact of stress on the way parents care for children, why should there be any association between support and parenting when there is little or low stress? The answer may be that there is a certain amount of stress inherent in the course of daily living and in parenting any child. Those stresses, or "hassles," as Crnic and Greenberg (1985) refer to them, can accumulate and be expressed in the family interaction. Presumably, social support could serve the same mediating or buffering role in this context as it does with the stresses that characterize the lives of "high-risk" families.

3.3. Professional Support

Thus far this review has focused on the parent's informal support network and the support provided by that network. There are also professional services available to families that are intended to support parents and, specifically, to provide mothers with information and advice about children and parenting practices. A complete review of the studies evaluating the effectiveness of these services is beyond the scope of this chapter. Instead, several studies selected for their methodological rigor and for their different approaches to the provision of professional support will be considered. Three types of study design will be included in the reviewed studies: a correlational design in which naturally occurring professional support is considered as one among several sources of social support provided parents (Crnic, Greenberg, & Slough, 1986; Crockenberg, in press); a design in which the parenting of mothers is compared across national groups that differ in the professional services they provide mothers (Crockenberg, 1985); and a design in which a special program of support services has been developed and the parenting of mothers participating in the program is compared with that of a control group (Lyons-Ruth, Botein, & Grunebaum, 1984; Lyons-Ruth & Karl, 1986; Unger & Wandersman, 1985).

3.3.1. Correlational Studies of Naturally Occurring Professional Support

Results of the Crnic et al. (1986) study relating to informal support were reported earlier. The sample included 52 mothers of preterm infants studied at 1, 8, and 12 months after birth. To study the independent contribution of professional support to differences in parenting behavior, a measure of professional support was constructed by combining responses to two questions concerning the availability of support from physicians, nurses, and social service providers and the mothers' satisfaction with that support. This measure was then added to a multiple regression equation after predictability associated with informal sources of support was partialed out. Professional support added significantly to the prediction of several aspects of parenting behavior and parenting satisfaction. From this finding we may conclude that, at least for mothers with special needs babies, support from professionals can have a beneficial impact on parenting that is independent of the impact of social support available through the mothers' informal support network.

In contrast, a study by Crockenberg (1987b) found no effect of professional support on the maternal behavior of adolescent mothers, despite the finding that professionals were mentioned by nearly half the mothers as frequent or very frequent sources of support (primarily in the area of listening, encouragement, and advice giving). On the assumption that frequent professional support tends to occur in the more at-risk families whose behavior may be more deviant than low-risk families even with professional support, the impact of professional support was tested separately within each risk classification. Professional support was considered high if a mother mentioned at least one professional who helped frequently or very frequently and low if professional help was less frequent. There was no evidence that professional support was associated with more sensitive and responsive mothering within either high- or low-risk groups.

The discrepancy in the results of these two studies may have to do with the nature of the support available to mothers of preterm babies in comparison with what is available to adolescent mothers. Boukydis, Lester, and Hoffman (1987) emphasize the importance that parents of preterm infants place on medical staff as sources of support, extending beyond hospitalization. Parents of preterm infants listed their pediatrician, pediatric nurse, and spouse as most helpful; and the intensive-care nursery staff, other parents of premature babies, and their child's pediatrician as the most important sources of information about child care. In Seattle, where the Crnic et al. (1986) study was carried out, good support services exist for parents of preterm babies. It can be expected that mothers who receive these services will benefit from them and that there will be differences in the behavior of mothers who do and do not receive sufficient professional support. The services available to adolescent mothers in the Crockenberg (1987b) sample were considerably more fragmented. Although 74% of the mothers indicated that they had received parenting advice from some professional source, 90% said they would have liked more advice and information (Crockenberg, 1986). It is unclear, therefore, whether the professional support these adolescent mothers received would have been sufficient to have affected their parenting.

3.3.2. A Cross-National Approach to the Study of Professional Support

Evidence that a certain type of professional support can contribute to differences in maternal behavior comes from a comparative study of English and American adolescent mothers (Crockenberg, 1985).

Through the National Health Service, England incorporates community-based social support for parents in a comprehensive program of health care that is free to families with limited incomes (Economic Models Limited, 1976; Davie, Butler, & Goldstein, 1972; Gill, 1980). The care begins before the child's birth and continues through the school years. Special attention is given to parents considered in need of parenting assistance. Midwives provide postnatal care for mothers and babies after they leave the hospital following delivery and home health visitors see new mothers on a regular basis, with frequency of home visits dependent on assessed need. These health professionals provide health information, advise mothers on the care of their infants, and refer families to other agencies when the problems encountered are outside their scope.

It is not surprising, then, that while English and American mothers report help from physicians with near identical frequency, English mothers experienced significantly more help from other professional sources (Crockenberg, 1985). In addition, when the English and American samples were combined, professional support was associated with more smiling and eye contact and with less routine contact in the interactive behavior of the adolescent mothers with their 3-month old babies. The effect of professional support was apparent, moreover, after differences associated with infant characteristics, maternal education and attitudes, stress, and family support were partialed from the regression equation, indicating that the association was not an artifact of these other differences. It appears from this study that certain types of professional support affect some aspects of the care young mothers provide their babies during the postnatal period.

3.3.3. Professional Support as Part of a Planned Intervention Program

Evaluations of programs designed to deliver professional support to high-risk mothers provide additional support for the claim that professional support can influence the way mothers care for their babies.

In the Unger and Wandersman (1985) study, adolescent mothers of low socioeconomic status were randomly assigned to an intervention ($n = 70$) or a control group ($n = 17$). In the intervention group, experienced mothers and paraprofessionals visited each mother once a month throughout her pregnancy and the baby's first year. These visitors provided emotional help, informational assistance, and instrumental support. They focused on the strengths of each mother and her environment, frequently involved the teen's family and friends, and they encouraged the teen mother to use the resources in her network. In addition, a structured curriculum emphasized the importance of a mother in influencing her baby's development. In the control group, teen mothers were contacted approximately once every three months to note the progress of mother and baby and to provide referral when needed; no structured curriculum was followed and no support services were offered other than referral.

At eight months postpartum, visited mothers demonstrated more knowledge about babies, greater satisfaction with mothering, and more responsive attitudes toward their babies than did comparison mothers. They were more likely to seek medical care for illness and a higher proportion remained in school. It is noteworthy that although professionals designed this program of service delivery, and selected and trained the paraprofessional staff, it was the nonprofessional staff that had direct contact with the adolescent mothers.

Another program that provided support to mothers through the use of professional and paraprofessional home visitors also reported beneficial effects of the intervention (Lyons-Ruth et al., 1984, Lyons-Ruth & Karl, 1986). The 34 mothers in the sample were considered at risk for developmental disadvantage because of poverty and stresses in the family and in addition were referred for possible parenting problems. Many had ongoing psychiatric problems or were suspected or known abusers. The mothers were randomly assigned to one of two intervention services: in one, weekly visits were made to mothers by paraprofessionals—experienced mothers from the community; and in the other, weekly visits were made by trained psychologists.

The paraprofessionals sometimes focused on both the babies and the mothers. Sometimes they actively attempted to change the parent's behavior by making recommendations or modeling alternative means of discipline. At other times they shared their own experience as parents. In their mother-centered role, they served as sympathetic listeners or as helpful friends, for example, by accompanying the client to pediatric appointments, to neurological evaluations, and to welfare agency appointments. The home-visiting format used by the professionals differed from that of the paraprofessionals, primarily with respect to less sharing of personal experience and more probing of intimate topics by the professionals.

During the evaluation phase of the project the behavior of the infants and mothers in the two groups was compared between groups and with a matched control group of mothers and infants from the community who had never been referred for parenting difficulties or been psychiatrically hospitalized. The results showed no differences between the two visited groups. However, there were fewer insecurely attached babies in the intervention groups than in the matched control group. In addition, the longer the mothers had been in treatment, the more sensitive and less angry they were toward their babies.

In sum, these studies indicate that social support delivered by professionals *or* trained paraprofessionals can be effective in encouraging sensitive and responsive caregiving in high-risk mothers. This is an important finding both because it suggests that social support can be provided at a lower cost than if high-paid professionals delivered services and because paraprofessionals may be better suited than professionals to the nontraditional service delivery model that appears to be particularly effective with certain groups of mothers. In the English setting, as well as in the two intervention studies, services were delivered in a way that minimally inconvenienced the mothers. Visitors came to the mothers in their homes. Not only did this reduce the amount of planning and organization required of the mothers in order to receive professional support, but it also meant that the support was provided in familiar settings, which research has shown underusers of formal health care services to prefer (McKinlay, 1970, cited in Gill, 1980). Other intervention projects reporting beneficial effects for mothers and/or babies have also used home visitors to provide services (Field, Widmayer, Stringer, & Ignatoff, 1980; Olds, 1983; Nurcombe et al., 1984).

4. SUMMARY

The primary conclusions of this review can be summarized as follows:

1. Social support is associated with a better adjustment to parenting or more appropriate parenting as indicated by greater responsiveness and sensitivity to infant needs, more interaction and stimulation, and less use of power assertion as a method of controlling child behavior. The benefits of social support are apparent for families under consider-

able and unusual stress and for families experiencing the everyday hassles of modern life.

2. Social support is associated also with adaptive child development as indicated by secure infant–mother attachments and competent child behavior. The impact of social support on the child may be direct—from the support person to the child—or indirect—mediated through the mother's behavior.

3. Emotional support and assistance with child care are identified as important types of social support and are frequently associated with the way mothers care for their children. However, the type of social support most encouraging of sensitive, responsive, and involved parenting likely depends on the specific needs of individual families.

4. Social support from family members, and in particular from the mother's partner, is typically most predictive of the type of parenting behavior described above.

5. There are instances, however, in which friends or professionals are better sources of support than are relatives, or simply necessary additional sources of support given the specific needs of the family. In particular, parents of children with unusual or atypical characteristics and needs may benefit from contact with other parents who have had similar experiences.

6. Professional support can be effective in promoting sensitive and responsive parenting. Moreover, paraprofessionals can be as effective as professionals in working with certain high-risk groups. An extensive outreach component, through which continuity of services to the family is assured, appears to be an important component of professional support services with certain at-risk groups.

To the extent that social support facilitates parenting practices associated with normal child development, it is important that health professionals work with families to develop their informal sources of support and to provide direct support for parenting when it is appropriate.

4.1. Strengthening Parents' Informal Sources of Social Support

To know how they might be useful, professionals need first to assess the social support a parent receives—how much and what type and how the parent views the adequacy of that support. From the research reviewed above we know that the needs of parents are quite individual and that they vary with the parent's developmental history, the child's age, and other characteristics. A mother with a history of abuse may require extensive mother–child therapy of the sort described by Fraiberg (1980), while a mother of twins may benefit most from another pair of hands to help with housework and child care (Glaser, 1987). Parents with a premature baby may need specialized information that is best provided by other parents with premature babies (Boukydis et al., 1987). It is essential, therefore, that the health professional have no preconceived notion of what a family will need or who should provide it.

Although social support is viewed as something beneficial for the parent, its receipt can involve costs and conflicts only the recipient is aware of. In the example given earlier, a grandmother caring for her granddaughter while the mother worked at the same time criticized the mother's working and mothering. Adolescent mothers report with some frequency that their mothers take over the role of primary parent or insist that their advice be followed (Crockenberg, in press). Parents of premature babies report that sometimes the fear and concern immediate family express about the baby make reliance on their help stressful (Boukydis et al., 1987). These may be instances of "support" that is not worth the emotional cost. A professional might explore the possibility of alternative child-care arrangements with the working mother and other sources of assistance for the parents of the premature baby. Alternately, she or he might help the parents develop strategies for getting what they need emotionally while maintaining the supportive aspects of the help they are receiving. Mothers can be encouraged, for example, to set limits on an intrusive helper in ways that leave supportive relationships intact.

One way to help families work out the conflicts that arise in supportive relationships is to include significant people in a parent's support network in services often targeted primarily, if not exclusively, on the mother (Crockenberg, 1986; Ooms, 1981). Not only does this type of approach to service delivery provide an arena for dealing with conflicts, it may obviate the need for conflict resolution by assuring that parents and the people who support them are exposed to the same information and advice. If, for example, a physician advises a mother to feed her baby on a "demand" schedule, it may be crucial that the baby's father, who may have another perspective on when the baby should be fed, be included in the advice-giving session.

Scheduling appointments to suit the needs of more than one adult will require some flexibility on the part of the professional, a requirement that translates also into the need for better funding of certain programs. In a report for the Ford Foundation, McGee (1984) noted that very few programs for adolescent mothers include a significant number of fathers or other family members. Although staff members in those programs understand that young mothers with family support fare better as parents, limited resources often result in working most closely with their primary client, the young mother.

4.2. Formal Sources of Social Support: Professional and Nonprofessional

When the parent's informal support system is limited, or when it is extensive but still insufficient in view of the parent's needs, a health professional may need to step in and provide support to the parent or family. This can be given directly in the form of emotional support to the parent and information about the child and his or her care. For example, a family physician or nurse practitioner can confirm that a baby is unusually irritable, suggest alternative methods for dealing with the crying, and convey to the parents how well they are doing under the circumstances.

When the support needed is very specialized, as in the case of a child with a specific disability or a mother whose background and current functioning suggests the need for intensive therapy, or when it requires extensive outreach to the family, health professionals may want to refer parents to other services. This referral may be to other professionals or professionally organized programs or it may be to a specific type of parent group with only limited ties to professionals (Wandersman, 1987). Depending on the size of the community, parenting groups may be available for adolescent mothers, parents of premature or otherwise high-risk infants, and parents identified as abusers. Parenting classes offer information and advice on child development and childrearing and they provide a context in which parents can learn from one another. Again, the parent's needs will determine what type of referral is appropriate.

To act effectively as a a referral agent, a health professional must know what services are available. Often this information can be obtained locally, through county health departments, universities, or professional organizations. The Family Resource Coalition,[1] a national federation that promotes development of community-based programs to strengthen families, offers a national parent referral service to link parents with programs.

Acknowledgments

This chapter was written during the time I was a visiting scholar in the Child Development Unit, Harvard Medical School and Children's Hospital. I would like to thank Dr. T. Berry Brazelton, chief of the Unit,

---

[1]Information can be obtained by writing the Family Resource Coalition, 230 N. Michigan Avenue, Suite 1625, Chicago, IL 60601.

for providing the physical and psychological space that allowed me to complete this chapter, and Dr. Zachariah Boukydis for reading and commenting on several earlier drafts.

5. REFERENCES

Abramson, L. Y., Seligman. M. E. P., & Teasdale, J. D. (1978). Learned helplessness in humans: Critique and reformulation. *Journal of Abnormal Psychology, 87,* 49–74.

Affleck, G., Tennen, H., Allen, D. A., & Gershman, K. (1986). Perceived social support and maternal adaptation during the transition from hospital to home care of high-risk infants. *Infant Mental Health Journal, 7*(1), 6–18.

Belsky, J. (1984). The determinants of parenting: A process model. *Child Development, 55,* 83–96.

Boukydis, C. F. Z., Lester, B. M., & Hoffman, J. (1987). Parenting and social support networks for parents of preterm and full-term infants. In C. F. Z. Boukydis (Ed.), pp. 61–83. *Research on support for parents and infants in the postnatal period.* New York: Ablex.

Bowlby, J. (1958). The nature of the child's tie with his mother. *International Journal of Psychoanalysis, 24,* 190–194.

Bryant, B. K. (1985). The neighborhood walk: Sources of support in middle childhood. *Monographs of the Society for Research in Child Development, 50*(3, Serial No. 210).

Cobb, S. (1976). Social support as a moderator of life stress. *Psychosomatic Medicine, 38*(5), 300–314.

Crittenden, P. (1985). Social networks, quality of child rearing, and child development. *Child Development, 56.* 1299–1313.

Crnic, K. A., & Greenberg, M. T. (1985, April). *Parenting daily hassles: Relationships among minor stresses, family functioning and child development.* Paper presented at the meetings of the Society for Research in Child Development, Toronto.

Crnic, K. A., Greenberg, M. T., & Slough, N. M. (1986). Early stress and social support influences on mothers' and high-risk infants' functioning in late infancy. *Infant Mental Health Journal, 7*(1), 19–33.

Crockenberg, S. B. (1981). Infant irritability, mother responsiveness, and social support influences on the security of infant–mother attachment. *Child Development, 52,* 857–865.

Crockenberg, S. B. (1985). Professional support and care of infants by adolescent mothers in England and the United States. *Journal of Pediatric Psychology, 10,* 413–428.

Crockenberg, S. (1986). Professional support for adolescent mothers: Who gives it, how adolescent mothers evaluate it, what they would prefer. *Infant Mental Health Journal, 7,* 49–58.

Crockenberg, S. (1987a). Predictors and correlates of anger toward and punitive control of toddlers by adolescent mothers. *Child Development, 58,* 964–975.

Crockenberg, S. (1987b). Support for adolescent mothers during the postnatal period: Theory and research. In C. F. Z. Boukydis (Ed.), *Research on support for parents and infants in the postnatal period.* New York: Ablex.

Crockenberg, S. (in press). English teenage mothers: Attitudes, behavior and social support. In E. J. Anthony (Ed.), *Yearbook of the International Association for Child Psychiatry and Allied Professions.* New York: Wiley.

Crockenberg, S., & McCluskey, K. (1986a). Change in maternal behavior during the baby's first year of life. *Child Development, 57,* 746–753.

Crockenberg, S., & McCluskey, K. (1986b). *Predicting infant attachment from early and current maternal behavior.* Paper presented at the biennial meeting of the Society for Research in Child Development, Toronto.

Cutrona, C. (1986). Objective determinants of perceived social support. *Journal of Personality and Social Psychology, 50,* 349–355.

Cutrona, C., & Troutman, B. (1986). Social support, infant temperament, and parenting self-efficacy: A mediational model of postpartum depression. *Child Development, 57,* 1507–1518.

Davie, R., Butler, N., & Goldstein. H. (1972). *From birth to seven: The second report of the National Child Development Study (1958 cohort).* London: Longman.

Dean, A., & Lin, N. (1977). The stress-buffering role of social support. *Journal of Nervous and Mental Disease, 165*(6), 403–417.

Dunst, C. J. (1985). Rethinking early intervention. *Analysis and Intervention in Developmental Disabilities, 5,* 165–201.

Dunst, C. J., & Trivette, C. M. (1986). Looking beyond the parent–child dyad for the determinants of maternal styles of interaction. *Infant Mental Health Journal, 7*(1), 69–81.

Economic Models Limited. (1976). *The British health care system.* Prepared for the American Medical Association.

Epstein, A. (1980). *Assessing the child development information needed by adolescent parents with very young children.* Final report of Grant OCD-90-C-1341, Office of Child Development, Department of Health, Education, and Welfare, Washington, DC (ERIC Document Reproduction Service No. ED 183 286)

Epstein, E., & Erskine, N. (1983). The development of personal theories of reality from an interactional perspective. In M. Magnussen & V. Allen (Eds.), *Human development: An interactional perspective* (pp. 133–147). New York: Academic Press.

Epstein, S. (1986). Implications of cognitive self-theory for psychopathology and psychotherapy. In N. Cheshire & H. Thomas (Eds.), *Self-esteem and psychotherapy.* New York: Wiley.

Erickson, E. (1959). Identity and the life cycle. *Psychological Issues* (Monograph 1). New York: International Universities Press.

Feiring, C., & Taylor, J. (1982). *The influence of the infant and secondary parent on maternal behaviors.* Unpublished manuscript, Educational Testing Service.

Field, T., Widmayer, S., Stringer, S., & Ignatoff, E. (1980). Teenage, lower-class, black mothers and their preterm infants: An intervention and developmental follow up. *Child Development, 51,* 526–436.

Flesock, M. W. (1985). Parental practices and attitudes in single parent families: The influence of family structure, social class and social support. *Dissertation Abstracts International, 45*(9-B), 3068.

Fraiberg, S. (1980). *Clinical studies in infant mental health: The first year of life.* New York: Basic Books.

Gaudin, J. M., & Pollane, L. (1983). Social networks, stress and child abuse. *Children and Youth Services Review, 5*(1), 91–102.

Gill, D. (1980). *The British National Health Service* (Public Health Service NIH Publication No. 80-2054). Washington DC: U.S. Department of Health and Human Services.

Glaser, K. (1987). A comparative study of social support for new mothers of twins. In C. F. Z. Boukydis (Ed.), *Research on support for parents and infants in the postnatal period.* New York: Ablex.

Gottlieb, B. (1983). Opportunity for collaboration with informal support systems. In S. Cooper & W. E. Hodges (Eds.), *The mental health consultation field* (pp. 181–204). New York: Human Science Press.

Herrenkohl, E., Herrenkohl, R., & Toedter, L. (1983). Perspectives on the intergenerational transmission of abuse. In D. Finkelor, R. Gelles, G. Hotaling, & M. Straw (Eds.), *The dark side of families: Current family violence research* (pp. 305–316). Beverly Hills, CA: Sage.

Hickson, G. B., Altemeier, W., & O'Connor, S. (1983). Concerns of mothers seeking care in private pediatric offices: Opportunities for expanding services. *Pediatrics, 72,* 619–624.

Lamb, M. E. (1981). The development of father–infant relationships. In M. E. Lamb (Ed.), *The role of the father in child development* (pp. 459–488). New York: Wiley.

Lamb, M. E., & Elster, A. B. (1985). Adolescent mother–infant–father relationships. *Developmental Psychology, 21*(5), 768–773.

Lee, D., & Collette, N. (1983, April). *Family support for adolescent mothers: The positive and negative impact.* Paper presented at the biennial meetings of the Society for Research in Child Development.

Leung, E. (1985). Family support and postnatal emotional adjustment. *Bulletin of the Hong Kong Psychological Society, 14,* 32–46.

Levine, L., Garcia-Coll, C. T., & Oh, W. (1985). Determinants of mother–infant interaction in adolescent mothers. *Pediatrics, 75*(1), 23–29.

Levitt, M. J., Weber, R. A. & Clark, M. C. (1986). Social network relationships as sources of maternal support and well-being. *Developmental Psychology, 22*(3), 310–316.

Longfellow, C., Zelkowitz, P., Saunders, E., & Belle, D. (1979, March). *The role of support in moderating the effects of stress and depression.* Paper presented at the biennial meeting of the Society for Research in Child Development, San Francisco.

Lowenthal, M. J., & Haven, C. (1968). Interaction and adaptation: Intimacy as a critical variable. *American Sociological Review, 33,* 20–30.

Luster, T. (1986, April). *Influences on maternal behavior: Childrearing beliefs, social support and infant temperament.* Paper presented at the International Conference on Infant Studies, Los Angeles.

Lyons-Ruth, K., Botein, S., & Grunebaum, H. U. (1984). Reaching the hard-to-reach: Serving isolated and depressed mothers with infants in the community. In B. Cohler & J. Musick (Eds.), *Intervention with psychiatrically disturbed parents and their young children: New directions for mental health services, 24.* San Francisco: Jossey-Bass.

Lyons-Ruth, K., & Karl, D. (1986, November). *Neighborhood support systems for infants.* Paper presented at the Harvard Family Research Project Seminar Series, Issues in the Implementation and Evaluation of Home Visit Programs, Cambridge.

Main, M., & Goldwyn, R. (1984). Predicting rejection of her infant from mother's representation of her own experience: Implications for the abused-abusing intergenerational cycle. *Monographs of Child Abuse and Neglect: The International Journal, 8.*

Main, M., Kaplan, N., & Cassidy, J. (1985). Security of attachment in infancy, childhood and adulthood: A move to the level of representation. In I. Bretherton & E. Waters (Eds.), Growing points of attachment theory and research (pp. 66–106). *Monographs of the Society for Research in Child Development, 50*(No. 1–2).

McGee, E. (1984). *Too little, too late: Services for teenage parents.* New York: Ford Foundation.

McKinlay, J. B. (1970). *Some aspects of lower class utilization behavior.* Unpublished doctoral dissertation, University of Aberdeen, Scotland.

Mercer, R. T., Hackley, K. C., & Bostrom, A. (1984). Social support of teenage mothers. *Birth Defects: Original Article Series, 20,* 245–290.

Newberger, E., Reed, R. B., Daniel, J. H., Hyde, J. N., & Kotelchuck, M. (1977). Pediatric social illness: Toward an etiologic classification. *Pediatrics, 60*, 178–185.

Nurcombe, B., Howell, D., Rauh, V., Teti, D., Ruoff, P., & Brennan, J. (1984). An intervention program for mothers of low birth weight infants: Preliminary results. *Journal of the American Academy of Child Psychiatry, 23*, 319–325.

Olds, D. (1983). An intervention program for high-risk families. In R. A. Hoekelman (Ed.), *A round table on minimizing high-risk parenting.* Media, PA: Harwal.

Ooms, T. (Ed.) (1981). *Teenage pregnancy in a family context.* Philadelphia: Temple University Press.

Polansky, N., Chalmers, M., Buttenweiser, C., & Williams, D. (1979). The isolation of the neglectful family. *American Journal of Orthopsychiatry, 49*, 149–152.

Quinton, D., & Rutter, M. (1985). Parenting behavior of mothers raised "in care." In R. Nicol (Ed.), *Longitudinal studies in child psychology and psychiatry.* Chichester, England: Wiley.

Roberts, W. L. (1986). *Parental stress and social networks: Relations with parenting and children's competence.* (ERIC Document Reproduction Service No. ED 271 228)

Rossi, A. S. (1968). Transition to parenthood. *Journal of Marriage and the Family, 30*, 26–39.

Ryan, K., Ullman, D., Adamakos, H., Diaz, R., Pascoe, J., & Chessare, J. (1985). *Environmental correlates of optimal child development: A look at the maternal social support system moderating levels of mother/child stress and home stimulation.* Paper presented at the spring convention of the Ohio Psychological Association. (ERIC Document Reproduction Service No. ED 261 771)

Seligman, M. E. P. (1975). *Helplessness: On depression, development, and death.* San Francisco: Freeman.

Shea, E. M., & Tronick, E. Z. (1982, August). *Maternal self-esteem as affected by infant health and family support.* Paper presented at the meeting of the American Psychological Association, Washington DC.

Tinsley, B. R., & Parke, R. D. (1983). Grandparents as support and socialization agents. In M. Lewis (Ed.), *Beyond the Dyad.* New York: Plenum Press.

Turner, R. J., & Avison, W. R. (1985). Assessing risk factors for problem parenting: The significance of social support. *Journal of Marriage and the Family, 47*(4), 881–892.

Unger, D. G., & Wandersman, L. P. (1985). Social support and adolescent mothers: Action research contributions to theory and application. *Journal of Social Issues, 41*(1), 29–45.

Wandersman, L. (1987). Parent–infant support groups: Matching programs to needs and strengths of families (pp. 139–160). In C. F. Z. Boukydis (Ed.), *Research on support for parents and infants in the postnatal period.* New York: Ablex.

Weinraub, M., & Wolf, B. M. (1983). Effects of stress and social supports on mother–child interactions in single and two-parent families. *Child Development, 54*, 1297–1311.

Werner, E. E., & Smith, R. S. (1982). *Vulnerable but invincible: A study of resilient children.* San Francisco: McGraw-Hill.

Young, L. (1964). *Wednesday's children: A study of child neglect and abuse.* New York: McGraw-Hill.

Zur-Szpiro, S., & Longfellow, C. (1983). Fathers support to mothers and children. In D. Belle (Ed.), *Lives in stress.* Beverly Hills, CA.: Sage.

5

Multimodal Treatment of Attention Deficit Hyperactivity Disorder in Children

WADE F. HORN AND NICHOLAS IALONGO

1. INTRODUCTION

Attention Deficit Hyperactivity Disorder (ADHD), often referred to as childhood hyperactivity or simply attention deficit disorder (ADD), is one of the most common referral complaints to child mental health services in the United States (Ross & Ross, 1982; Rubinstein & Brown, 1984). Indeed, it accounts for between 40% and 50% of all child referrals to outpatient mental health clinics, or approximately 200,000 cases annually (O'Malley & Eisenberg, 1973; Trites, Dugas, Lynch, & Ferguson, 1979; LaGreca & Quay, 1984). According to the most recent revision of the *Diagnostic and Statistical Manual of Mental Disorders* (DSM-III-R) (American Psychiatric Association, 1987), the essential features of ADHD are developmentally inappropriate degrees of inattention, impulsiveness, and hyperactivity of six or more months duration with an onset before age 7. Children with ADHD generally display some disturbance in each of these areas, but to varying degrees.

Wade F. Horn • Department of Psychiatry, Children's Hospital National Medical Center, Washington, D.C., and George Washington University Medical School, Washington, D.C. **Nicholas Ialongo** • Department of Psychology, University of Virginia, Charlottesville, Virginia 22903.

Much research over the past several decades has been dedicated toward both the understanding and treatment of this disorder. Yet, despite over 50 years of research evaluating the effectiveness of a variety of treatment approaches with ADHD children, the discovery of a single treatment approach that effectively normalizes the behavioral and learning problems of these children and that significantly alters the poor long-term prognosis associated with the disorder continues to allude clinical researchers. Consequently, over the past decade, clinicians have become increasingly interested in the use of various combinations of treatments as a means of addressing the multiple problem areas presented by ADHD children. Most commonly, the components of these multimodal intervention packages are psychostimulant therapy, behavioral parent training, cognitive-behavioral self-control therapy, and school consultation. Unfortunately, empirical research regarding the comparative and combined effectiveness of such multimodal treatments has been relatively sparse.

The present chapter will first review the literature pertaining to children with ADHD in order to facilitate an understanding of the magnitude and diversity of problems associated with ADHD children. Following this, a review of the most common treatment approaches for ADHD and their demonstrated effectiveness will be presented along with a rationale for employing a multimodal treatment approach. We will then review the published literature on multimodal treatment approaches with ADHD children. Finally, we will provide an overview of a series of comparative and combined clinical research studies conducted by our research laboratory over the past five years and provide suggestions for future research.

2. PREVALENCE OF ADHD

Estimates of the prevalence of ADHD in school-age children vary widely, with some estimates as low as 1% and others as high as 20% (Barkley, 1981; Safer & Allen, 1976). Discrepancies in prevalence estimates are in large part attributable to the lack of agreement as to the best means for diagnosing the disorder. In particular, prevalence estimates are often quite high when ratings of a child's behavior from a single source are used as the defining criterion. For example, Trites and Laprade (1983) found that 14% of 14,038 children in the Ottawa public schools were rated by their classroom teachers as evidencing ADHD as measured by the Conners Teacher Rating Scale (Conners, 1969). However, prevalence estimates drop dramatically when agreement across ratings from different observers, particularly across different settings, is required to diagnose a child as evidencing problems indicative of

ADHD. For example, Sandoval, Lambert, and Sassone (1980) compared behavioral ratings of children made by teachers, parents, and physicians. Twelve percent of their sample was rated as evidencing ADHD by at least one of the raters. However, when agreement across all three observers was required to establish a diagnosis, only 1.9% were found to evidence ADHD.

Different rating scales also yield different prevalence estimates for ADHD. Holborow, Berry, and Elkins (1984) compared ratings made on nearly 2,000 children in the public schools in Queensland, Australia, using the Conners Teacher Rating Scale (Conners, 1969), the Queensland Scale (adapted from Davids, 1971), and the Pittsburgh Adjustment Scale (Miller, Palkes, & Stewart, 1973). Of this sample, 12% were rated as evidencing significant ADHD problems by at least one of the scales. However, when agreement of significant ADHD problems on all three rating scales was required to establish a diagnosis, only 3.5% of this sample was found to evidence ADHD.

Given these problems in establishing a good prevalence estimate, Barkley (1981) in his authoritative text suggests that the best prevalence estimate for ADHD is between 3% and 4% of school-age children, or about one in every classroom in the United States. Hence, even this relatively conservative prevalence estimate indicates the great magnitude of this childhood disorder.

Epidemiological studies have consistently found more males than females to evidence ADHD. Male-to-female prevalence ratios have been variously estimated from 3:1 to 9:1 in favor of males (Whalen & Henker, 1980). A number of hypotheses have been offered to explain this sex difference, including genetic, prenatal, developmental, and cultural explanations (Eme, 1979; Preis & Huessey, 1979). No single hypothesis, however, has yet to receive adequate empirical support. It is also unclear whether the symptomatology of the disorder varies by sex—with some studies finding sex differences (DeHaas & Young, 1984; Kashani, Chapel, Ellis, & Shekim, 1979) and others finding few or no sex differences (Befera & Barkley, 1985; Wagner, 1986). A recent investigation by Wagner (1986) suggests that studies employing cross-situational criteria (i.e., agreement across multiple observers) for diagnosing ADHD are less likely to find differences in symptomatology across the sexes compared with studies relying upon the ratings made by a single observer.

3. PRIMARY SYMPTOMATOLOGY

A cardinal feature of ADHD is difficulty focusing and sustaining one's attention to a task (Douglas, 1972; Preis & Huessey, 1979; Ross &

Ross, 1982; Safer & Allen, 1976). At home, parents describe ADHD children as having difficulty attending to commands, completing chores and homework assignments, and playing alone for prolonged periods of time. At school, these children are described by their teachers as having difficulty paying attention in class, completing in-seat assignments in a timely manner, and remembering directions.

ADHD children are also often described by parents and teachers as more distractible than other children. Recent research, however, indicates that the latter characteristic may not actually be the case. For example, Prinz, Tarnowski, and Nay (1984) found that while their sample of ADHD children did make more errors than their nonclinic control sample on a simulated academic task, the ADHD sample was not more distracted by a videomonitor of simulated classroom distractions than was the control group of children. Similar results have been reported by McMahon (1984) and earlier by Campbell, Douglas, and Morganstern (1971). Hence, while it is clear that ADHD children are less efficient in their attentional strategies and have more difficulty than non-ADHD children sustaining their attention to a task, they may not be more distracted than other children by stimuli external to the task being performed. This may account for the failure to increase academic productivity when intervention strategies are employed that attempt to manage the inattention of ADHD children by placing them in isolated and barren cubicles in order to minimize the amount of external distractions.

A second symptom of ADHD is difficulty inhibiting impulses. ADHD children often react before thinking adequately about the consequences of their actions. This impulsiveness is often more a problem with delaying a response than it is with knowing the proper response. Indeed, after an impulsive act many ADHD children will realize what it is they have done wrong and may even know what the correct response should have been. Douglas and her colleagues (1972) have conceptualized this difficulty as a failure to "stop, look, and listen." Such impulsivity leads to tremendous conflict with parents, teachers, and peers. At home and at school, these children repeatedly violate even the most basic of rules and social conventions resulting in their being more frequently admonished and punished than other children (Klein & Young, 1979). Their impulsiveness also leads them to place themselves in riskier situations more frequently than other children. This results in their suffering more physical injuries than other children. Indeed, parents often describe their ADHD children as being more "accident prone" compared with siblings (Barkley, 1981).

A third symptom considered by some to be central to a diagnosis of ADHD is motoric overactivity. Research, however, suggests that overactivity is not always present in ADHD children, and when it does occur, it is often situation specific rather than pervasive. For example, overactivity is most likely to be present in highly structured, group situations in which sustained attention and delay of impulses are required for successful performance. These children may not appear overactive in one-on-one situations or in free-play situations, such as on the playground. Hence, when motoric overactivity is present, it may be more the result of a difficulty adjusting activity level to situational demands than due to a pervasive biological "drive." In addition, research suggests that attention deficits and impulse control problems, compared with motoric overactivity, are more stable over time (August, Stewart, & Holmes, 1983) and more predictive of school failure (Weithorn, Kagan, & Marcus, 1984). For these reasons, motoric overactivity is probably best considered to be an often-associated, but not essential, feature of children with ADHD. Indeed, in the most recent revision of the *Diagnostic and Statistical Manual of Mental Disorders* (DSM-III-R) (American Psychiatric Association, 1987), overactivity is considered to be a frequent, but not required, feature of ADHD.

4. SECONDARY SYMPTOMATOLOGY

In addition to inattention, impulsivity, and overactivity, there are also several additional symptoms that are often associated with, but are not necessary for, a diagnosis of ADHD. Primary among these secondary characteristics is poor school performance. Indeed, ADHD children are two to three times more likely than non-ADHD children to be retained at least once during their academic careers (Barkley, 1981). In some cases, this underachievement at school is secondary to the inattention and impulsivity problems exhibited by these children. That is, ADHD children are often less available for academic instruction either because they are so frequently off-task in the classroom or because disciplinary measures by their teachers result in their being removed from the classroom. However, ADHD children are also more at risk than non-ADHD children for information processing problems as well. Barkley (1981) estimates that 60% to 80% of all ADHD children have diagnosable learning disabilities, and these learning problems are not likely to improve substantially with age. For example, Weiss, Minde, Werry, Douglas, & Nemeth (1971) found that only 20% of their adolescent sample of ADHD children had made a satisfactory academic adjustment in high school.

A second major associated characteristic of ADHD children is aggressive conduct problems. Ratings of ADHD and conduct problems are often correlated in factor analytic studies of childhood behavioral problems (e.g., Lahey, Green, & Forehand, 1980). Indeed, there are some authors who argue that ADHD is so consistently correlated with conduct problems that these two syndromes might best be considered to be a single childhood disorder (e.g., Stein & O'Donnell, 1985). However, recent research suggests that differentiation of ADHD children into subgroups on the basis of aggressive symptomatology does have prognostic significance. August et al. (1983) conducted a four-year follow-up study of a group of ADHD boys with aggressive conduct problems and a second group of ADHD boys without aggressive conduct problems. In adolescence, the group of ADHD boys with aggressive conduct problems was found to be frequently noncompliant, aggressive, antisocial, and egocentric, and to abuse alcohol. The group of ADHD boys without aggressive conduct problems continued to evidence inattention and impulse control problems in adolescence, but did not exhibit antisocial and aggressive behavior.

Given the difficulties ADHD children have with inattention, impulsiveness, and aggression, it is not surprising that a third major associated problem is poor peer relationships. When placed in socially frustrating situations, ADHD children are more likely than their non-ADHD peers to respond impulsively without considering the consequences of their actions. Often these impulsive decisions lead to aggressive or otherwise socially inappropriate behaviors. This often leads to social isolation, if not outright social rejection. Possibly as a defense against rejection, ADHD children are often described as being more comfortable with younger playmates who may be more forgiving or tolerant of social improprieties. Furthermore, peer relationship difficulties are often severe and chronic. For example, Waddell (1984) in a retrospective follow-up study of 30 adolescents diagnosed as ADHD in childhood found his sample of ADHD adolescents to be significantly less well socialized and to have fewer interpersonal interactions compared with a matched control group. This chronic history of poor peer relationships also appeared to have exacted a great toll from the self-esteem of these ADHD children. They were more likely to describe themselves as inadequate and to be more dissatisfied with their own behavior and their social relationships than were the adolescents in the matched control group. Peer relationship problems, when present, are particularly significant since poor peer relationships have been found to be predictive of poor adult adjustment (Cowen, Pederson, Badigian, Izzo, & Trost, 1973; Robins, 1966; Roff, 1961).

Children with attention deficit hyperactivity disorder are also often described as clumsy and poorly coordinated (Barkley, 1981). These problems may involve fine motor control, gross motor control, or both. For boys in particular, motor incoordination problems may further exacerbate their difficulties with forming effective peer relationships because they are often left out of or held in poor regard when participating in latency-age or adolescent sporting activities.

There is also evidence that ADHD children are more likely than non-ADHD children to have an external (Linn & Hodge, 1982) and/or unknown (Lopez, 1986) locus of control. It has been suggested that one reason for the more external and/or unknown locus of control in ADHD children is that their inattention problems make it difficult for them to accurately perceive behavior-consequence linkages. Hence, while other children are making the developmental shift from an external to an internal locus of control, ADHD children continue to externalize blame often in nonsensical ways or to have little understanding as to any source of control for their behavior. The importance of this variable lies in preliminary evidence from our research laboratory that ADHD children with an external locus of control are less likely to benefit from treatment than ADHD children with a more internal locus of control (Horn, Ialongo, Popovich, & Peradotto, 1987).

5. PROGNOSIS

The list of primary and secondary symptoms of ADHD reflects the tremendous pervasiveness and diversity of problems presented by ADHD children. In addition, research evidence increasingly suggests that ADHD is a chronic disorder as well. Whereas there may be decreases in the severity of motoric overactivity in adolescence, problems with inattention and impulse control have often been found to persist (Hoy, Weiss, Minde, & Cohen, 1978) and underachievement problems at school may become even more prominent (Wender, 1983). In addition, ADHD adolescents have been described as having a more rebellious attitude and to be more often in conflict with authorities than non-ADHD adolescents (Mendelson, Johnson, & Stewart, 1971). Furthermore, there is evidence that social and emotional problems persist into early adulthood, including increased incidences of alcohol abuse, sociopathy, and depression (Blouin, Bornstein, & Trites, 1978; Borland & Hechman, 1976; Weiss, Hechtman, & Perlman, 1978). It is important to note, however, that long-term outcome is not uniformly poor; rather there appears to be great variation within ADHD samples with regard to outcome. For example, in his review of the literature, Barkley (1981) estimates that 50% to 60% of ADHD children have an "adequate" adjustment in adulthood.

Given this variation in the long-term outcome of ADHD children, recent research has begun to investigate whether there are variables at the time of initial diagnosis that may be associated with particular adolescent and adult outcomes. Most notable among these recent studies is a five-year follow-up study of children initially diagnosed in childhood and later assessed in adolescence carried out by Loney, Kramer, and Milich (1981). The Loney et al. (1981) study is notable in that a prospective multivariate design was employed and ecologically valid assessments of cognitive and behavioral functioning were performed. Results indicated that prediction of cognitive and behavioral outcome was dependent upon the class of behaviors being assessed. For example, aggressive symptoms in adolescence were largely predicted by childhood aggression and to a lesser degree by adverse response to drug treatment and a disturbed parent–child relationship (i.e., a rejecting and punitive parent). Hyperactive symptoms in adolescence were predicted by socioeconomic status, aggressiveness in earlier childhood, and perinatal complications. Adolescent delinquency was predicted by childhood aggression, family variables, and an ecological variable (urban residence). These results were essentially replicated by this same research group in a second prospective follow-up study of 21-year-old males diagnosed as ADHD in childhood (Loney, Whaley-Klahn, Kosier, & Conboy, 1985).

Hechtman, Weiss, Perlman, and Amsel (1984) also attempted to determine whether variables at time of initial diagnosis predicted adult outcome. In this study children originally diagnosed as ADHD between the ages of 6 and 12 years were followed into early adulthood (ages 17 to 24 years). Although no single initial variable was associated with a particular adult outcome, several personality, ecological, and familial variables interacted to predict adult status. Similar to the Loney et al. studies, socioeconomic status (SES), mental health status of family members, IQ, aggressivity, and emotional adjustment assessed during childhood were found to be significant predictors of a variety of adult outcome measures, including adult psychiatric status, educational achievement, occupational status, and antisocial behavior.

While it seems undeniable that the problems of ADHD children often persist into adolescence and adulthood, there exist significant methodological shortcomings in many of these follow-up studies. Foremost among these issues is the fact that inattention, impulsivity. and overactivity are seen in many childhood psychiatric disorders and consequently are not specific to ADHD. Unfortunately, many of the follow-up studies of children whose clinical picture included symptoms of inattention, impulsivity, and/or overactivity failed to adequately define the diagnostic criteria used in subject selection. Consequently, one is unable to conclude in many cases if, in fact, a population of ADHD children was followed up. Additional shortcomings of the existing follow-up literature as it pertains to ADHD children is the frequent use of retrospective follow-up designs, reliance on case histories in lieu of objective assessment of current and past functioning, the absence of adequate control samples, and the failure to assess environmental and organismic variables other than the core symptoms of ADHD that may be related to long-term outcome.

Nonetheless, the available literature does suggest that the view (e.g., Laufer & Denoff, 1957; Wender, 1971) that ADHD is a disorder of early childhood that largely dissipates as the child grows into adolescence is unfounded. Rather, the core symptoms of chronic inattention and impulsiveness for many ADHD children continue to result in social and emotional dysfunction both in adolescence and adulthood.

6. TREATMENT APPROACHES

6.1. Psychostimulant Medication

The most frequently employed method of treatment for children with attention deficit hyperactivity disorder is psychostimulant medication, primarily methylphenidate, dextroamphetamine, or pemoline (Safer & Krager, 1983). Indeed, Sprague and Sleator (1977) reported that over 500,000 children in the United States were being treated with methylphenidate at the time of their survey. However, in biannual school surveys from 1971 through 1981, Safer and Krager (1983) found the rate of medication treatment of ADHD students increased two- to threefold, which suggests the Sprague and Sleator figure may actually *under*estimate the number of school-age children in the United States currently receiving stimulant therapy for ADHD.

The most common school period for medication use appears to be in grades 1 through 4, with entrance into the first grade and secondary school corresponding to an increased use of medication for ADHD (Safer & Krager, 1983). The median duration of psychostimulant therapy for elementary school students is one to two years, whereas for middle/junior high school students, the median duration of treatment is five to six years (Safer & Krager, 1983). Medication for ADHD problems in adulthood is apparently relatively rare; however, on the basis of long-term follow-up studies suggesting that ADHD difficulties often persist into adulthood, the therapeutic use of stimulant therapy with adults seems to be on the rise.

Methylphenidate is considered to be the stimulant of choice for children 6 years of age and older. Indeed, in a survey by Safer and Krager (1983), methylphenidate accounted for 91% of the stimulant medication prescribed for ADHD. The widespread selection of methylphenidate in school-age children appears to be tied to evidence that in contrast to dextroamphetamine, it is less likely to produce anorexia or adverse cardiovascular effects. Methylphenidate has also been found to be somewhat more effective in clinical trials than pemoline (Bassuk, Schoonover, & Gelenberg, 1983), although pemoline has the advantage of a longer half-life than methylphenidate, allowing for less frequent administrations of the medication.

While its manufacturer recommends dextroamphetamine for use in children with ADHD problems between the ages of 3 and 5 years, there exist no empirical studies indicating its superiority to methylphenidate in this age group (Bassuk et al., 1983). Consequently, the use of dextroamphetamine is typically limited to those cases in which a child exhibits a poor response or adverse side effects to methylphenidate. When neither methylphenidate or dextroamphetamine appears helpful, a trial of pemoline may be indicated.

A complete understanding of the neurophysiology and pharmacokinetics underlying the beneficial effects of the psychostimulants with ADHD children awaits further inquiry. What appears clear, however, is that there is no single mechanism that can explain the ameliorating effects of the psychostimulants, as a number of cortical areas have been shown to be differentially affected by these agents. It is known that amphetamines are sympathomimetics and act primarily on the midbrain, the reticular activating system, the hypothalamus, and the limbic structures. Methylphenidate, which has a similar biochemical structure and pharmacological action, also probably acts in the lower brain. Pemoline has a pharmacological action similar to both dextroamphetamine and methylphenidate, but without sympathomimetic activity (Bassuk et al., 1983).

The widespread use of stimulant therapy in the treatment of ADHD is undoubtedly a function of its cost efficiency and the fact that in well-designed, double-blind placebo-controlled studies, psychostimulants are more effective than placebo in decreasing the core symptoms of ADHD. Numerous studies have demonstrated psychostimulants to be effective in reducing the behavioral hyperactivity and impulsiveness and increasing the attention spans of about 70% of children with this disorder (Barkley, 1977; Brown & Sleator, 1979; Douglas & Peters, 1979; Porrino et al., 1983; Rapport, DuPaul, Stoner, & Jones, 1986). Furthermore, psychostimulants have also been found to improve some of the secondary symptoms of ADHD, such as classroom deportment (Conners & Taylor, 1980; Gittelman-Klein et al., 1976) and academic performance (Rapport, Murphy, & Bailey, 1980, 1982; Rapport, Stoner, DuPaul, Birmingham, & Tucker, 1985; Rapport et al., 1986).

Although currently the most widely employed intervention for ADHD, the psychostimulants are not without their limitations. First, up to 40% of ADHD children respond poorly or not at all to stimulant medication (Barkley, 1981; Barkley & Cunningham, 1978). Moreover there currently exists no empirically validated way of determining *a priori* which ADHD children will be medication responders.

Second, the psychostimulants can have unwanted side effects, including blood pressure elevation, gastrointestinal irritability, nausea, vomiting, anorexia, and weight loss. Untoward effects of a more behavioral nature include irritability, restlessness, insomnia, and alteration of mood. Psychostimulant medication may also give rise to the development of facial and body tics, with several documented cases of the development of Gilles de la Tourette's syndrome following the onset of psychostimulant therapy.

The emergence of increasingly severe side effects typically occurs with dosages of methylphenidate exceeding 0.7 mg/kg. At 1.0 mg/kg of methylphenidate, 20% to 50% of children display severe side effects. Along with these untoward side effects, there is some data to suggest that linear growth may be adversely affected by prolonged use of psychostimulants. However, the literature is ambiguous in this regard. What appears to be the case is that some children may be at greater risk for growth suppression than others (Campbell, Green, & Deutsch, 1985). Hence, careful longitudinal monitoring of growth parameters is warranted whenever psychostimulants are prescribed.

A third criticism of the use of psychostimulants is that it does little to improve academic performance (e.g., Barkley & Cunningham, 1978). However, as pointed out by Sprague (1983), this is not unexpected in that all stimulants can do is facilitate the learning process by increasing attention span and decreasing impulsivity. For these children to make up often severe academic underachievement problems, concomitant and appropriate remedial and special education services are required. There has also been the suggestion that the lack of improvement in academic skills with psychostimulant therapy is due to state-dependent learning effects. That is, once children learn a task or academic material under the influence of a psychostimulant, they will most efficiently recall that task or learned material only when again under the influence of that particular psychostimulant (Douglas, 1980; Swanson & Kinsbourne, 1976). More recent research, however, has concluded that such state-dependent learning is not always found, and where it is found the degree of state-dependent learning is not clinically significant (see Gittleman, 1983; Gittleman, Klein, & Feingold, 1983).

A fourth criticism of the use of psychostimulants is that it has not been found to be successful in improving the poor social relations and problem-solving skills of these children (Ayllon, Layman, & Kandel, 1975; Barkley & Cunningham, 1978). Indeed, recent studies suggest that stimulant medication alone is only modestly effective in reducing the frequency of peer conflict in ADHD children (Hinshaw, Henker, & Whalen, 1984a, b). Again, the failure of psychostimulant therapy to improve social relationships and problem-solving skills is not unexpected. Simply taking a pill will not cause others to want to make friends with the child, nor will it "teach" the child cognitive strategies that the child does not already possess.

A fifth criticism of the use of psychostimulants with ADHD children is that it reinforces the notion, on the part of both the child and the child's caretakers, that the child is not responsible for or in control of his or her behavior. Whalen and Henker (1976) were among the first to describe the potentially negative attributional set acquired by many ADHD children following the onset of psychostimulant therapy. These authors noted that some children would begin to state rather unequivocally that the reason they misbehaved on a particular day was because they didn't take their pill. Parents and teachers also often acquire the attribution that the "pill" ultimately controls the child's behavior and consequently there is little the parent, teacher, or child can do to enhance a child's self-control. Indeed, there is preliminary evidence from our research laboratory that the dose level of methylphenidate predicts degree of parent "resistance" in behavioral parent training groups, with higher doses being associated with greater resistance to the parent training (Packard, 1986). It seems that the parents whose children responded well to medication came to believe that their child's problems were all biological, and hence the parent training was really superfluous. If this finding is substantiated in further research, it may be important in clinical interventions combining parent training and psychostimulants to delay psychostimulant therapy until after the family has begun behavioral parent training.

Finally, and perhaps most important, long-term follow-up studies have failed to demonstrate that ADHD children provided with long-term psychostimulant treatment have significantly better adult outcomes than nontreated ADHD children (Weiss, Kruger, Dnielson, & Elman, 1975). A promising note was found in a more recent study by Hechtman et al. (1984). In contrast to their untreated counterparts, ADHD children treated long-term with stimulant medication were less likely to experience social ostracism and low self-esteem as adults. Unfortunately, there was no evidence that stimulant medication resulted in improved educational, work, or mental health outcomes.

6.2. Parent Training

The limitations of psychostimulant therapy alone, combined with the rejection of psychostimulants by some parents of ADHD children as an acceptable form of treatment, has spurred clinical researchers to explore additional treatment approaches with chronically inattentive and impulsive children. One alternative approach has been the use of parent training based on social learning theory principles (e.g., Barkley, 1981; Forehand, 1977; Patterson, 1974). In general, this approach teaches parents to become more systematic in their manipulation of environmental contingencies applied to their child's behavior in order to reduce the probability of maladaptive behavior and increase the probability of adaptive behavior. Parents are often taught to first monitor their child's behavior in a systematic fashion and then to rearrange environmental contingencies so as to promote more appropriate behavior. The use of star charts as a means of systematizing the delivery of positive reinforcement and the use of timeout as a mild form of punishment contingent upon inappropriate behavior are frequently included in behavioral parent training programs.

Also frequently incorporated has been instruction in the development and management of home-based reinforcement systems for school problems, such as daily home report card systems. More recently, behavioral parent training programs have also begun to focus on the enhancement of the parent–child relationship through the use of "special time" techniques during which a parent is instructed to spend time each day with the child in a nondirective, attentive, and supportive manner. Detailing behavioral parent training programs, however, is beyond the scope of the present chapter. Interested readers are referred to Barkley (1981), Forehand (1977), and Patterson (1974).

Clinical research on the effectiveness of behavioral parent training has found therapeutic value while therapy is in process (see reviews by Berkowitz & Graziano, 1972; Graziano, 1977; Johnson & Katz, 1973;

Moreland, Schwebel, Beck, & Wells, 1982; Wells & Forehand, 1980).
Indeed, Graziano (1983) has stated that ". . . utilizing parents as cooperative change agents in therapeutic skills may be the single most important development in the child therapy field" (p. 49). Nonetheless, there
is less evidence for generalization and long-term maintenance of treatment gains obtained with traditional behavioral parent training (O'Dell,
1974; Phillips & Ray, 1980). Furthermore, there is little evidence to
suggest that behavioral parent training alone results in substantially
more improved outcomes than psychostimulant therapy alone (e.g., Git-
telman et al., 1980).

One explanation for the difficulty in obtaining generalization and
maintenance of the effects of behavioral parent training involves subject
attribution effects. The training of parents to manipulate a child's environment may cause a child to attribute behavioral change to external
forces and decrease the child's intrinsic motivation to engage in adaptive
modes of functioning (Deci & Chandler, 1986; Dollinger, 1979). Experimental evidence for this formulation has been reported by Ross (1975),
who found that increasing the salience of external rewards resulted in
reductions in subjects' intrinsic motivation to engage in a task. However,
negative results have also been reported (Fisher et al., 1978).

6.3. Cognitive-Behavioral Intervention

Partly in response to the limitations of parent training, clinical researchers over the past 15 years have explored the use of "cognitive–
behavioral" interventions with ADHD children, such as training in attentional skills (Douglas, Parry, Marton, & Garson, 1976; Egeland,
1974), self-instruction (Meichenbaum & Goodman, 1971), and problem
solving (Camp & Bash, 1981; Shure & Spivack, 1972). Working from
Luria's (1961, 1969) model of cognitive development, proponents of the
cognitive behavioral approach argue that ADHD children have failed to
develop age-appropriate cognitive mediational skills. According to this
view, it is through the development of these mediational skills or covert
"self-talk" that the normal child learns to regulate his or her own
behavior.

The proponents of the cognitive–behavioral approach contend that
the maintenance of treatment gains can only be obtained through the
teaching of a generalized set of cognitive mediational ("self-talk") skills
that the ADHD child can internalize. More specifically, it has been hypothesized that when children successfully use the self-control and problem-solving skills they have been taught, they can only attribute success
to themselves and not to an external agent (Kendall & Braswell, 1985;

Meichenbaum, 1977; Whalen & Henker, 1976). Consequently, internalization occurs as the child attributes behavior change to the acquisition of new problem-solving and self-control skills, rather than to the effort of others.

In the typical self-control therapy, the child is taught a series of self-talk steps for use when confronted with problem situations. For example, in our clinical research laboratory (Horn, Ialongo, Popovich, & Peradotto, 1987; Horn, Ialongo, Greenberg, Packard, & Smith-Winberry, 1985), we teach ADHD children a "Problem Solving Plan" incorporating the following self-instructional steps: (1) "Do I have a problem?"; (2) "Take a deep breath and get myself calm"; (3) "What is my problem?"; (4) "How many alternative solutions can I think of?"; (5) "How good is each solution?"; (6) "Pick the best solution and try it"; and (7) "How did my solution work?". Other approaches to problem solving and self-instructional training are available in excellent texts by Meichenbaum (1977) and Kendall and Braswell (1985).

Unfortunately, the empirical investigation of the effects of self-instructional and problem-solving training with ADHD children has generally found significant treatment effects on cognitive laboratory measures but with little generalization to either the home or classroom environment (see review by Abikoff, 1985). This lack of generalization of treatment effects from the laboratory may reflect the fact that while the child has adequately learned the self-control strategies (as evidenced by the intervention effects on the laboratory measures), the behavioral contingencies in the classroom and home environments maintaining maladaptive behavior have remained unchanged. Indeed, there is evidence that the effectiveness of cognitive–behavioral self-control therapy is enhanced when classroom token economies are included that are designed to reinforce the use of the self-control strategies (Horn, Chatoor, & Conners, 1983).

6.4. Multimodal Treatment Approaches

Increasingly, clinicians and researchers alike have begun to advocate the use of multimodal treatment approaches in order to successfully intervene across the broad range of problems presented by ADHD children. The multimodal treatment approach that has received the most empirical study has been the combination of psychostimulants with traditional behavior therapy.

Perhaps the most methodologically sound study to evaluate the comparative and combined effectiveness of behavioral therapy and psychostimulants with ADHD children is that of Gittleman-Klein et al.

(1980). The children in this study were carefully selected from cutoff scores on the Conners Teacher Rating Scale (1969), parent reports, and classroom observations before they were considered eligible for the study. After entering the study, the children were randomly assigned to one of three eight-week interventions: behavior therapy plus placebo, behavior therapy plus methylphenidate, and methylphenidate alone. The behavior therapy component involved the training of both the child's parents and his or her teachers in the application of social learning theory principles to child behavior management. A number of pre- and posttreatment measures were taken, including teacher rating scales, teacher evaluations of academic performance, observational data from the classroom, global improvement ratings from a psychiatrist and the classroom teacher, and parent ratings.

Results indicated that the combination of methylphenidate and behavior therapy was the most effective treatment, followed by methylphenidate alone. Behavior therapy plus placebo was the least effective treatment. Hence, this study established the superiority of a combination treatment approach with ADHD children. Indeed, the combination of methylphenidate and behavior therapy was the only treatment approach that resulted in improvement such that the children treated were indistinguishable from a normal control group on virtually all measures at posttest. It is also important to note, however, that while behavior therapy alone was the least effective treatment, it did produce clinically significant treatment gains. Thus, behavior therapy alone may provide an effective alternative to stimulant therapy in cases in which the child's parents refuse stimulant therapy or the child develops intolerable side effects or fails to show a favorable response to medication.

Several other more recent investigations have also found the combination of stimulant therapy and behavior therapy to be superior to either treatment alone (Pelham, Schnedler, Bologna, & Contreras, 1980; Pelham et al., 1986). There are other studies, however, that have found no clear advantage of a combination approach over stimulant therapy or behavior therapy alone (Firestone, Crowe, Goodman, & McGrath, 1986; Woolraich, Drummond, Salomon, O'Brien, & Sivage, 1978).

A distinguishing feature between studies that did find a combination approach superior and studies that did not is the scope and intensity of the behavioral therapy. In studies that did find the combination approach superior, the behavior therapy component provided both school- *and* home-based behavior therapy. Studies that did not find additive effects of methylphenidate and behavior therapy invariably included only a clinic-based or a school-based behavior therapy intervention component. Furthermore, in some studies there was a limit on the amount of direct contact allowed for the behavior therapy component. In the more successful combined intervention approaches, such as in the Gittleman-Klein et al. (1980) study, there tended to be no limit set on the amount of direct contact between the behavioral therapist, parents, and teachers.

A second multimodal treatment approach that has been increasingly investigated in the empirical literature is the combination of psychostimulants and cognitive–behavioral self-control therapy. Several single-case studies demonstrated an additive impact of combining psychostimulants with cognitive–behavioral self-control therapy. For example, Horn, Chatoor, and Conners (1983) investigated the impact of adding two dosage levels of dexedrine or placebo to a self-control intervention with an ADHD child on a psychiatric inpatient unit. Teacher reports, direct classroom observations, and psychometric testing were used to assess treatment effectiveness. The combination of high dose of dexedrine with the self-control therapy resulted in the greatest improvement as noted in the teacher reports and the systematic classroom observational data. However, it was not until a direct reinforcement contingency was added to the intervention package that there was an increase in the academic performance of this ADHD child.

Similarly, Wells, Conners, Imber, and Delamater (1981) found that a combination of methylphenidate and a behavioral self-control program was more effective than dexedrine alone, methylphenidate alone, or the behavioral self-control program plus placebo in decreasing the gross motor and off-task behavior of an elementary-school-age ADHD boy on a psychiatric inpatient unit.

Unfortunately, recent group research has been unable to replicate these early findings. For example, Abikoff and Gittleman (1985) published the results of their large clinical research program examining the potential additive effectiveness of self-control therapy and methylphenidate. In this study, ADHD children were randomly assigned to one of three treatment conditions: (1) methylphenidate alone, (2) methylphenidate plus self-control therapy, or (3) self-control therapy plus placebo. At the end of the 16-week intervention, few significant group differences emerged for any of the teacher and parent measures of behavior, and there was no evidence that the methylphenidate plus self-control therapy was superior to methylphenidate alone. Similar findings have recently been reported by Brown, Borden, Wynne, Schlesser, and Clingerman (1986). Hence, while it may be that certain ADHD children benefit from a combination of psychostimulants and cognitive–behavioral self-control therapy, the data are not convincing that for the major-

ity of ADHD children this combination is more effective than psychostimulants alone.

A third multimodal treatment strategy is to combine psychostimulant therapy with behavioral parent training and instruction in self-
control strategies. Such an approach might first provide maximal benefit
by altering those contingencies in the child's home that have previously
helped maintain the child's maladaptive behavior patterns, while also
helping the child focus on the development of more adaptive behavioral
skills presented through instruction in self-control strategies. Secondly,
the potential fostering of external attributions by the stimulant therapy
and behavioral parent training might be countered by self-control training designed to facilitate the child's acquisition of new self-control and
problem-solving skills. Consequently, when behavior change does occur,
the child sees himself or herself as an active participant in the behavior
change process and not merely a passive recipient of externally controlled treatments. Third, the stimulant therapy might facilitate the acquisition of the problem-solving and self-control skills through the enhancement of the child's attentional skills. Finally, the stimulant therapy
might also facilitate the child's recognition of the connection between
response and consequences (see Barkley, 1981; Pelham, 1983), thus
increasing the probability that the parents will be successful in the
use of the behavioral techniques they have learned. Parental success in
using the behavioral management techniques should militate against
parent discouragement and failure to continue with the behavioral intervention.

Satterfield and his colleagues (Satterfield, Satterfield, & Cantwell,
1981; Satterfield, Cantwell, & Satterfield, 1979) have published the results of a prospective three-year mutimodality treatment of 100 ADHD
boys. Individual psychotherapy for the child and/or parents, group
therapy, family therapy, and remedial education for the child were provided as needed. All subjects received stimulants and families were given
as much treatment time as they required. Fifty percent of their ADHD
sample continued in therapy, while the remainder dropped out of treatment. At three-year follow-up, the children who continued in therapy
were more advanced educationally and were less antisocial than those
who dropped out of treatment. This study, however, is compromised by
the fact that the families most motivated to continue in treatment may be
nonrepresentative of the whole group and that their better outcomes
may be more a function of their level of motivation than the multimodal
treatment employed (Weiss & Hechtman, 1986). In addition, Satterfield
et al. failed to fully describe their treatment components (Sprague,

1983), making replication of the study difficult. Nevertheless, in contrast to the extant ADHD intervention literature, maintanence of treatment gains over a three-year period in the 50% of the sample that continued in therapy represents a significant advance.

Pelham, Schnedler, Bologna, and Contreras (1980) also studied the impact of a multimodal treatment including behavioral parent training, child therapy, and psychostimulants. Consistent with the results of the Satterfield studies, Pelham et al. also found that the combination treatment was effective in reducing the multiple symptoms of their sample of ADHD children. Unfortunately, they did not study the comparative impact of the various treatment components, and the psychostimulant therapy consisted of week-long medication probes only, rather than the prolonged use of the medication. Consequently, there are no well-controlled empirical studies regarding the possible combined and comparative effects of psychostimulants, behavioral parent training, and self-control therapy.

7. STUDY 1: SHORT-TERM COMPARATIVE AND COMBINED EFFECTIVENESS OF BEHAVIORAL PARENT TRAINING AND SELF-CONTROL THERAPY

It was from this theoretical background and review of prior research that our laboratory began to study the comparative and combined effectiveness of behavioral parent training, cognitive–behavioral self-control therapy, and psychostimulants with ADHD children. There had been no published studies up to that time that had investigated the potential additive effects of behavioral parent training and cognitive–behavioral self-control therapy with ADHD children. Consequently, in our initial study we decided to investigate whether combining behavioral parent training with self-control therapy resulted in greater treatment effectiveness than either treatment alone. Details of this study are published elsewhere (Horn, Ialongo, Popovich, & Peradotto, 1987), and only a summary is included here.

A randomized design with repeated measures and multiple outcome criteria was employed with 24 ADHD children between the ages of 7 and 11 years old, comparing parent training only, cognitive–behavioral self-control therapy only, and a combination of the two treatments. All subjects were blindly assessed at pretest, posttest, and one-month follow-up. Each intervention program met for eight weekly, 90-minute sessions at a university-based psychological clinic. The focus of the behavioral parent training groups was on teaching parents to apply social learning theory principles to the management of their child's behavior. The self-control groups instructed the children in the "Problem Solving Plan" adapted from Camp and Bash (1981) and outlined earlier in this chapter. No school intervention component, however, was included in order to allow the use of the classroom as a test for generalization of treatment effects from the clinic to the school setting. Pretest, posttest, and one-month follow-up assessments included parent and teacher behavior ratings, clinic psychometric testing, and direct observations of classroom behavior.

The results of this study are reported in detail by Horn et al. (1987) and will only be summarized here. First, whereas all three treatment groups did evidence significant behavioral improvements in the home as assessed by the Conners Parent Rating scale at posttest and follow-up, there was little evidence for differential improvement across treatment conditions. Second, the children in all three treatment groups evidenced significant improvements in self-concept, assessed by the Piers-Harris Self-Concept Scale (Piers & Harris, 1964), as well as significant increases in perceived self-control behavior, assessed by the Humphrey's Self-Control Scale (Humphrey, 1982). Once again, however, there was no evidence for differential improvements across treatment conditions on any of these child self-report measures. Third, no treatment produced significant treatment effects on any of the measures of classroom behavior or academic performance.

The failure of the combined treatment condition to produce generalization of treatment effects from the home to the classroom, though disappointing, was not totally unexpected. Kendall and Braswell (1982) in an evaluation of a school-based self-control instruction program failed to find significant generalization of treatment effects to the home. They point out the potentially critical nature of the context of training in achieving generalization across settings. Indeed, in this initial study the contingencies in the classroom maintaining maladaptive behavior were not changed. Consequently, although the children may have learned the self-control instructions, the classroom environment was not programmed to prompt or reinforce the child's use of these new behaviors.

This initial study was limited by some methodological shortcomings. First, the sample size was relatively small ($n = 8$ subjects in each treatment condition). Second, the follow-up component was relatively brief (i.e., one month), which may not have allowed for an adequate examination of the long-term maintenance of the treatment effectivenss of the respective treatment conditions. Third, in the interest of including a "pure" generalization setting, no school consultation component was incorporated in the design. Consequently, a second study was designed to attempt to both replicate and extend the results of Horn et al. (1987).

8. STUDY 2: LONG-TERM COMPARATIVE AND COMBINED EFFECTIVENESS OF BEHAVIORAL PARENT TRAINING AND SELF-CONTROL THERAPY

On the basis of the results of the first study, all treatment conditions in this second study (Horn, Ialongo, Greenberg. Packard, & Smith-Winberry, 1985) were expanded to include a teacher consultation component. In addition, both the parent and the child groups were lengthened to 12 weeks and a fourth treatment condition was included in which the parents received the parent training but the children were simultaneously seen in a behavioral play group rather than in a self-control instruction treatment group. The behavioral play group was similar to the self-control training child group in that it did include a token reinforcement system for appropriate behavior and training in relaxation skills, but it did not include instruction in specific self-control strategies. This latter control group was included to determine the independent contribution of the specific self-instructional strategies to the combined treatment condition.

8.1. Subjects

Subjects were 56 (43 males, 13 females; 49 Caucasian, 5 Blacks, 1 Hispanic, 1 Oriental) elementary-school-age children referred for treatment of chronic inattention and impulsivity problems. Referrals were received from pediatricians, psychiatrists, school and mental health personnel, community nurses, and the parents themselves. Each child then underwent an evaluation for the presence of an attention deficit hyperactivity disorder in accordance with DSM-III-R criteria. This evaluation included obtaining a developmental history from the parents and the administration of the Conners Parent and Teacher Questionnaires (Conners, 1969; Goyette, Conners, & Ulrich, 1978). In addition, the child was administered a visual Continuous Performance Test (CPT) (Rosvold, Mirksy, Sarason, Bransome, & Beck, 1956), the Matching Familiar Figures Test (MFF) (Kagan, Rosman, Day, Albert, & Phillips, 1964), and the Peabody Picture Vocabulary Test-Revised (PPVT-R)

(Dunn & Dunn, 1981). The developmental history interview and psychological testing were conducted by research assistants kept blind to subject status (i.e., ADHD vs. non-ADHD).

The study inclusion criteria were (1) the identified problem child is between the ages of 6 years, 6 months, and 11 years, 6 months; (2) a score on the Hyperactivity Index of the Conners Parent Questionnaire two or more standard deviations above published means (Goyette et al., 1978); (3) parental reports of an early onset and chronic history of ADHD symptoms; (4) a pattern of scores on the CPT and MFF suggestive of problems with inattention and impulsivity; and (5) the absence of gross physical impairments, intellectual deficits, or psychosis in either the child or parent(s).

In addition, a sample of 9 waiting list control subjects (7 males, 2 females; 9 Caucasian) was also included all of whom had met the inclusion criteria outlined above for a diagnosis of ADHD. However, rather than receiving treatment immediately following the initial assessment, these subjects were placed on a waiting list for six weeks. Following the six-week period, subjects were retested and treatment was provided immediately following this second testing. This wait-list control group was included in order to assess the effects of repeated testing and regression artifacts. The six-week waiting list control period was selected because it was considered both unethical and impractical to require these subjects to wait the entire length of the study (i.e., one year) before offering treatment.

Finally, a sample of 9 non-ADHD normal controls (4 males, 5 females; 8 Caucasian, 1 Black) was included. This normative comparison group was included to allow for the identification of clinically significant improvements—changes that return deviant subjects to within nondeviant limits—as well as statistically significant changes (Kendall & Norton-Ford, 1982).

Prior to posttesting, 11 families dropped out of the study, 2 from the Parent Training (PT) Only group, 2 from the Child Self-Control (SC) Only group, 3 from the PT + SC group, and 4 from the PT + Behavioral Play group. Analysis of the demographics of the subjects who dropped out of the study compared with the treatment subjects who remained in the study revealed no significant differences ($p > .05$) for age of child, family income, child IQ, pretest Parent Conners Hyperactivity Score, pretest Parent Conners Total Problems Score, pretest Teacher Conners Hyperactivity Score, and pretest Teacher Conners Total Problems Score. Final subject characteristics for each treatment group, the wait-list group, the dropout group, and the normal control group are presented in Table 1. Univariate ANOVAs for each of the demographic

TABLE 1. Demographic Characteristics of Each Treatment Group

Group	n	Mean age	Mean IQ	Pretest Hyperactivity Index Score		Family income (Thous.)
				Mother	Teacher	
Behavioral Parent	12	8.66	103.91	22.50	15.75	26.81
Training Only (PT)		(1.55)	(15.95)	(4.01)	(6.79)	(7.78)
Self-Control	12	9.00	100.41	22.25	17.50	33.30
Training Only (SC)		(1.41)	(13.44)	(4.02)	(7.30)	(18.63)
PT + SC	11	8.45	114.72	22.09	17.10	27.18
		(1.91)	(10.11)	(3.61)	(5.58)	(13.28)
PT + Behavioral	10	8.80	101.60	23.70	19.20	24.33
Play Group		(1.98)	(12.80)	(3.12)	(4.91)	(9.01)
Wait-list controls	9	8.88	110.77	19.0	20.11	35.11
		(1.53)	(16.28)	(6.63)	(2.84)	(14.54)
Treatment dropouts	11	9.09	103.63	22.37	19.72	22.60
		(1.44)	(12.15)	(4.57)	(7.45)	(9.74)
Normal controls	9	9.44	115.11	3.44	3.66	18.25
		(1.74)	(21.47)	(2.12)	(1.73)	(14.52)
Overall means:		8.89	106.79	19.33	16.34	26.97
		(1.61)	(15.26)	(7.42)	(7.49)	(13.40)

Note Standard deviations are presented in the parentheses below each mean. All differences between means are nonsignificant ($p > .05$), except for analysis of Conners pretest Hyperactivity Index scores where the mean scores of the normal controls are significantly lower than the mean scores of any other group.

and pretest outcome variables indicated that all differences between means were nonsignificant, except that the Conners Hyperactivity Index scores for the normal controls were significantly lower than the Conners Hyperactivity Index scores for the ADHD subjects. In addition, chi-square analyses indicated no significant differences in group composition for sex, race, and marital status of the parents.

8.2. Independent Variable

The 56 subjects who had been diagnosed as ADHD by the inclusion criteria were randomly assigned to one of the following four treatment conditions: (1) behavioral parent training alone, (2) self-control therapy alone, (3) behavioral parent training plus self-control therapy, and (4) behavioral parent training plus a behavioral play group. Two sets of groups were conducted for each treatment condition with seven families included in each treatment group—for a total of 14 families assigned to each treatment condition.

Each intervention group met for 12 weekly, 90-minute sessions. The parent group sessions were co-led by two advanced-level graduate students in an APA-approved clinical psychology training program. The self-control therapy groups were co-led by two graduate students also in an APA-approved clinical psychology training program. The behavioral play group, however, was co-led by two advanced undergraduate students. While it is recognized that choosing to use undergraduates as the group leaders for the play group introduces differences in level of training of the therapist across child group conditions, it was felt that it would be easier to keep the undergraduate group leaders from incorporating "implicit" self-control instruction into the behavioral play group than it would be if graduate students were used as group leaders.

Neither the parents nor the children were informed of this difference in group leader status, and as a check on the effectiveness of the group leaders, a posttest consumer satisfaction questionnaire (Forehand & McMahon, 1981) was administered to determine how well liked and "professional" each of the group leaders was perceived to be. Subsequent analysis revealed no significant differences between therapists on this questionnaire. In addition, extensive training in each of the clinical procedures was provided prior to the start of the treatment groups by the senior author, as well as weekly supervision throughout the intervention phase of the study. The weekly supervision and use of a structured treatment manual helped to ensure that treatment implementation was equivalent across treatment groups.

8.3. Dependent Variables

All dependent measures were administered at three points in time: pretest, posttest, and eight-month follow-up. All dependent measures were administered by either clinical psychology graduate students or advanced undergraduates. The child assessors received approximately 20 hours of training and were periodically monitored throughout the study from behind a one-way mirror in order to ensure continued proficiency with the assessment instruments. All examiners were kept blind as to subject status (i.e., ADHD vs. normal), treatment condition, and treatment period (i.e., pre-, post-, or follow-up).

The home behavior of each child was assessed by the Conners Parent Rating Scale (Conners, 1969; Goyette et al., 1978) and the Achenbach Child Behavior Profile (Achenbach, 1978; 1979). Each child's school behavior was assessed by the Conners Teacher Rating Scale (Conners, 1969; Goyette et al., 1978) and the Kendall-Wilcox Teacher's Self-Control Rating Scale (Kendall & Wilcox, 1979). In addition, each child's academic performance was assessed by performance on the Wide Range Achievement Test-Revised (WRAT-R) (Jastak & Wilkinson, 1984). An index of each child's attentional skills and impulse control was again obtained by administering a visual CPT and the MFF. The PPVT-R was once again administered as a measure of the child's level of general cognitive development and was used primarily to screen out children with gross intellectual deficits.

Several children's self-report measures were also administered. The Nowicki-Strickland Locus of Control Scale for Children (1973) was given to assess each child's attributions of causality. To assess the child's view of his or her own behavior, Humphrey's Children's Self-Control Scale (1982) was administered. The Piers-Harris Self-Concept Scale (Piers & Harris, 1964) was administered to assess each child's self-esteem.

8.4. Results

In order to determine whether the randomization procedure was successful in minimizing pretest group differences, one-way univariate ANOVAs were initially computed for all dependent variables using the four treatment groups and the wait-list control group as the independent variable. None of the 22 one-way ANOVAs were statistically significant, indicating that there were no pretest differences between the ADHD subject groups. Following this analysis, one-way repeated measures univariate ANOVAs were computed for each of the dependent variables in order to determine whether there were any differences over time in either the wait-list control or normal control groups. There were no significant differences over time for either the normal controls or the wait-list controls. Hence, the scores of the normal controls remained remarkably stable over the one-year period encompassed by this study, and the scores of the untreated ADHD subjects evidenced no changes from pretest to posttest.

The data were then analyzed for pretest to posttest and pretest to follow-up differences for the four treatment groups. At posttest, while all four treatment groups did evidence gains on both the parent and teacher report measures, there was little difference in outcome between any of the four treatment conditions—essentially replicating the results of the first study. However, significant differences in outcome as a function of treatment group did emerge at eight-month follow-up. The data consistently showed that *both* the parent training plus the cognitive–behavioral self-control therapy and the parent training plus the behavioral play group treatments were significantly superior to the parent training alone and the self-control training alone in reducing the severity of the parent behavioral ratings, and that there were no significant differences on any of the outcome measures between either of the two combination treatments. Summaries of these findings comparing the combination treatments with parent training alone and self-control training alone at posttest and follow-up are shown in Tables 2 and 3.

Since mean group differences in small samples may or may not accurately reflect meaningful differences at the individual level, an individual case analysis of changes on the Conners Parent Rating Scale was also performed. For this analysis a case was defined as a success if the subject's score on the Conners Parent Rating Scale improved by at least five points *and* was no longer above the cutoff for a score indicative of an attention deficit hyperactivity disorder. These two criteria were chosen to ensure that only subjects exhibiting a clinically meaningful magnitude of change (five points on the Conners Hyperactivity Index is roughly equivalent to one standard deviation unit on this scale) *and* who were no

TABLE 2. Contrasts Comparing Parent Training + Self-Control Training (PT + SC) with Parent Training Alone (PT) and Self-Control Training Alone (SC) at Posttest and Follow-up

Parent report measure	Posttest	Follow-up
Mother Conners Total Problems Score	ns	$t = -2.62$, $df = 28.2$ $p < .01$
Mother Conners Hyperactivity Index	ns	$t = -2.13$, $df = 29.2$ $p < .05$
Mother Conners Conduct Problems Score	ns	$t = -1.82$, $df = 24.9$ $p = .08$
Mother CBCL Total Problems Score	ns	$t = -2.36$, $df = 0.28$ $p < .05$
Mother CBCL Internalizing Problems Score	ns	$t = -2.03$, $df = 22.8$ $p < .05$
Mother CBCL Externalizing Problems Score	ns	$t = -2.19$, $df = 21.2$ $p < .05$
Mother CBCL Hyperactivity Subscale Score	ns	$t = -2.31$, $df = 27.9$ $p < .05$
Overall Satisfaction with Treatment	$t = 3.77$, $df = 40$ $p < .01$	$t = 2.10$, $df = 37.0$ $p < .05$
Satisfaction with Therapists	ns	ns
Teacher Conners Hyperactivity Index	ns	ns
Teacher Conners Conduct Problems	ns	ns
Teacher Kendall Self-Control Scale	ns	ns
Nowicki-Strickland Locus of Control	ns	ns

Note. ns = nonsignificant. In all instances, significant differences indicate better functioning in the PT + SC therapy group.

TABLE 3. Contrasts Comparing Parent Training + Behavioral Play Group (PT + PLAY) with Parent Training Alone (PT) and Self-Control Training Alone (SC) at Posttest and Follow-up

Parent report measure	Posttest	Follow-up
Mother Conners Total Problems Score	ns	$t = -2.30$, $df = 47$, $p < .05$
Mother Conners Hyperactivity Index	$t = -1.51$, $df = 57$, $p = .09$	$t = -2.44$, $df = 47$, $p < .05$
Mother Conners Conduct Problems Score	ns	ns
Mother CBCL Total Problems Score	ns	$t = -2.08$, $df = 47$, $p < .05$
Mother CBCL Internalizing Problems Score	ns	$t = -2.53$, $df = 47$, $p < .05$
Mother CBCL Externalizing Problems Score	ns	ns
Mother CBCL Hyperactivity Subscale Score	ns	$t = -1.66$, $df = 25$, $p = .11$
Overall Satisfaction with Treatment	$t = 4.10$, $df = 40$, $p < .01$	$t = 3.53$, $df = 37$, $p < .01$
Satisfaction with Therapists	ns	ns
Teacher Conners Hyperactivity Index	$t = 2.98$, $df = 52$, $p < .01$	ns
Teacher Conners Conduct Problems	ns	ns
Teacher Kendall Self-Control Scale	ns	ns
Nowicki-Strickland Locus of Control	ns	ns

Note. ns = nonsignificant. In all instances, significant differences indicate better functioning in the PT + PLAY therapy group.

longer above the cutoff for a diagnosis of an attention deficit hyperactivity disorder were considered as a clinical success. All other cases were considered to be clinical failures. This case analysis was performed on the Conners Parent Rating Scale at posttest and again at follow-up.

As depicted in Table 4, at posttest there is no statistically significant difference in case improvement rates between groups. At follow-up, however, differential success rates did attain statistical significance (chi-square = 7.48, $df = 3$, $p < .05$). Visual inspection of this table indicates that the two combination treatments had nearly identical success rates at follow-up (73% and 78%, respectively). In contrast, only 27% of the children receiving self-control therapy alone and 42% of the children receiving parent training alone were classified as successes at follow-up. This finding mirrors the findings in Tables 2 and 3 indicating greater improvement in parent ratings at follow-up for the children receiving either PT + SC or PT + Behavioral Play Group compared with either PT alone or SC alone.

TABLE 4. Analysis of Parent and Teacher Conners Hyperactivity Index Scores

Treatment group	n	Mean Parent Conners Hyperactivity Scores			Mean Teacher Conners Hyperactivity Scores		
		Pre	Post	Follow-up	Pre	Post	Follow-up
SC Only	12	22.3	18.2	16.0	17.5	13.6	19.6
PT Only	12	22.5	17.6	15.3	15.8	12.1	13.2
PT + SC	11	22.1	16.0	12.2	17.1	14.7	16.2
PT + PLAY	10	23.0	14.4	11.2	19.2	19.2	16.1
Dropouts	11	22.2	—	—	17.8	—	—

Treatment group	Posttest		Follow-up	
	Success	Failure	Success	Failure
SC Only	3 (25.0%)	9 (75.0%)	3 (27.3%)	8 (72.7%)
PT Only	3 (25.0%)	9 (75.0%)	5 (41.7%)	7 (58.3%)
PT + SC	4 (36.4%)	7 (63.6%)	8 (72.7%)	3 (27.3%)
PT + PLAY	6 (60.0%)	4 (40.0%)	7 (77.8%)	2 (22.2%)
	chi square = 3.77		chi square = 7.48	
	$df = 3$, ns		$df = 3$, $p < .05$	

Note. ns = nonsignificant. Success at both posttest and follow-up was defined as (1) an improvement of at least five points on the Conners Parent and Teacher Hyperactivity Index and (2) a score that is no longer above the clinical cutoff for a diagnosis of ADHD.

While the results appeared to establish the superiority of the parent training combined with either self-control therapy or a behavioral play group compared with either PT alone or SC alone in terms of parent ratings of their children's behavior, further analyses were performed to establish whether either combination treatment "normalized" the behavior of these ADHD children. Unfortunately, in nearly every instance in which the treated ADHD subjects were significantly different from the normal controls at pretest, the ADHD subjects remained significantly different from the normal controls at posttest and follow-up. Thus, it appears that while the combination treatments were more effective than either self-control therapy alone or parent training alone, no treatment resulted in improvement that made these ADHD children as a group indistinguishable from nonclinc-referred children.

These results of this second study, using a larger sample size than was the case in the initial study, both replicated and extended the findings of Horn et al. (1987). In both Horn et al. (1987) and this second study, all treatment conditions resulted in similar improvement rates as measured immediately upon treatment termination. In the Horn et al. (1987) study, however, there was no differential treatment impact as measured at one-month follow-up. This contrasts with the greater home improvement found at six- to eight-month follow-up in the second study for children receiving both behavioral parent training and a child therapy component. Thus, it appears that there are "sleeper effects" when combining parent training with a child therapy component that are not detectable immediately after treatment. Rather, it is only when behavioral status is measured at six to eight months following treatment that greater improvement is found with the combination treatment. This suggests a long-term spiral of positive interactions in which the children in the combined treatment conditions display better interpersonal interactional skills at the same time that the parents are prompting and reinforcing the display of greater self-control and interactional skills.

It is surprising, however, that both the self-control therapy and the behaviorally managed play group when combined with the behavioral parent training resulted in greater improvement rates at follow-up compared with either parent training alone or self-control therapy alone and that these two combination treatments had nearly identical improvement rates at follow-up. There appear to be at least two possible explanations for this finding. First, it is possible that the self-instructional steps are not the critical ingredient in cognitive–behavioral self-control therapy. Rather, it may be that the opportunity to practice socially appropriate interactional skills, encouraged by the use of reinforcement contingencies for appropriate behavior in the child therapy groups, is the critical treatment ingredient.

A second possible explanation for the fact that both combined treatments resulted in greater improvement rates than either parent training alone or self-control therapy alone and that the two combined treatments had nearly identical improvement rates at follow-up may relate to *parent* attribution variables. Although no explicit data were collected on this variable, anecdotal evidence suggests that the parents in the behavioral parent training only treatment condition were suspicious of the reason given for their having been assigned to the parent training only treatment condition. Although all families were informed of the random nature of assignment to treatment condition, the families in the behavioral parent training only groups believed that the therapists had looked at the pretest assessment information and had come to the conclusion that they were the "bad parents" in particular need of parent training. And the "proof" for this belief was that their children were not simultaneously involved in therapy as well. In the parent training only treatment groups, time needed to be spent convincing the parents that we did, indeed, believe their children had behavioral problems and that we did not view them as "bad parents."

The parents in the combined treatment conditions did not display any similar suspicions. Rather, they readily accepted our view that both the parent and child needed help and neither was to blame for the current difficulties; after all, their children were also in treatment in an adjoining room. If it is true that "resistant" parents are less likely to implement the ideas presented in the parent training groups, it may be that an important function served by the addition of a child therapy component to behavioral parent training is that it reduces the parents' resistance to the parenting instructional materials by providing conclusive evidence to the parent that the therapist does believe their child has difficulties and that the parent is not viewed as the only one in need of treatment.

The context of training, however, still appeared to have a considerable impact on the degree of generalization of treatment effects. While three-quarters of the ADHD children at follow-up were no longer evidencing behavioral symptoms of ADHD in the home, at school many of these same children were still scoring above the clinical cutoff on the Conners Hyperactivity Index for a diagnosis of ADHD. Given the often-presumed biological nature of the attentional difficulties in ADHD children (Conners & Wells, 1986), it is possible that the improvements that did occur in the home were more in terms of conduct improvements than attentional improvements. It may be that in order to address the attentional problems evidenced by ADHD children, one must add a medication component designed to enhance attentional skills, such as the use of methylphenidate or d-amphetamine.

Evidence for the above postulation comes from an earlier study reported by Horn, Chatoor, and Conners (1983). Using a single-case design methodology, a combination of dexedrine and self-control training was shown to be effective in decreasing the behavioral problems of an ADHD child in the classroom. However, only dexedrine was successful in decreasing inattention problems as measured by a visual Continuous Performance Test. In addition, a tentative finding was that a lower dose of dexedrine was maximally effective in reducing errors on the visual Continuous Performance Test, while a higher dose produced maximal benefit in the behavioral sphere.

Such differential dose effects are consistent with the dual-dose response curves for psychostimulant medication reported by Sprague and Sleator (1975–1976). Consequently, a third study (Horn et al., 1986) was planned to examine the impact of adding psychostimulant medication to a clinic-based intervention program including behavioral parent training and cognitive-behavioral self-control training, particularly as it relates to generalization of treatment effects to the classroom. The possibility of differential dose effects was also examined by including a high and low dose of psychostimulant medication.

9. STUDY 3: COMPARATIVE AND COMBINED EFFECTIVENESS OF PSYCHOSTIMULANTS, BEHAVIORAL PARENT TRAINING, AND SELF-CONTROL THERAPY

Our first two studies had thus far determined that the combination of parent training and child therapy was superior to either treatment alone. Consequently, in this third study we decided to examine the possible additive effects of psychostimulant medication with the combination of parent training and self-control therapy. The self-control therapy was chosen rather than the behavioral play group because of the greater face validity of the self-control therapy to the parents of the ADHD children. However, the agenda of the cognitive–behavioral self-control groups were altered to allow the child participants greater opportunity to interact with one another with a concomitant reduction in the amount of time spent in didactic presentations.

For this third study, a randomized, controlled trial design with repeated outcome measures was employed comparing placebo alone, low dose (0.4 mg/kg) of methylphenidate alone, high dose (0.8 mg/kg) of methylphenidate alone, placebo plus parent and child therapy, low dose of methylphenidate plus parent and child therapy, and high dose of methylphenidate plus parent and child therapy. Different levels of methylphenidate were employed on the basis of previous research indicating dual-dose response curves for behavioral and cognitive improvement (Sprague & Sleator, 1977). Preliminary analyses of pretest to posttest changes are available and will be presented in some detail here. We are currently in the process of collecting eight-month follow-up data on this sample of ADHD children.

9.1. Subjects

A total of 119 children between the ages of 7 and 11 years were evaluated for the presence of ADHD. This third study was housed in a university-based medical facility that serves a socioeconomically and geographically diverse population of children, families, and adults. Referral sources included the families themselves, pediatricians, psychiatrists, teachers, mental health professionals, and school nurses. The diagnosis of ADHD was made in accord with DSM-III-R criteria and was based upon (1) a psychoeducational assessment of the child, including laboratory measures of inattention and impulsivity, (2) a structured interview with the parents, and (3) teacher and/or parent ratings of the child on the Abbreviated Teacher and Parent Conners Rating Scales that were two or more standard deviations above published norms. Data obtained from the parent interview, psychological assessment, and the teacher and parent ratings were reviewed independently by the principal investigators—a licensed clinical psychologist and a board-certified pediatrician—to determine whether the data supported a diagnosis of ADHD. Only those subjects diagnosed independently by both investigators as ADHD were included in the study.

Twelve of these 119 children were determined ineligible and referred for other services, and 11 families elected not to continue as participants in the research program following the initial assessment. The remaining 96 children participated as the research subjects in the study. In addition, a sample of 31 non-ADHD normal controls matched for age, IQ, sex, SES, and race were recruited. These children and their families completed the same assessment battery administered to the ADHD subjects both at pretest and at posttest.

9.2. Method

Sixteen families with children diagnosed as ADHD were then randomly assigned to each of the following six treatment groups: (1) high dose (0.8 mg/kg) of methylphenidate alone, (2) low dose (0.4 mg/kg) of methylphenidate alone, (3) medication placebo alone, (4) high dose of methylphenidate plus behavioral parent training and self-control instruction, (5) low dose of methylphenidate plus behavioral parent training and self-control instruction, and (6) medication placebo plus parent training and self-control instruction.

All medication was dispensed in a double-blind fashion. The children were monitored for side effects of the medication by board-certified pediatricians. Children who experienced intolerable side effects of the medication had their dose reduced by one-half. This procedure allowed both the family and the medical staff to continue to be blind to actual medication dose. Four of the thirty-two (12.5%) children randomly assigned to the high dose of methylphenidate and one of thirty-two (3%) children randomly assigned to the low-dose condition experienced intolerable side effects and had their respective dosage levels reduced in the fashion described above. The side effects experienced by the children requiring a reduction in their medicine involved frequent stomach upset and increased irritability.

Each intervention group receiving the behavioral parent training and self-control instruction met for 12 weekly, 90-minute sessions. The parent group sessions were co-led by two advanced-level graduate students in an APA-approved clinical psychology training program. The child group sessions were co-led by two graduate students and one advanced undergraduate helper. Extensive training in the clinical procedures was provided prior to the start of treatment by the senior author, as well as a weekly supervision session during the intervention. The behavioral parent training was modeled after the work of Patterson (1974) and Barkley (1981), whereas the work of Kendall and Braswell (1985) and Camp and Bash (1981) provided the basis for the self-control training.

Similar to the first two studies, a multimethod strategy for assessing treatment outcome was employed including measures of (1) the secondary features of ADHD (academic problems, low self-concept, poor peer relations, conduct problems), (2) the presence of co-occurring child psychopathology as reflected in parent and teacher report, and (3) family functioning. All dependent measures were administered once before treatment and once immediately after the 12-week treatment period. In addition, an eight-month follow-up is being conducted. Training and assessment procedures were the same as described in the second study. All examiners were again kept blind as to subject status (i.e., ADHD vs. normal), treatment condition (i.e., medication and therapy status), and treatment period (i.e., pre-, post-, or follow-up).

9.3. Results

Preliminary data analysis are available for (1) the parent Conners Hyperactivity Index, (2) the parent PIC-R, (3) the teacher Conners Hyperactivity Index, (4) the teacher Kendall Self-Control Scale, (5) the Piers-Harris Self-Concept Scale, (6) the Ford Social Desirability Scale for Children, (7) the Matching Familiar Figures Test, and (8) the visual Continuous Performance Test. The remainder of the data are currently being analyzed. To be included in the data analysis, families must have attended all of the periodic pediatrician visits for medication monitoring, and families receiving parent training and self-control instruction must have attended 75% of the therapy sessions. Separate $2 \times 3 \times 2$ analyses of variance (presence or absence of parent and child therapy groups $\times$ methylphenidate dose level $\times$ time) were performed on the parent and teacher outcome variables listed above. The results of these analyses are shown in Table 5.

Unfortunately, 37.5% ($n = 6$) of the placebo only families dropped out of the study prior to posttesting. In every case, the families reported

TABLE 5. Period and Period by Group Interaction Effects for Parent, Teacher, and Child Measures

Measure	Period effects			Period by group interaction effects		
	F	df	p	F	df	p
Mom's Conners Hyperactivity Index	46.25	1,79	<.01		ns	
Mom's PIC Factor I (Undisciplined)	46.38	1,79	<.01		ns	
Mom's PIC Factor II (Social Incompetence)	46.25	1,79	<.01		ns	
Mom's PIC Factor IV (Cognitive Dev.)	13.38	1,79	<.01		ns	
Mom's PIC Factor XIV (Family Relations)	5.33	1,79	<.05		ns	
Teacher Conners Hyperactivity Index	73.81	1,79	<.01	5.05	5,79	<.01
Teacher Kendall Self-Control Scale	66.68	1,79	<.01	3.32	5,79	<.05
Continuous Performance Test total errors	8.30	1,79	<.01		ns	
Matching Familiar Figures Test errors		ns			ns	
Piers-Harris Self-Concept Scale	23.48	1,79	<.01	3.31	5,79	<.05

Note. ns = nonsignificant. Sample size for each treatment condition is as follows: (1) placebo alone ($n = 10$), (2) low dose of methylphenidate alone ($n = 16$), (3) high dose of methylphenidate alone ($n = 16$), (4) placebo plus therapy ($n = 15$), (5) low dose of methylphenidate plus therapy ($n = 13$), and (6) high dose plus therapy ($n = 15$). All main effects for group were nonsignificant indicating that there were no significant differences on any of the dependent variables at pretest.

that the reason they were terminating their participation in the program was that there was no evidence of improvement in their child and that they were seeking alternative services. This 37.5% attrition rate prior to posttesting is significantly higher than the attrition rate of no more than 12.5% ($n = 2$) in any other treatment condition. It is, therefore, unclear how comparable the placebo-only families are to the families in the other treatment conditions at posttest. Indeed, given the fact that nearly 40% of ADHD children administered a placebo show significant clinical improvement (see Barkley, 1981), it is likely that the families remaining in the placebo-only condition at posttest represent a biased sample of families highly influenced by expectancy effects. Although families in the other treatment conditions are also likely to have been influenced to some extent by expectancy effects, it is not as likely that these subsamples are biased toward overinclusion of families sensitive to expectancy effects since very little attrition was found in any of the other treatment conditions. The high differential attrition rate found for the placebo-only treatment condition renders the scores for these families at posttest highly suspect. Consequently, when interpreting the data in Table 5, we will not include further discussion of the scores from the placebo-only families.

In examining the parent reports of home behavior, all treatment conditions resulted in improvement over time, with no treatment condition being significantly more effective compared with any other treatment condition. Examination of the teacher report data (see Figures 1 and 2), however, indicates that high dose of methylphenidate alone is superior to low dose of methylphenidate alone in reducing chronic inattention and impulsivity problems in the classroom. Among those families also receiving parent and child therapy, methlyphenidate regardless of dose appears superior to placebo, with no significant difference between low- and high-dose conditions.

It appears that when intervening with methylphenidate alone, 0.8 mg/kg of methylphenidate is superior to 0.4 mg/kg in reducing chronic inattention and impulse control problems in the school. However, when intervening with a combination of methylphenidate, parent training, and child self-control therapy, a comparable reduction in inattention and impulse control problems is achieved by either 0.8 mg/kg or 0.4 mg/kg of methylphenidate. Hence, the major effect of combining methylphenidate with parent and child therapy may be that similar effects

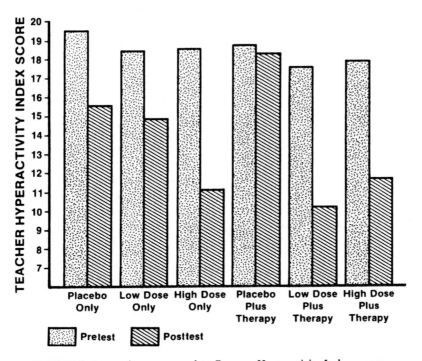

FIGURE 1. Pre- and posttest teacher Conners Hyperactivity Index scores.

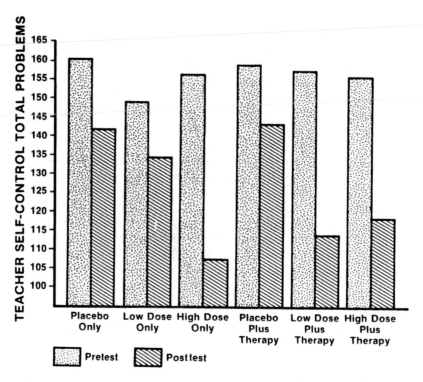

FIGURE 2. Pre- and posttest teacher Kendall Self-Control Rating Scale.

can be achieved with a *lower* dose of methylphenidate. This finding may be particularly important for children who experience intolerable side effects at higher dose levels of methylphenidate. Indeed, in the present study 4 of 32 (12.5%) children at the high-dose level experienced intolerable side effects. It is also noteworthy that when placebo was combined with parent and child therapy, a reduction in hyperactive symptomotology was achieved in the parent, but not the teacher, report data comparable to either medication condition. It seems that methylphenidate may be a necessary part of a clinic-based treatment when the focus is on altering hyperactive symptoms in the classroom.

10. CONCLUSIONS

The available literature on the treatment of attention deficit hyperactivity disorder suggests that single-modality treatments are generally not effective in ameliorating the myriad of difficulties experienced by many ADHD children. Although the literature is more sparse in regard to the empirical evaluation of multimodal treatments, several conclusions based upon our work and the work of others appears warranted.

First, there does appear to be a synergistic impact of combining psychostimulants with a treatment package of behavioral parent training and cognitive-behavioral self-control therapy. Our work suggests that such a combination allows for the use of lower doses of psychostimulants compared with using psychostimulants alone. This finding seems particularly important in view of the fact that many children experience intolerable side effects on doses as high as 0.8 mg/kg of methylphenidate and must consequently have the dose of the stimulant reduced and perhaps the effectiveness of the medication as well. The failure of some researchers to find synergistic effects of psychostimulants and behavioral treatments may be due to their exclusion of a concomitant child therapy component. Indeed, all three reports (i.e., Horn et al., 1986; Pelham et al., 1980; Satterfield et al., 1981) of the simultaneous use of psychostimulants, behavioral parent training, and child therapy in the treatment of ADHD have found not only statistically significant but also clinically significant improvements in the behavioral symptomatology of ADHD children.

Second, there also appears to be some synergistic effect of combining behavioral parent training with a child therapy component. However, this additive impact does not appear to be evident at the end of treatment. Rather, there is a "sleeper effect" of combining these two treatments such that it is not until six to eight months after treatment that one is able to detect a significant and clinically meaningful synergistic effect. It is also important to note that the combination of parent training and child therapy was able to reduce the severity of the ADHD symptomotology in the home to the point where three-quarters of the children were no longer diagnosable as ADHD on the basis of parent reports. Teacher reports of inattention at school, however, remained at high levels. Hence, it may be that with "situational" ADHD, where the primary difficulties are in the home but not at school, these children can be well managed through the use of nonmedical interventions.

Third, the question being addressed should *not* be which treatment is the best for ADHD children, but rather which treatments may be necessary to intervene with a particular symptom picture in a particular child. Our research, as well as the work of others, suggests that the chronic inattention problems of ADHD children may best be ameliorated by the use of psychostimulants. In contrast, the impulse control problems of ADHD children, often resulting in tremendous social conflict and improprieties, can be well managed by either environmental/behavioral interventions, psychostimulants, or a combination of the two treatments. Remediation of academic underachievement, on the other hand, may require a combination of psychostimulants, behavioral therapy, and educational interventions.

Hence, the goal of an assessment for ADHD should be to clearly delineate the needs of a particular child and then to choose the best intervention strategies for dealing with the problems of a given child. For example, if a child presents primarily with attentional problems in school but whose parents or teachers do not report a history of noncompliant or acting out behavior, psychostimulant therapy alone may be a reasonable starting point for intervention. Alternatively, if a child also presents with impulse control problems resulting in chronic social conflict with parents and teachers, a combination of parent training, child therapy, and psychostimulants may be useful. If a child presents primarily with inattention and impulsivity in the home with little or no difficulty at school, behavior therapy may be the treatment of choice without the need for psychostimulants. Finally, should a child also evidence underachievement problems, special education assistance would be mandatory.

Fourth, it appears from the evaluations of multimodal treatments of ADHD children that cognitive–behavioral self-control therapy is the least efficacious of the three most widely used treatments for ADHD problems in childhood. By itself, cognitive-behavioral self-control therapy has not proven to be particularly helpful in the management of ADHD (see review by Abikoff, 1985). In addition, research examining the combination of psychostimulants and cognitive–behavioral self-control therapy indicates that little improvement, if any, is obtained through this combination of treatments compared with the use of psychostimulants alone (Abikoff & Gittleman, 1985). In contrast, we found evidence that cognitive-behavioral self-control therapy does result in greater effectiveness when combined with parent training compared with either treatment alone. However, the additive impact of combining self-control therapy and parent training may be less a function of the specific self-instruction steps and more a function of either nonspecific effects of the child therapy group or the lessening of parents' resistance to parent training.

There remain, however, many unanswered questions regarding the use of multimodal treatment approaches. First, while it seems reasonable to speculate on which children may require which components of a multimodal treatment package, there is as yet no empirically validated method for predicting *a priori* a particular child's response to psychostimulants, behavioral parent training, and self-control therapy, either singly or in various combinations. Research is direly needed to determine which children and families do, in fact, require the entire multimodal treatment and which children and families may only need various components of the treatment package. This is an important issue since it is very costly, both in financial and personnel terms, to provide all three treatments. It would be extremely useful to be able to predict which children can be managed with a relatively low-cost intervention, such as the psychostimulants, and which children require the more expensive combination treatments.

A second issue requiring further investigation relates to timing when introducing psychostimulants in combination with other therapies. As noted earlier, our research laboratory has found preliminary evidence suggesting that dose level of psychostimulants predicted level of parental resistance in behavioral parent training—with higher dosages of methylphenidate predictive of higher levels of resistance (Packard, 1986). It may be that parents will be more likely to attempt to implement the ideas presented in behavioral therapy if the stimulant therapy is provided *after* the advent of the parent training. That is, initial and often times dramatic improvement with psychostimulants may cause the parent and/or teacher to believe they need not do anything differently in the management of the child because the child's problems are all "biological." Indeed, prior research finding little additive impact of psychostimulants and behavior therapy may have inadvertently made their parents more "resistant" to the potential for additive effects if the medication was provided at the onset of the behavior therapy.

Another issue generally neglected in the empirical literature is the acceptability of the use of psychostimulants with ADHD children. Kazdin (1980, 1981) has published a series of studies on the acceptability of various behavioral techniques with clinic-referred children. However, there is a dearth of information on what factors lead some parents to reject out-of-hand the use of psychostimulants for their ADHD children. This issue is of critical importance since no treatment is effective that is not adhered to by the consumer. Research is also needed to determine whether or not the manner of presenting the use of psychostimulants for ADHD problems predicts parental acceptance or rejection of the use of psychostimulants with their child. The acceptability of the use of psychostimulants to the ADHD children themselves would also seem to be an important topic for future investigations.

In summary, it appears that multimodal treatment packages incorporating psychostimulants, parent training, teacher consultation, and child therapy show great promise in ameliorating many of the difficulties of ADHD children. While psychostimulants may be the "core" of any such program, many ADHD children seem to benefit from combining psychostimulants with other treatments. Nonetheless, there is little evidence that any multimodal treatment results in a "cure" for ADHD. Rather, it appears that such multimodal treatments can be an effective "coping" package resulting in clinically significant improvements in the cognitive and behavioral problems presented by ADHD children.

11. REFERENCES

Abikoff, H. (1985). Efficacy of cognitive training interventions in hyperactive children: A critical review. [Special issue] Attention deficit disorder: Issues in assessment and intervention, *Clinical Psychology Review. 5*, 479–512.

Abikoff, H., & Gittleman, R. (1985). Hyperactive children treated with stimulants: Is cognitive training a useful adjunct? *Archives of General Psychiatry, 42*, 953–961.

Achenbach, T. M. (1978). The Child Behavior Profile: I. Boys aged 6–11. *Journal of Consulting and Clinical Psychology, 46*, 478–488.

Achenbach, T. M. (1979). The Child Behavior Profile: An empirically based system for assessing children's behavioral problems and competence. *International Journal of Mental Health, 7*, 24–42.

American Psychiatric Association. (1987). *Diagnostic and statistical manual of mental disorders* (3rd ed., revised). Washington, DC: Author.

August, G. J., Stewart, M. A., & Holmes, C. S. (1983). A four-year follow-up of hyperactive boys with and without conduct disorders. *British Journal of Psychiatry, 143*, 192–198.

Ayllon, T., Layman, D., & Kandel, H. J. (1975). A behavioral–educational alternative to drug control of hyperactive children. *Journal of Applied Behavior Analysis, 8*, 137–146.

Barkley, R. A. (1977). Review of stimulant drug research with hyperactive children. *Journal of Child Psychology, Psychiatry and Allied Disciplines, 18*, 1–31.

Barkley, R. A. (1981). *Hyperactive children: A handbook for diagnosis and treatment.* New York: Guilford Press.

Barkley, R. A., & Cunningham, C. E. (1978). Do stimulant drugs enhance the academic performance of hyperactive children? *Clinical Pediatrics, 17*, 85–92.

Bassuk, E., Schoonover, S., & Gelenberg, A. (1983). *The practitioner's guide to psychoactive drugs* (2nd ed.). New York: Plenum.

Befera, M. S., & Barkley, R. A. (1985). Hyperactive and normal girls and boys: Mother–child interactions, parent psychiatric status, and child psychopathology. *Journal of Child Psychology and Psychiatry, 26*, 439–452.

Berkowitz, B. P., & Graziano, A. M. (1972). Training parents as behavior therapists: A review. *Behavior Research and Therapy, 10*, 297–317.

Blouin, A. G. A., Bornstein, R. A., & Trites, R. L. (1978). Teenage alcohol use among hyperactive children: A five-year follow-up study. *Journal of Pediatric Psychology, 3*, 188–194.

Borland, B., & Hechman, H. K. (1976). Hyperactive boys and their brothers. *Archives of General Psychiatry, 33*, 669–675.

Brown, R. T., Borden, K. A., Wynne, M. E., Schlesser, R., & Clingerman, S. R. (1986). Methylphenidate and cognitive therapy with ADD children: A metholodological consideration. *Journal of Abnormal Child Psychology, 14*, 481–497.

Brown, R. T., & Sleator, E. K. (1979). Methylphenidate in hyperkinetic children: Differences in dose effects on impulsive behavior. *Pediatrics, 64*, 408–411.

Camp, B. W., & Bash, M. A. (1981). *Think aloud: Increasing social and cognitive skills—A problem-solving program for children.* Champaign, IL: Research Press.

Campbell, M., Green, W. H., & Deutsch, S. I. (1985). *Child and adolescent psychophar- macology: Vol. 2. Developmental clinical psychology and psychiatry.* Beverly Hills, CA: Sage.

Campbell, S. W., Douglas, V. I., & Morganstern, G. (1971). Cognitive styles of hyperactive children and the effect of methylphenidate. *Journal of Child Psychology and Psychiatry,* 18, 239–249.

Conners, C. K. (1969). A teacher rating scale for use in drug studies with children. *American Journal of Psychiatry, 126,* 884–888.

Conners, C. K., & Taylor, E. (1980). Pemoline, methylphenidate, and placebo in children with minimal brain dysfunction. *Archives of General Psychiatry, 37,* 922–930.

Conners, C. K., & Wells, K. C. (1986). *Hyperkinetic children: A neuropsychological approach.* Beverly Hills, CA: Sage.

Cowen, E. L., Pederson, A., Babigian, J., Izzo, L., & Trost, M. A. (1973). Long-term follow- up of early detected vulnerable children. *Journal of Consulting and Clinical Psychology, 41,* 438–446.

Davids, A. (1971). An objective instrument for assessing hyperkinesis in children. *Journal of Learning Disabilities, 4,* 35–37.

Deci, E. L., & Chandler, C. L. (1986). The importance of motivation for the future of the LD field. *Journal of Learning Disabilities, 19,* 577–640.

de Haas, P. A., & Young, R. D. (1984). Attention styles of hyperactive and normals girls. *Journal of Abnormal Child Psychology, 12,* 531–546.

Dollinger, S. J. (1979). Extrinsic rewards, reward-associated messages, and intrinsic moti- vation. *Cognitive Therapy and Research, 3,* 367–370.

Douglas, V. I. (1972). Stop, look and listen: The problem of sustained attention and impulse control in hyperactive and normal children. *Canadian Journal of Behavioral Science, 4,* 283–217.

Douglas, V. I. (1980). Treatment and training approaches to hyperactivity: Establishing internal and external control. In C. K. Whalen & B. Henker (Eds.), *Hyperactive chil- dren: The social ecology of identification and treatment.* New York: Academic Press.

Douglas, V. I., Parry, P., Marton, P., & Garson, C. (1976). Assessment of a cognitive training program for hyperactive children. *Journal of Abnormal Child Psychology, 4,* 389–410.

Douglas, V. I., & Peters, K. G. (1979). Toward a clearer definition of the attentional deficit disorder of hyperactive children. In G. A. Hale & M. Lewis (Eds.), *Attention and cognitive development.* New York: Plenum Press.

Dunn, L. M., & Dunn, L. M. (1981). *Peabody Picture Vocabulary Test-Revised.* Circle Pines, MN: American Guidance Service.

Egeland, B. (1974). Training impulsive children in the use of more efficient scanning techniques. *Child Development, 45,* 165–171.

Eme, R. F. (1979). Sex differences in childhood psychopathology: A review. *Psychological Bulletin, 86,* 574–593.

Firestone, P., Crowe, D., Goodman, J. T., & McGrath, P. (1986). Vicissitudes of follow-up studies: Differential effects of parent training and stimulant medication with hyperac- tives. *American Journal of Orthopsychiatry, 56,* 184–194.

Fisher, E. B., Winkler, R. C., Krasner, L., Kagel, J., Battalio, R. C., & Basmann, R. L. (1978). Economic perspectives in behavior therapy: Complex interdependence in token economies. *Behavior Therapy, 9,* 391–403.

Forehand, R. (1977). Child compliance to parental requests: Behavioral analysis and treat- ment. In M. Hersen, R. M. Eisler, & P. M. Miller (Eds.), *Progress in behavior modification* (Vol. 5). New York: Academic Press.

Forehand, R., & McMahon, R. J. (1981). *Helping the non-compliant child: A clinician's guide to parent training.* New York: Guilford Press.

Gittleman, R. (1983). Hyperkinetic syndrome: Treatment issues and principles. In M. Rutter (Ed.), *Developmental neuropsychiatry.* New York: Guilford Press.

Gittleman, R., Klein, D. F., & Feingold, I. (1983). Children with reading disorders: II. Effects of methylphenidate in combination with reading instruction. *Journal of Child Psychology and Psychiatry, 24,* 193–212.

Gittleman-Klein, R., Abikoff, H., Pollack, E., Klein, D. F., Katz, S., & Mattes, J. (1980). A controlled trial of behavior modification and methylphenidate in hyperactive children. In C. Whalen & B. Henker (Eds.), *Hyperactive children: The social ecology of identification and treatment.* New York: Academic Press.

Gittleman-Klein, R., Klein, D. F., Abikoff, H., Katz, S., Gloisten, A. C., & Kates, W. (1976). Relative efficacy of methylphenidate and behavior modification in hyperactive children: An interim report. *Journal of Abnormal Child Psychology, 4,* 361–379.

Goyette, C. H., Conners, C. K., & Ulrich, R. F. (1978). Normative data on Revised Conners Parent and Teacher Rating Scales. *Journal of Abnormal Child Psychology, 6,* 221–236.

Graziano, A. M. (1977). Parents as behavior therapists. In M. Hersen, R. M. Eisler, & P. M. Miller (Eds.), *Progress in behavior modification* (vol. 4, pp. 251–298). New York: Academic Press.

Graziano, A. M. (1983). Behavioral approaches to child and family systems. *Counseling Psychologist, 11,* 47–56.

Hechtman, L., Weiss, G., Perlman, T., & Amsel, R. (1984). Hyperactives as young adults: Initial predictors of adult outcome. *Journal of the American Academy of Child Psychiatry, 23,* 250–260.

Hinshaw, S. P., Henker, B., & Whalen, C. K. (1984a). Self-control in hyperactive boys in anger-inducing situations: Effects of cognitive-behavioral training and of methylphenidate. *Journal of Abnormal Child Psychology, 12,* 55–77.

Hinshaw, S. P., Henker, B., & Whalen, C. K. (1984b). Cognitive–behavioral and pharmacologic intervention for hyperactive boys: Comparative and combined effects. *Journal of Consulting and Clinical Psychology, 52,* 739–749.

Holborow, P. W., Berry, P., & Elkins, J. (1984). Prevalence of hyperkinesis: A comparison of three rating scales. *Journal of Learning Disabilities, 17,* 411–417.

Horn, W. F., Chatoor, I., & Conners, C. K. (1983). Additive effects of dexedrine and self-control training: A multiple assessment. *Behavior Modification, 7,* 383–402.

Horn, W. F., Ialongo, N., Greenberg, G., Packard, T., & Smith-Winberry, C. (1985). *Behavioral parent training and cognitive-behavioral self-control therapy with ADD children: A follow-up study.* Paper presented at the annual meeting of the Association for the Advancement of Behavior Therapy, Houston, TX.

Horn, W. F., Ialongo, I., Pascoe, J. M., Greenberg, G., Lopez, M., Wagner, A., Puttler, L., & Packard, T. (1986). *Additive effects of psychostimulants, parent training, and self-control therapy.* Paper presented at the 94th meeting of the American Psychological Association, Washington, DC.

Horn, W. F., Ialongo, N., Popovich, S., & Peradotto, D. (1987). Behavioral parent training and cognitive–behavioral self-control therapy with ADD-H children: Comparative and combined effects. *Journal of Clinical Child Psychology, 16,* 57–68.

Hoy, E., Weiss, G., Minde, K., & Cohen, N. (1978). The hyperactive child at adolescence: Cognitive, emotional, and social functioning. *Journal of Abnormal Child Psychology, 67,* 311–324.

Humphrey, L. L. (1982). Children's and teachers' perspectives on children's self-control:

The development of two rating scales. *Journal of Consulting and Clinical Psychology, 50,* 624–633.

Jastak, S., & Wilkinson, G. S. (1984). *The Wide Range Achievement Test-Revised.* Wilmington, DE: Jastak Associates.

Johnson, S. A., & Katz, R. C. (1973). Using parents as change agents for their children: A review. *Journal of Child Psychology and Psychiatry, 4,* 181–200.

Kagan, J., Rosman, B. L., Day, D., Albert, J., & Phillips, W. (1964). Information processing in the child: Significance of analytic and reflective attitude. *Psychological Monographs, 78*(1, Serial No. 578).

Kashani, J., Chapel, J. L., Ellis, J., & Shekim, W. D. (1979). Hyperactive girls. *Journal of Operational Psychiatry, 10,* 145–148.

Kazdin, A. E. (1980). Acceptability of time out from reinforcement procedures for disruptive child behaviors. *Behavior Therapy, 11,* 329–344.

Kazdin, A. E. (1981). Acceptability of child treatment techniques: The influence of treatment efficacy and adverse side effects. *Behavior Therapy, 12,* 493–506.

Kendall, P. C., & Braswell, L. (1982). Cognitive–behavioral self-control therapy for children: A components analysis. *Journal of Consulting and Clinical Psychology, 50,* 672–689.

Kendall, P. C., & Braswell, L. (1985). *Cognitive–behavioral therapy for impulsive children.* New York: Guilford Press.

Kendall, P. C., & Norton-Ford, J. D. (1982). Therapy outcome research methods. In P. C. Kendall & J. N. Butcher (Eds.), *Handbook of research methods in clinical psychology.* New York: Wiley.

Kendall, P. C., & Wilcox, L. E. (1979). Self-control in children: Development of a rating scale. *Journal of Consulting and Clinical Psychology, 47,* 1020–1029.

Klein, A. R., & Young, R. D. (1979). Hyperactive boys in their classroom: Assessment of teacher and peer perceptions, interactions, and classroom behaviors. *Journal of Abnormal Child Psychology, 7,* 425–442.

LaGreca, A. M., & Quay, H. C. (1984). Behavior disorders of children. In N. S. Endler & J. McV. Hunt (Eds.), *Personality and the behavior disorders.* New York: Wiley.

Lahey, B. B., Green, K. D., & Forehand, R. (1980). On the independence of ratings of hyperactivity, conduct problems, and attention deficits in children: A multiple regression analysis. *Journal of Consulting and Clinical Psychology, 48,* 566–574.

Laufer, M. W., & Denhoff, E. (1957). Hyperkinetic behavior syndrome in children. *Journal of Pediatrics, 50,* 463–474.

Linn, R. I., & Hodge, G. K. (1982). Locus of control in childhood hyperactivity. *Journal of Consulting and Clinical Psychology, 50,* 592–593.

Loney, J., Kramer, J., & Milich, R. (1981). The hyperkinetic child grows up: Predictors of symptoms, delinquency and achievement at follow-up. In K. D. Gadow & J. Loney (Eds.), *Psychosocial aspects of drug treatment for hyperactivity.* Boulder, CO: Westview Press.

Loney, J., Whaley-Klahn, M., Kosier, T., & Conboy, J. (1985). Hyperactive boys and their brothers at 21: Predictors of aggressive and antisocial outcomes. In S. Mednick & K. Van Dusen (Eds.), *Prospective studies in delinquent and criminal behavior.* Boston: Kluiver-Nijhoff.

Lopez, M. L. (1986). *Locus of control in hyperactive vs. normal children.* Unpublished master's thesis, Michigan State University, East Lansing.

Luria, A. (1961). *The role of speech in the regulation of normal and abnormal behaviors.* New York: Liveright.

Luria, A. (1969). Speech and formation of mental processes. In M. Cole & I. Maltzman (Eds.), *A handbook of contemporary Soviet psychology.* New York: Basic Books.

McMahon, R. C. (1984). Hyperactivity as a dysfunction of activity, arousal or attention: A study of research related to DSM-III's attention deficit disorder. *Journal of Clinical Psychology, 40,* 50–58.

Meichenbaum, D. (1977). *Cognitive-behavior modification: An integrative approach.* New York: Plenum Press.

Meichenbaum, D., & Goodman, J. (1971). Training impulsive children to talk to themselves: A means of developing self-control. *Journal of Abnormal Psychology, 77,* 115–126.

Mendelson, W., Johnson, N., & Stewart, M. A. (1971). Hyperactive children as teenagers: A follow-up study. *Journal of Nervous and Mental Disease, 153,* 237–279.

Miller, R. G., Palkes, H. S., & Stewart, M. A. (1973). Hyperactive children in suburban elementary schools. *Child Psychiatry and Human Development, 4,* 121–127.

Moreland, J. R., Schwebel, A. I., Beck, S., & Wells, R. T. (1982). Parents as therapists: A review of the behavior therapy parent training literature 1975 to 1981. *Behavior Modification, 6,* 250–276.

Nowicki, S., Jr., & Strickland, B. R. (1973). A locus of control scale for children. *Journal of Consulting and Clinical Psychology, 40,* 148–154.

O'Dell, S. (1974). Training parents in behavior modification: A review. *Psychological Bulletin, 81,* 418–433.

O'Malley, J., & Eisenberg, L. (1973). The hyperkinetic syndrome. *Seminars in Psychiatry, 5,* 95–103.

Packard, T. N. (1986). *The effects of psychosocial stress and parental adjustment on engagement in behavioral parent training.* Unpublished doctoral dissertation, Michigan State University, East Lansing.

Patterson, G. R. (1974). Interventions for boys with conduct problems: Multiple settings, treatments, and criteria. *Journal of Consulting and Clinical Psychology, 42,* 471–481.

Pelham, W. E. (1983). The effect of psychostimulants on academic performance in hyperactive and learning-disabled children. *Thalamus, 3,* 1–47.

Pelham, W. E., Schnedler, R. W., Bologna, N. C., & Contreras, J. A. (1980). Behavioral and stimulant treatment of hyperactive children: A therapy study with methylphenidate probes in a within-subjects design. *Journal of Applied Behavior Analysis, 13,* 221–236.

Pelham, W. E., Schnedler, R. W., Miller, J., Ronnei, M., Paluchowski, C., Budrow, M., Marks, D., Nilsson, D., & Bender, M. E. (1986). The combination of behavior therapy and psychostimulant medication in the treatment of hyperactive children: A therapy outcome study. In L. Bloomingdale (Ed.), *Attention deficit disorders.* New York: Spectrum Books.

Phillips, J. S., & Ray, R. S. (1980). Behavioral approaches to childhood disorders: Review and critique. *Behavior Modification, 4,* 3–34.

Piers, E., & Harris, D. (1964). Age and other correlates of self-concept in children. *Journal of Educational Psychology, 55,* 91–95.

Porrino, L. J., Rapoport, J. L., Behar, D., Sceery, W., Ismond, D. R., & Bunney, W. E., Jr. (1983). A naturalistic assessment of the motor activity of hyperactive boys. *Archives of General Psychiatry, 40,* 681–687.

Preis, K., & Huessey, H. R. (1979). Hyperactive children at risk. In M. J. Cohen (Ed.), *Drugs and the special child.* New York: Gardner Press.

Prinz, R. J., Tarnowski, K. J., & Nay, S. M. (1984). Assessment of sustained attention and distraction in children using a classroom analogue task. *Journal of Clinical Child Psychology, 13,* 250–256.

Rapport, M. D., DuPaul, G. J., Stoner, G., & Jones, J. T. (1986). Comparing classroom and clinic measures of attention deficit disorder: Differential, idiosyncratic, and dose-response effects of methylphenidate. *Journal of Consulting and Clinical Psychology, 54,* 334–341.

Rapport, M. D., Murphy, A., & Bailey, J. S. (1980). The effects of a response cost treatment tactic on hyperactive children. *Journal of School Psychology, 18,* 98–111.

Rapport, M. D., Murphy, A., & Bailey, J. S. (1982). Ritalin vs. response cost in the control of hyperactive children: A within subject comparison. *Journal of Applied Behavior Analysis, 15,* 205–216.

Rapport, M. D., Stoner, G., DuPaul, G. J., Birmingham, B. K., & Tucker, S. (1985). Methylphenidate in hyperactive children: Differential effects of dose on academic learning and social behavior. *Journal of Abnormal Child Psychology, 13,* 227–244.

Robins, L. (1966). *Deviant children grown up.* Baltimore: Williams & Wilkins.

Roff, M. (1961). Childhood social interactions and young adult bad outcomes. *Journal of Abnormal and Social Psychology, 63,* 333–337.

Ross, D., & Ross, S. (1982). *Hyperactivity: Current issues, research and theory.* New York: Wiley.

Ross, M. (1975). Salience of reward and intrinsic motivation. *Journal of Personality and Social Psychology, 32,* 245–254.

Rosvold, H. D., Mirksy, A. S. F., Sarason, I., Bransome, E. L., & Beck, L. H. (1956). A continuous performance test of brain damage. *Journal of Consulting Psychology, 20,* 343–350.

Rubinstein, R. A., & Brown, R. T. (1984). An evaluation of the validity of the diagnostic category of attention deficit disorder. *American Journal of Orthopsychiatry, 54,* 398–414.

Safer, D. J., & Krager, J. M. (1983). Trends in medication treatment of hyperactive children. *Clinical Pediatrics, 22,* 500–504.

Safer, R., & Allen, D. (1976). *Hyperactive children: Diagnosis and management.* Baltimore: University Park Press.

Sandoval, J. S., Lambert, N. M., & Sassone, D. (1980). The identification and labelling of hyperactivity in children: An interactive model. In C. K. Whalen & B. Henker (Eds.), *Hyperactive children: The social ecology of identification and treatment* (pp. 145–171). New York: Academic Press.

Satterfield, J. H., Cantwell, D. P., & Satterfield, B. (1979). Multimodality treatment. *Archives of General Psychiatry, 36,* 965–974.

Satterfield, J. H., Satterfield, B., & Cantwell, D. P. (1981). Three-year multi-modality treatment study of 100 hyperactive boys. *Journal of Pediatrics, 98,* 650–655.

Shure, M. B., & Spivack, G. (1972). Means–end thinking, adjustment and social class among elementary school-aged children. *Journal of Consulting and Clinical Psychology, 37,* 389–394.

Sprague, R. L. (1983). Hyperkinetic/attentional deficit syndrome: Behavior modification and educational techniques. In M. Rutter (Ed.), *Developmental neuropsychiatry.* New York: Guilford Press.

Sprague, R. L., & Sleator, E. K. (1975–1976). What is the proper dose of stimulant drugs in children? *International Journal of Mental Health, 4,* 75–104.

Sprague, R. L., & Sleator, E. K. (1977). Methylphenidate in hyperkinetic children: Differences in dose effects on learning and social behavior. *Science, 198,* 1274–1276.

Stein, M. A., & O'Donnell, J. P. (1985). Classification of children's behavior problems: Clinical and quantitative approaches. *Journal of Abnormal Child Psychology, 13,* 269–280.

Swanson, J. M., & Kinsbourne, M. (1976). Stimulant-related state-dependent learning in hyperactive children. *Science, 192,* 1354–1357.

Trites, R. L., Dugas, F., Lynch, G., & Ferguson, B. (1979). Incidence of hyperactivity. *Journal of Pediatric Psychology, 4,* 179–188.

Trites, R. L., & Laprade, K. (1983). Evidence for an independent syndrome of hyperactivity. *Journal of Child Psychology and Psychiatry, 24,* 573–586.
Waddell, K. J. (1984). The self-concept and social adaptation of hyperactive children in adolescence. *Journal of Clinical Child Psychology, 13,* 50–55.
Wagner, A. E. (1986). *Gender differences in hyperactive school-age children.* Unpublished master's thesis, Michigan State University, East Lansing.
Weiss, G., & Hechtman, L. (1986). *Hyperactive children grown up.* New York: Guilford Press.
Weiss, G., Hechtman, L., & Perlman, T. (1978). Hyperactives as young adults: School, employer, and self-rating scales obtained during ten-year follow-up evaluation. *American Journal of Orthopsychiatry, 48,* 438–445.
Weiss, G., Kruger, E., Danielson, U., & Elman, M. (1975). Effects of long-term treatment of hyperactive children with methylphenidate. *Canadian Medical Association Journal, 112,* 159–165.
Weiss, G., Minde, K., Werry, J. S., Douglas, V. I., & Nemeth, E. (1971). Studies on the hyperactive child, VIII: Five-year follow-up. *Archives of General Psychiatry, 24,* 409–414.
Weithorn, C. J., Kagen, E., & Marcus, M. (1984). The relationship of activity level ratings and cognitive impulsivity to task performance and academic achievement. *Journal of Child Psychology and Psychiatry, 25,* 587–606.
Wells, K. C., Conners, C. K., Imber, L., & Delameter, A. (1981). Use of single-subject methodology in clinical decision-making with hyperactive children on the psychiatric inpatient unit. *Behavioral Assessment, 3,* 359–369.
Wells, K. C., & Forehand, R. (1980). Child behavior problems in the home. In S. M. Turner, K. Calhoun, & H. E. Adams (Eds.), *Handbook of behavior therapy.* New York: Wiley.
Wender, E. H. (1983). Hyperactivity in adolescence. *Journal of Adolescent Health Care, 4,* 180–186.
Wender, P. (1971). *Minimal brain dysfunction in children.* New York: Wiley.
Werry, J. A., & Hawthorne, D. (1976). Conners' Teacher Questionnaire—norms and validity. *Australian and New Zealand Journal of Psychiatry, 10,* 257–262.
Whalen, C. K., & Henker, B. (1976). Psychostimulants and children: A review and analysis. *Psychological Bulletin, 83,* 1113–1130.
Whalen, C. K., & Henker, B. (1980). *Hyperactive children: The social ecology of identification and treatment.* New York: Academic Press.
Wolraich, M., Drummond, T., Salomon, M. K., O'Brien, M. C., & Sivage, C. (1978). Effects of methylphenidate alone and in combination with behavior modification procedures on the behavior and academic performance of hyperactive children. *Journal of Abnormal Child Psychology,* 1978, *6,* 149–161.

## 6

Sleep Disturbances in Childhood and Adolescence

MARY A. CARSKADON, THOMAS F. ANDERS, AND WILLIAM HOLE

1. INTRODUCTION

A primary effort of current sleep researchers is to define the normal development of sleep and to find meaningful normative measures. The study of sleep disturbances is difficult, therefore, because such disturbances are interruptions of this incompletely described normal course of events. Thus, few comprehensive theories are currently available to illuminate the mechanisms of most pediatric sleep disorders. The problems in children are confounded by the fact that children—particularly young children, but even those well into adolescence—rarely complain about sleep disturbances. Complaints usually come second-hand from a concerned parent or from a teacher who observes disruptive classroom behavior in an older child or adolescent.

Thus, the sleep disturbances of which we are commonly aware in children and adolescents are those that—for whatever reason—come to the attention of someone other than the child. In infants and younger children, the most frequently reported sleep disturbances are those involving nighttime wakefulness or those associated with "abnormal," unusual, or noteworthy behaviors during sleep. Parental perceptions of sleep disturbances, however, are influenced by many factors, including

---

Mary A. Carskadon, Thomas F. Anders, and William Hole • Department of Psychiatry and Human Behavior, Division of Child Psychiatry, Bradley Hospital, Brown University Program in Medicine, East Providence, Rhode Island 02915.

their expectations, the environmental conditions, their own responsiveness, and the way the child signals. In the most extreme cases, parents may perceive common sleep behaviors as problematic; conversely, they may see nothing worrisome in a child's most bizarrely abnormal sleep disturbance. Disentangling these factors and identifying and characterizing causative or perpetuating interactions is a difficult problem, particularly in the youngest children.

In older children and adolescents, the sleep disturbances noted most often are those associated with disruptive behavior frequently associated with excessive daytime sleepiness. Thus, in addition to many of the same factors influencing perception of disturbed sleep in younger groups, there is the added difficulty that the symptoms of interest become manifest in a context removed from nighttime sleep. The shift in the nature of the sleep disturbances from childhood to adolescence also suggests that a number of the childhood sleep problems are developmental and that many children may simply "outgrow" them before reaching adolescence.

Much research remains to be done in the assessment of sleep and waking function in youngsters, particularly in the following areas: development of the circadian organization of state in normal and disordered sleep; impact of disordered sleep on alertness and sleepiness and impact of excessive somnolence in children on learning, behavior, and so forth; therapeutic approaches and outcomes; sleep disturbances in organic and psychiatric diseases; and the role of dysfunctional parent–child interactions in the etiology of sleep disorders.

Despite the limitations of current knowledge, significant progress can be seen. A start has been made toward understanding normal developmental progress, and efforts to establish a nosology of pediatric sleep disturbances have identified many problems specific to the pediatric population. This chapter will therefore highlight pediatric sleep disturbances using a developmental framework. At each stage, an attempt will be made to summarize certain of the common notions regarding etiology and to outline appropriate approaches to treatment.

2. INFANCY AND EARLY CHILDHOOD

2.1. Sleep Patterns of Infants

A major task of the newborn is to organize behavior, both in terms of coalescing behavioral functioning into discrete states—e.g., wake, nonrapid eye movement (NREM), and rapid eye movement (REM) sleep—as well as organizing states into a rhythmic daily pattern of distribution. Most studies of infant sleep, however, have been carried out only during partial segments of the 24 hours, and few have examined sleep–wake patterns across many cycles. Therefore, questions remain about the early development of circadian organization in infants. There is some evidence that the newly developing sleep–wake pattern exists within a circadian framework from a very early age, but that entrainment to 24 hours does not occur until several weeks of age (Kleitman & Englemann, 1953). Such a "free-running" pattern may, for example, lead parents to report that the child who had begun to "sleep at night" no longer does so.

It is not clear to what extent early sleep problems may result from abnormalities of this type of developmental adjustment, nor is it clear what environmental cues are important to establish entrainment or to what extent prematurity, medical illness, birth injury, or other stresses may disrupt or delay circadian organization of behavioral state. Preliminary findings from sleep–wake diaries kept by parents over the first month of a child's life suggest that prematurity may convey a risk for delayed entrainment of circadian rhythms (Hole, Lamoureaux, & Anders, 1987). Although, further studies promise to provide additional insights regarding this fundamental developmental process, a general pattern of development can be described.

In most infants, a clear diurnal/nocturnal distribution of wake and sleep emerges by 6 weeks of age (Anders & Keener, 1985; Anders, Keener, & Kraemer, 1985; Coons, 1987); by 3 months, clearly defined, discrete EEG sleep stages are present (Hoppenbrouwers 1987; Coons, 1987); and by 6 to 9 months, the majority of children have "settled" into a pattern of well-consolidated nocturnal sleep (Moore & Ucko, 1957; Jenkins, Owen, Bax, & Hart, 1984; Richman, 1987).

The two most frequent complaints made by parents of infants and toddlers have to do with not sleeping through the night and problems in falling asleep at bedtime. These two "insomnias" can be extremely unsettling for parents and disruptive to family life. When studied with polysomnography in the sleep laboratory (Coons, 1987) or at home using time-lapse video (Anders & Keener, 1985), it is very clear that infants do not sleep continuously through the night. To "sleep like a baby" is to wake, at least briefly, at fairly frequent intervals. In 2- to 3-week-olds, the longest sustained daily sleep period averages only about four hours (Anders & Keener, 1985; Coons, 1987); in infants aged 6 months to a year, the longest sustained sleep period has an average length of approximately seven hours. Thus, when parents assume that their infant has slept for 10 or 12 hours through the night, this assumption is likely to be considerably off the mark. What varies notably from infant to infant is the child's response to arousals from sleep: many babies are able to put themselves back to sleep with no intervention and without parents even realizing they have awakened; other infants fuss and cry when they wake in the night and thereby provoke parental notice and usually a parental response.

2.2. Settling and Night Waking

Some definitions of terms are in order. Moore and Ucko (1957) define "settling" as an infant's ability to sleep uninterrupted from midnight until 5:00 a.m. for four weeks, waking less often than once a week. From a biological perspective, the infant's ability to consolidate such long, sustained sleep periods is important because even by the end of the first year, the *total* hours of sleep per 24 hours does not shift dramatically from birth. Thus the developmental achievement of the infant is to attain a behavioral reorganization consisting of consolidated sleep periods at night and sustained waking episodes during the daytime. Settling reflects this consolidation. Settling usually begins by 5 to 6 months of age, and survey data suggest that 90% of infants have settled by their first birthday (Richman, 1987).

Although most infants achieve well-consolidated nocturnal sleep patterns by 6 to 9 months of age and are "self-soothers," that is, able to put themselves back to sleep without parental assistance following the inevitable and universal arousals, many tend to develop a problem with "night waking" at about this age. Night waking is defined as occurring when sleep disruptions during the night take place for more than a week in an infant who has already settled (Moore & Ucko, 1957). In other words, after at least a month of untroubled nighttime sleep ("settled"), the infant begins to wake and signal distress between the hours of midnight and 5:00 a.m. Night waking has been reported to occur in as many as 50% of infants who have successfully settled. A number of reports (Moore & Ucko, 1957; Ragins & Schachter, 1971; Anders & Keener, 1985) confirm a rise in night waking as a fairly consistent trend during the first two years of life, emerging at about age 6 months and often persisting beyond the first year. Anders and colleagues (1985) speculate that whether or not an infant becomes a night waker depends in part upon the infant's temperament or native irritability—a constitutional factor—and in part upon the way in which parents respond to the arousals—an environmental or interactional factor.

Both settling and night waking need to be differentiated from the difficulties many parents have putting their child to bed at night. These bedtime struggles (described below) begin to appear around the first birthday and may persist through the age of 5 or 6 years.

Factors that have been reported in infants with problems settling or sleeping through the night suggest that such difficulties are more likely than night waking to have a biological basis. For example, premature infants with low birth weight, infants in whom there have been medical complications during pregnancy and delivery, brain-damaged infants, and certain nursing infants have all been noted to experience delays in achieving settling. Night waking, by contrast, may at times be associated with biological factors but is more likely to be related to acute disruptions in the child's life. Thus, a well-settled infant may begin to experience night waking when the family takes a vacation and the child must sleep in a strange bed or when unexpected family stresses develop. Whether night waking persists beyond the acute situation, however, is usually related more to the parents' response than to the infant's behavioral adjustment.

Most night wakings are transient disturbances, perhaps associated with such events as a "bad dream" or a cold. After 15 to 18 months of age, night waking may recur frequently or persistently. In the latter circumstance, causal factors can generally be discerned within the parent–child relationship or in the context of family stresses. Persistent night waking, unfortunately, is difficult to define with any great precision. Because parental response thresholds for night waking vary enormously, it is not a simple matter to determine a normative pattern. It is nevertheless probably true that parental concerns during early childhood expressed to family physicians and pediatricians most often relate to issues of night waking and difficulties falling asleep. Only the most serious and protracted cases, however, reach the attention of a sleep expert. Persistent night waking in the first year of life is likely to lead to difficulties falling asleep by age 18 months. By two years of age, night waking and falling asleep problems are usually linked in a pattern of parent–child struggle that is evident both at bedtime and during the middle of the night after an awakening.

Ferber (1987a), too, posits a number of environmental/interactional factors that are associated with "excessive wakefulness" problems of young children. The following factors are among those he cites. *Feeding:* breast or bottle feeding at night tends to reinforce the arousals; in addition, if large quantitities are ingested, the frequency and volume of voiding may have an impact on night waking. *Co-sleeping:* beyond the first few months, co-sleeping in Western cultures may be associated with night waking; this interactional pattern may also suggest serious family problems, depending upon the parent's motivation for continuing the pattern. *Alacrity of parental response:* for example, with an "oversolicitous" response, which may be common in the case of parents whose infants have histories of neonatal distress, bad habits may become conditioned response patterns. *Inappropriate associations to falling asleep:* the infant whose parent holds and rocks and sings a lullaby to induce sleep or the toddler who drifts off nightly in the family room with the television blaring comes to associate these circumstances with the process of falling asleep. Then, when the child wakes in the night—as all children do—the dark and quiet and stillness of the bedroom to which the parent transported the sleeping child are incompatible with a smooth return to sleep because the child has not learned to associate these conditions with falling asleep.

The sleep problems of infancy may also be of medical origin. Those conditions causing pain have the most clearcut association with disturbed sleep, though Ferber (1987a) cautions that chronic serous otitis is frequently overlooked in this regard. Although controversial, there is increasing evidence that food allergy, specifically allergy to cow's milk, may be associated with disturbed and reduced sleep (Kahn et al., 1987). Kahn and his colleagues found evidence of immunologic reactions to milk in infants (mean age 25 weeks) whose average sleep time was approximately five hours at night and one hour in the daytime. Colic has an obvious association with disturbed sleep (Weissbluth, 1987); significantly, however, the sleep disturbance may persist even after the colic condition has resolved. The brain-damaged child may also have disturbed sleep (Okawa & Sasaki, 1987), which may manifest as the inability to achieve a stable, 24-hour rhythm of sleep and wakefulness (Okawa et al., 1987). Sleep disturbances in mentally retarded or brain-damaged infants tend to persist and to be resistant to the types of behavioral therapy that are quite useful in an unimpaired child.

2.3. Difficulties Falling Asleep

When parent–child bedtime problems are present, they frequently have the following pattern. Typically, a child and parent will do "battle" at bedtime. The child "demands" some kind of recurring comfort and these persistent requests upset the parents. Soon, both the child and parents are upset and struggling. Finally, the parent will give in to the child's demands and the child will fall asleep. Often, however, the child reawakens after a relatively brief episode of sleep and the struggle resumes.

This kind of sleep problem seems to reflect a perturbation of the parent–child relationship and the parent's ability to regulate and modulate the child's needs. These bedtime battles usually occur in the context of the separation–individuation stage of the child's psychological development. During the first year, maintenance of conditions enhancing physiological homeostasis and provision of psychological comfort and security have been the chief tasks of the primary caregivers, and this has been the basis for formation of attachment relationships between the child and the caregiver. During the separation–individuation stage, however, the infant needs to achieve some autonomy from the primary caregiver. Such autonomy requires brief periods of separation that progressively lengthen as the child engages in the wider world of other adults and children. Insofar as falling asleep is a rehearsal for such separation, it often becomes a time of "separation struggle." Because night waking problems themselves involve recurrent falling asleep problems, the two types of disturbance quickly become intertwined.

2.4. Consequences of Disturbed Sleep

There is currently no evidence to suggest that these common perturbations of falling asleep and waking up in the middle of the night have long-lasting effects on the development of personality. Similarly, there are no data to suggest that these disturbances are related to sleep–wake state pathophysiology. The proportionate relationship and the organizational structure of REM and NREM sleep are normal in these children. The major disturbance seems to be the stress that the sleep problem causes the family. As the problem worsens, with more awakenings and more complicated rituals to return to sleep, parents' sleep patterns become disrupted as well. Family stress increases as opinions regarding cause and cure conflict and as professional advice either disagrees with parental practice or is not helpful in resolving the problem.

Whether the sleep habits and patterns of infancy and early childhood become the sleep habits of older childhood or adulthood remains a question for future research. That is, are short and "light" sleepers as infants more prone to develop patterns of insomnia as adults? Conversely, do children who fall asleep quickly, easily, and unmindful of the environment develop into adults with undisturbed, restful sleep? One might also speculate whether the diurnal patterns of "owls" (people whose productivity peaks in late evening) versus "larks" (those who are early morning risers) have their origins in the sleep–wake patterns of infancy and early childhood. Each of these questions is of more than passing interest; unfortunately, data bearing on these issues are unavailable.

2.5. Managing Sleep Problems

For the present, recommendations for treatment of these disturbances vary from professional to professional. Although a quarter century of permissiveness in pediatrics has successfully reduced parental complaints of feeding and toileting disturbances in their young children, the lack of scheduling and limit setting in the management of sleeping and waking behavior may account for the sharp rise of these complaints. The sleep–wake cycle in humans is regulated by the interaction of biological and social factors. The process of falling asleep is a cue for setting the biological clock, which is thought to be regulated by biological, environmental (light–dark), and social factors. Regularity in the timing of going to bed and falling asleep (as well as waking up) is essential if a robust daily cycle is to be established. Excessive permissiveness and lack of regularity in these processes is frequently associated with nighttime sleep problems. In infancy and young childhood, regularity of the daytime nap schedule is also important to establish the daily cyclicity.

Treatment of early-childhood sleep disturbances requires an individual approach that takes into consideration the child's needs as well as the family's concerns. In general, a consistent schedule of napping and bedtime, along with a predictable strategy for parental response to night wakings, need to be established. A regularly recurring pattern of pre-bedtime rituals, such as a bath, bedtime stories, and parental "good nights," should also be encouraged. Bottles should be discouraged before bedtime. Feeding and sleeping patterns should be independent. Holding and rocking the child to sleep should also be discouraged, since the child's ability to fall asleep by himself or herself in a consistent setting is a major goal of treatment. If necessary, parents might sit by the bedside, touching or stroking the child, but even this pattern should be gradually diminished. Naps are often an easy arena in which to begin developing the child's ability to fall asleep independently.

A falling-to-sleep problem is often more problematic with one parent than the other. When a treatment program begins, therefore, the parent with the fewest difficulties in this area should be involved most frequently. Occasionally, another caregiver—for example, a grandparent or babysitter—may be required to assist in instituting treatment. It is critically important in all cases, however, not to impose a treatment program until the professional understands the particular constellation of stresses and strains associated with the disturbance.

3. OLDER CHILDREN

3.1. Parasomnias

Another type of sleep problem affects children starting from approximately 18 months of age. These disturbances have been called "parasomnias" (ASDC, 1979) and include night terrors, sleepwalking, sleeptalking, and possibly NREM enuresis. Their etiology is unknown. Most often their course is short lasting and their occurrence infrequent. Males are more commonly affected than females, and there is a strong family history in many cases. Children who have symptoms of one of the parasomnias are likely to develop symptoms of another. Night terrors are more common in the second and third years of life, whereas the peak incidence of sleepwalking and bedwetting is in the primary school years.

The following features are common to the parasomnias: the child is amnesic for the event in the morning; the child is extremely difficult to waken during the episode; the parasomnia episode is characterized by autonomic arousal; events are more likely to occur if the child is sleep deprived or overtired; and the event occurs in the first hour or two of the night. This cluster of common signs can be explained by the fact that the parasomnias arise from stage 4 NREM sleep. Stage 4 sleep in youngsters is associated with a pattern of high-voltage, slow-wave activity in the EEG, and extremely high arousal threshold. Busby and Pivik (1983), for example, failed to discern any signs of arousal from this stage in children exposed to noise as loud as 123 db.

Broughton (1968) has suggested that parasomnias may be categorized as disorders of partial arousal from sleep. The behavioral manifestations would certainly seem to support this characterization. It is well known, for example, that sleep deprivation raises arousal threshold and thus may predispose to incomplete arousal. It has been suggested that perhaps even deprivation of an afternoon nap may precipitate the onset of parasomnias (Ferber, 1985). Ferber (1985) places the parasomnias on a continuum of arousal responses occurring at the NREM to REM transition early in the night. One extreme is the normal transition associated with a few body movements and perhaps a brief moan or groan and the other extreme is the night terror episode with its associated inconsolable agitation.

3.1.1. Diagnostic Issues

Because the first NREM to REM transition usually follows sleep onset by about one to three hours, a careful history regarding time of occurrence of the event is usually sufficient to make the diagnosis. Thus, an episode occurring in the early morning hours when REM sleep tends to predominate could not be considered a typical NREM parasomnia. Furthermore, if the child can relate a vivid dream experience during the event, parasomnias can be ruled out because stage 4 NREM sleep is rarely associated with recall of mental activity.

A useful aid in gathering information to make these assessments is to have the parent keep a diary of the child's sleep in which are noted bedtime, an estimate of time of sleep onset, the times when arousals or disruptive events occur, and morning wake-up time. (Such a diary can be very useful in the assessment of any sleep problem, not just for parasomnias.) With regard to parasomnias, parents should be encouraged to be especially diligent about reporting the child's behaviors during the first three hours of sleep. A parasomnia event may occasionally take place during the latter portion of the night when stage 4 may occur, but such timing is rare.

Because most parasomnia events occur only sporadically, a sleep laboratory polysomnographic recording is rarely useful to confirm the diganosis. Only in severe and intractable cases in which the parasomnia occurs almost nightly can the sleep laboratory aid in the diagnostic process. Rarely, seizure activity may have a presentation similar to parasomnias, though there are usually other features (daytime symptoms) that will suggest this diagnosis. If seizures are suspected, nocturnal polysomnography can be quite valuable.

Parasomnias that persist into adolescence are rare and merit more careful diagnostic evaluation, particularly as they may be associated with significant psychological impairment.

3.1.2. Management

Treatment of parasomnias is usually supportive. Reassurance to parents that the problem is temporary, that it runs in families, and that it has no significant long-term consequences usually suffices. When a parasomnia, especially bedwetting, inhibits the child from usual social interactions, such as sleeping over at a friend's house or attending summer camp, a trial of medication may be indicated. (It is common, however, for even a recurrent and persistent parasomnia to remit temporarily in such a novel setting.) Another indication for pharmacotherapy is when the nightly occurrence of an event begins to impair daytime function. Benzodiazepines (usually diazepam) are the drugs of choice for sleepwalking or night terrors (Guilleminault, 1987a). These compounds apparently reduce the events through their suppression of stage 4 sleep

(Fisher, Kahn, Edwards, & Davis, 1973). The tricyclics (usually imipramine) are used to control enuresis, presumably acting through anticholinergic mechanisms (Mikkelsen & Rapoport, 1980; Nino-Murcia & Kennan, 1987).

Special mention should be made about "safeproofing" the sleeping environment of the child who sleep walks. Sleepwalkers generally do not engage in purposeful activity during an event. A history of goal-directed behavior should lead the clinician to reject the diagnosis of sleepwalking. Most sleepwalking episodes are short lived. The child may just leave the bed and slump to the floor. Whereas a sleepwalking child may be capable of navigating a stairway, a fall is a likely result of such an attempt. Therefore, windows and doors should be secured, and alarms may be necessary to waken the parent if such precautions are not possible. Folklore cautions us against waking a sleepwalker. While catastrophe will not result from waking someone who is sleepwalking, it is generally recommended not to try to awaken children from any of the parasomnias. As we have noted, the disorders involve impaired arousal and attempts to waken the child only seem to prolong and intensify the episode (Ferber, 1985). It is usually possible to guide the child gently back to bed, where normal sleep will ensue.

3.2. Sleep-Disordered Breathing

Sleep-disordered breathing could be described with equal relevance at any age from infancy through adolescence. Sleep-related breathing disorder, chiefly the obstructive sleep apnea syndrome, has been reported in a number of case series in youngsters (see, for example, Guilleminault, Eldridge, Simmons, & Dement, 1976; Guilleminault, Korobkin, & Winkle, 1981). Sleep-disordered breathing poses a number of specific medical risks and is also associated with significant impairment of waking function. Among the medical risks of the obstructive sleep apnea syndrome are sudden infant death syndrome (Guilleminault, 1987b), cor pulmonale (Menashe, Farrehi, & Miller, 1965; Noonan, 1965), cardiac arrhythmias (Tilkian et al., 1976; Guilleminault, Connolly, & Winkle, 1983), pulmonary hypertension (Guilleminault, Eldridge, Simmons, & Dement, 1975; Loughlin, Wynne, & Victorica, 1981), systemic hypertension (Guilleminault et al., 1975), and growth abnormalities and failure to thrive (Guilleminault et al., 1981; Lind & Lundell, 1982; Brouillette, Fernbach, & Hunt, 1982). Sleep-related breathing disorders in children and adolescents have also been associated with excessive daytime sleepiness, impaired intellectual function, and poor behavioral adjustment (Dement, Carskadon, & Richardson,

1978; Weissbluth, David, Poncher, & Reiff, 1983; Guilleminault et al., 1981; Brouillette et al., 1984; and Frank, Kravath, Pollak, & Weitzman, 1983).

The most commonly reported cause of sleep-disordered breathing in children is adenotonsillar hypertrophy (see, for example, Menashe et al., 1965; Noonan, 1965; Guilleminault et al., 1976, 1981; Kravath, Pollak, & Borowiecki, 1977; Lind & Lundell, 1982; Richardson, Seed, Cotton, Bento, & Kramer, 1980; Reynolds, Stool, & Holzer, 1980). Obstructive sleep apnea has also been reported in Down's syndrome (Clark, Schmidt, & Schuller, 1980; Loughlin et al., 1981; Levine & Simpser 1982; Guilleminault et al., 1981; Guilleminault, Nino-Murcia, Heldt, Baldwin, & Hutchinson, 1986; Frank et al., 1983), nasal obstruction due to allergies (Lavie, Gertner, Zomer, & Podoshin, 1981; McNicholas et al., 1982), and with various craniofacial or neurologic abnormalities (Guilleminault et al., 1981).

Symptoms associated with sleep-disordered breathing include labored breathing or breathing pauses during sleep; snoring—often quite loud and disruptive, particularly in older children; mouth breathing while awake; and thrashing during sleep. Reappearance of bedwetting in a child who has been dry may also be a clue to this disorder, though the nighttime breathing difficulties are the critical phenomena (Guilleminault et al., 1976). The child with severely disrupted nocturnal sleep due to sleep-disordered breathing may also experience notable impairment of daytime function, including excessive sleepiness, which often manifests in children as behavior and conduct problems or even hyperactivity (Anders, Carskadon, & Dement, 1980).

The constellation of symptoms is generally unmistakable. The key issue is for the clinician to elicit them effectively. A child may appear grossly medically normal when awake, yet have serious disease while asleep. Questions regarding snoring and sleep-related breathing pauses and daytime functioning and behavior should be routine parts of the assessment of all children with any upper airway narrowing, particularly enlarged tonsils and adenoids. A proper sleep–wake history can be useful in determining therapeutic strategy. The sleep laboratory can also be helpful, primarily to determine the severity of the sleep apnea syndrome and the nocturnal impact on sleep structure and cardiopulmonary function. Again, such information has implications for therapy.

In the case of adenotonsillar hypertrophy, the treatment of choice is surgical removal of the excess tissue in the airway (Mangat, Orr, & Smith, 1977; Guilleminault et al., 1981; Brouillette et al., 1982). Chronic tracheostomy has been used where airway size is compromised by structural abnormalities, though other approaches are currently favored. In the case of craniofacial anomalies, surgical reconstruction of the mandible and/or hyoid has been used with some success in adults (Spire, Kuo, & Campbell, 1983). Issues concerning skeletal growth and development may complicate the decision to apply such techniques in youngsters. Older children and adolescents, even some who are mildly retarded, can tolerate the current nonsurgical treatment of choice, which has gained widespread use in adults with obstructive sleep apnea syndrome: continuous nasal positive airway pressure during sleep (Guilleminault et al., 1986).

4. ADOLESCENTS

Among the myriad changes—both physiological and psychological—that accompany adolescence, are changes in the ways disturbed sleep becomes manifest. As mentioned previously, much of the sleep disturbance that erupts during the adolescent years is first noted because of its impact on waking behavior. In many instances, the arousal disorders of younger children have disappeared by adolescence or will gradually diminish across the adolescent years. As with other types of developmental disorders, however, there are no clear lines of demarcation. Thus, certain of the disturbances discussed below may appear in youngsters before they reach the second decade, and others may appear in adults.

4.1. Insomnias

A "childhood-onset" type of insomnia has been described in adults who have long-standing difficulties initiating and maintaining sleep (ASDC, 1979); however, very little is known about the early diagnosis of this disorder. The insomnias that seem most likely to occur in adolescents are primarily associated with either psychiatric problems or with a circadian rhythm disorder. Interestingly, the distinction between these two etiologies is often blurred.

4.1.1. Depression

Several models of depression in adults include a component involving a circadian rhythm dysfunction (Wehr & Wirz-Justice, 1982; Kripke, 1983). To a certain degree, these models have arisen as a result of the sleep disturbances that are common symptoms of adult depression, as well as the polysomnographically described abnormal distribution of sleep states in depressed adults. Thus, the abnormal distribution of REM sleep in depressed adults, which has been suggested as a biological marker of the psychiatric disorder (Kupfer, 1976), is also thought to be a marker of a circadian phase disruption. REM sleep is commonly thought to be linked to the circadian oscillator controlling body temperature (Czeisler, Zimmerman, Ronda, Moore-Ede, & Weitzman, 1980) and hence normally has its peak distribution in the latter portion of a night's sleep. In depressed adults, REM sleep tends to accumulate more toward the beginning of the night (Kupfer, 1976), suggesting a phase advance of REM sleep. Patients with depression often complain of waking early in the morning with an inability to return to sleep, again a finding that has been noted as suggesting a phase advance.

The circadian rhythm models of depression in adults are unproved and encounter difficulties when applied to younger depressives. For one thing, a REM sleep abnormality has not been consistently reported in depressed children and adolescents (Taub, Hawkins, & Van de Castle, 1978; Puig-Antich et al., 1982; Puig-Antich et al., 1983; Lahmeyer, Poznanski, & Bellur, 1983). Second, many adolescents who are depressed complain of excessive sleep rather than insomnia (Hawkins, Taub, & Van de Castle, 1985). Brumback and Weinburg (1977) reported that disturbed sleep was present in 80% of depressed youngsters, and the disturbance manifested as "a child who may have great difficulty falling asleep until late at night, sleep restlessly, and awaken frequently during the night, have bad dreams, and have difficulty awakening in the morning." Thus, even though noted as a "sleep disturbance," a problem with waking in the morning is a common feature of depression in younger individuals. This symptom may be called hypersomnolence by others (Hawkins et al., 1985). In fact, it may be that a circadian rhythm dysfunction different from the adult type is present in adolescent depressives. A possible disorder of this kind, the delayed sleep phase syndrome, is discussed below.

4.1.2. Delayed Sleep Phase Syndrome

One of the most common features of adolescent sleep patterns is staying up late at night. One survey of eleventh and twelfth graders, for example, found that over 60% reported that they enjoyed staying up late (Price, Coates, Thoresen, & Grinstead, 1978). We have recently found in a survey of 250 tenth, eleventh, and twelfth grade boarding school students that 45% go to bed later than midnight on school nights and 90% later than midnight (38% later than 1:00 a.m.) on weekends (Carskadon

& Mancuso, 1987). This change in adolescent sleep habits may be attributed in part to the relaxation of parental restrictions on bedtime, as well as to the adolescent's desire for independence, which is often realized by taking control of this aspect of his or her life (Carskadon & Dement, 1987). Many adolescents cope quite well with arranging a sleep schedule, but problems may arise in a portion of the group. These problems may result in a delayed sleep phase syndrome (DSPS), as described here, or in a pattern of insufficient sleep, as described below.

The delayed sleep phase syndrome was first described in 1979 (Weitzman et al.) in a small number of young adult patients. DSPS is usually categorized as a disorder of sleep–wake cycle organization (ASDC, 1979), but purely in terms of chief complaint it could be classed as either an "insomnia" or a "hypersomnia." One of the features that distinguishes this disorder from many common sleep problems is that it tends to occur most frequently in adolescents and young adults (Weitzman et al., 1981). The extent to which the development of the disorder is related to adolescent changes in sleep habits is unknown, though it is likely that the manifestation of DSPS depends upon such a schedule change.

The key dysfunction in this disorder is thought to involve an abnormally shallow range of entrainment on the phase-advance portion of the phase response curve, a critical regulatory mechanism for circadian rhythms. While it is possible for a person with DSPS to entrain to a 24-hour period, it is not possible to readjust the phase position by advancing to an earlier time. Thus, the disturbance is called "phase delay," because the patient's circadian phase position lags behind the environmental phase. The most notable symptoms of this syndrome involve sleep and wakefulness.

4.1.2a. Symptoms.   Difficulty in school is often the first symptom to be noted, often because of tardiness and absenteeism. Parents will generally complain that it is "impossible" to wake the child in the morning, and the child will note that it is "impossible" to fall asleep at a decent hour at night. Hence, the child complains of difficulty falling asleep, the parents complain of difficulty waking the child, and the teachers complain that the child either misses or cannot stay awake in school. In the true DSPS, no matter how early the child tries to go to bed, he or she does not fall asleep until 2:00, 3:00, 4:00, or 5:00 a.m. or even later. And no matter when bedtime was, the child has great difficulty waking before 10:00 or 11:00 a.m. or later than noon. In a susceptible child, the syndrome may be triggered by one or two exceptionally late nights followed by sleeping late the next morning (Ferber, 1987b). Clearly, not every child gets into this trouble with a few late nights, but the vulnerable child can have serious problems after quite a short episode. The modern teenager's bedroom, with television, microcomputer, and other marvels, is a likely source of the initiating stimulus for DSPS.

The child or adolescent with DSPS sleeps quite well on weekends or holidays if permitted to stay up late and to sleep as late as desired. On week days, however, the conflict between sleeping and getting up for school becomes manifest. This conflict, with the parent struggling to wake the youngster whose circadian phase is at its nadir, can become a source of serious family stress. Ferber (1987b) notes that it is important to differentiate the true physiological delayed sleep phase syndrome from the "motivated" DSPS. The latter has similar sleep–wake symptoms; however, the child perpetuates the phase delay to derive secondary gain, usually an escape from having to go to school. Thus, youngsters with separation problems, school avoidance, and other psychological problems, frequently including depressed mood, may develop a form of "motivated DSPS" (Ferber, 1987b). In this group, the sleep–wake pattern tends to normalize during long vacations when going to school is no longer an issue.

4.1.2b. Treatment. The treatment of DSPS involves a technique called chronotherapy (Czeisler et al., 1981). In brief, this technique entails first stabilizing the child's schedule to the times that are phase appropriate, for example, sleeping from 4:00 a.m. until noon or 1:00 p.m. Then the day length is increased by three hours, and bedtime and rising time therefore delayed three hours, for five to ten days until bedtime coincides with the desired sleeping time. This program must be strictly reinforced and if performed in the home requires the cooperation of parents. Thus, for example, the child may sleep from 7:00 a.m. until 3:00 p.m. on the first day, from 10:00 a.m. until 7:00 p.m. on the second day, and so forth, until bedtime is 10:00 p.m. and rising time 6:00 or 7:00 a.m. on the sixth day. At this point, the new schedule must be rigidly adhered to in order to avoid reinstituting the problem. There is some indication that time of waking in the morning may be more important than bedtime to maintain synchrony of sleep–wake to the daily cycle (Webb & Agnew, 1974). It is usually recommended, however, that strict adherence to both bedtime and rising time be maintained in patients susceptible to DSPS (Czeisler et al., 1981).

Treatment of the "motivated DSPS" with this chronotherapeutic approach will not be effective, as the child will resist the prescribed program (Ferber, 1987b). Because the true cause of the sleep disturbance in this case is psychological, the treatment must first address those issues.

4.2. Hypersomnias

The term "hypersomnia" is used here to describe a problem with too much sleep, excessive daytime sleepiness, or both. In order to understand how such problems may manifest in adolescents, it is important to describe briefly our current understanding of normal sleep and waking function in this age group. Much of this understanding derives from longitudinal sleep laboratory data gathered across a six-year span in a group of normal boys and girls (Carskadon, 1979, 1982; Carskadon & Dement, 1987; Carskadon et al., 1980; Carskadon, Orav, & Dement, 1983; Carskadon, Keenan, & Dement, 1987). The longitudinal study included laboratory measures not only of sleep at night (from 10:00 p.m. until 8:00 a.m. for every child on every night in the lab), but also of daytime alertness, the latter using an operationally defined technique called the multiple sleep latency test (MSLT) (Carskadon & Dement, 1982a). The MSLT measures sleepiness/alertness at intervals across the day as the speed of falling asleep under standard low-stimulus conditions with an admonition not to resist sleep.

Pre- and early pubertal Tanner (1962) stage 1 and 2 children (ages 8 to 14 years) slept an average of 9.5 hours at night and were not sleepy at all during the daytime: they had no tendency to fall asleep on the MSLT. Mid- and late pubertal Tanner stage 3, 4, or 5 adolescents (ages 13 to 18 years) also slept an average of 9.5 hours at night, but showed a tendency for an increased sleep tendency (reduced speed of falling asleep) in the afternoons. Thus, adolescents became sleepier even though sleep at night remained constant. In subsequent experiments, it was found that reduction of nocturnal sleep to the "societal norm" (i.e., 8 hours) or less, increased the level of sleepiness in adolescents (Carskadon & Dement, 1981, 1982b, in press), at times to a "pathological" range (Carskadon et al., 1986). These findings have led us to the conclusion that few adolescents are optimally alert (Carskadon & Dement, 1987).

To distinguish this "normal" sleepiness from a "disorder of excessive somnolence" (ASDC, 1979), the best rule of thumb may be the perception on the part of the child, parents, or teacher that it has become a problem in school, at home, or in the child's social life. One special caution is that even "normal" adolescent sleepiness may be a factor predisposing to drug abuse (Carskadon & Dement, 1987), and this possibility should be explored in such cases.

4.2.1. Narcolepsy

Narcolepsy is a disorder that involves a dissociation from sleep of the components of REM sleep. The chief symptom is excessive daytime sleepiness, which in adults can be totally incapacitating (Zarcone, 1973). Another primary symptom of the disorder is cataplexy, which involves the flaccid paralysis of antigravity muscles in response to strong emotions, such as laughter, anger, startle, or hilarity. This paralysis may be partial, manifesting as muscle weakness particularly in the arms or legs, or total, and it is usually of short duration. Hypnagogic hallucinations and sleep paralysis complete the classic symptom tetrad of narcolepsy. The hypnagogic hallucinations are often frightening, particularly when they occur in association with sleep paralysis. Although this cluster of symptoms seems quite bizarre, each can be easily comprehended within the framework of a disorder of normal REM sleep (Dement, Rechtschaffen, & Gulevich, 1966).

The physiological signs of REM sleep, which occurs with a 90-minute cycle in all humans (past infancy) every single night, include an activated central nervous system (desynchronized EEG), bursts of rapid eye movements and other phasic activities, along with total paralysis of postural muscles. The latter arises from a pontine center, which in REM sleep activates the medullary inhibitory regions and results in postsynaptic hyperpolarization of brain stem and spinal motoneurons (Chase, 1983). Psychologically, REM sleep is associated with the vivid imagery of dreaming (Dement & Kleitman, 1957). Hence, when the components of REM sleep dissociate into wakefulness, strange symptoms occur. Cataplexy and presumably sleep paralysis involve the identical pattern of paralysis as is found in REM sleep. Hypnagogic hallucinations represent the abnormal occurrence of dream imagery in the waking state. The laboratory sign of narcolepsy—sleep-onset REM episodes—confirms the abnormal relationship of REM sleep to wakefulness. In noninfant humans, sleep-onset REM episodes never occur under normal circumstances.

Retrospective studies of adult patients with narcolepsy suggest that the onset of the disorder occurs overwhelmingly in the teenage years (Daniels, 1934; Sours, 1963; Kessler, Guilleminault, & Dement, 1974). Only very rarely is the diagnosis made before age 10 (Guilleminault, 1987c). Considerable evidence also exists to suggest that narcolepsy is a familial disorder (Daly & Yoss, 1959; Yoss & Daly, 1960; Kessler, 1976; Baraitser & Parkes, 1978). In canine narcolepsy, a clear genetic transmission of the disorder has been described (Baker, Foutz, McNerney, Mitler, & Dement, 1982). Recent findings from around the world have localized a major histocompatibility complex fragment (HLA DR2) in virtually 100% of adult narcoleptics (Juji, Satake, Honda, & Doi, 1984; Langdon, Welsh, vanDam, Vaughan, & Parkes, 1984; Billiard & Seignalet, 1985).

4.2.1a. Diagnosis. Diagnosis of narcolepsy in children and adolescents is somewhat difficult because the symptom of daytime sleepiness is often elusive in this age group, as described previously. In addition, because sleepiness is usually the first symptom and may precede the other symptoms by a number of years (Zarcone, 1973), the usual diagnostic criterion for narcolepsy may not be met. This criterion is the presence of some sign of a REM sleep dysfunction, which is usually a history of cataplexy or the documentation of sleep-onset REM episodes on laboratory recordings (Mitler et al., 1979). In a prospective study of children at risk for narcolepsy (Carskadon, Harvey, & Dement, 1981; Carskadon et al., 1983), we found that while sleep-onset REM episodes may be recorded before a youngster describes cataplexy, such episodes may not occur even when the child has reported sleepiness. Thus the diagnosis remains problematic. A family history of narcolepsy is certainly suggestive, and the presence of HLA DR2 in an at-risk child would also be indicative. Too few prospective data are available, however, to make a conclusive statement.

4.2.1b. Treatment. The disorder should be carefully explained to parents and child, with an emphasis that although it is life long, narcolepsy is not degenerative and can often be at least partially controlled with proper behavioral adaptations. Thus, the initial approach to treating narcolepsy in a child or adolescent should involve optimizing the sleep schedule, which generally means increasing the length of the nocturnal sleep period and scheduling one or two daytime naps of about 30 minutes. In some instances, explanations to school officials (i.e., nurses or teachers) are necessary to implement such a schedule. We have shown in one older adolescent that lengthening sleep at night from eight to ten hours not only reduced the sleepiness but also improved sleep structure (Carskadon, 1982).

If schedule changes are insufficient to alleviate the symptoms, drug therapy can be instituted. Guilleminault (1987c) recommends low doses of pemoline or methylphenidate to control sleepiness and protriptyline to control cataplexy. He does not recommend amphetamines or mazindol for children with narcolepsy. Side effects and symptom rebound upon withdrawal are important considerations with all of these compounds.

4.2.2. Periodic Hypersomnias

The periodic hypersomnias, Kleine-Levin syndrome and menstruation-related hypersomnolence, have been reported only very rarely and will be described briefly.

4.2.2a. Kleine-Levin Syndrome. The Kleine-Levin syndrome involves a recurrent pattern of excessive sleep, hyperphagia, and abnormal behaviors, usually occurring in pubertal teenage boys or postpubertal young adult males (Critchley & Hoffman, 1942). The episodes usually last about two weeks, though they may last as long as six weeks in some patients, and they recur at intervals of about one-half to four months. Fewer than 100 cases of Kleine-Levin syndrome have been reported in the literature, and only in a very few instances has the disorder been reported in females (Duffy & Davison, 1968; Gilligan, 1973; Lavie, Gadoth, Gordon, Goldhammer, & Bechar, 1979). Several reports have noted sleep-onset REM episodes during the hypersomnolent episodes (Wilkus & Chiles, 1975; Lavie et al., 1979; Reynolds et al., 1984), and in one reported case the patient later developed narcolepsy (Ceroni, 1968). The etiology of the disorder is unknown, and no effective treatments have been reported, including amphetamine (Gilligan, 1973; Parkes, 1981) or methylphenidate (Frank, Braham, & Cohen, 1974). Although the episodes of hypersomnolence and hyperphagia tend to cease after two or three years, they have been reported to persist for longer than ten years in several cases. Kleine-Levin syndrome is so rare as to be an unlikely cause of excessive somnolence in most teenagers yet so distinct in its symptomatology as to be easy to rule out.

4.2.2b. Menstruation-Related Periodic Hypersomnolence. Menstruation-realted periodic hypersomnolence occurs in adolescent females, usually within a year or two of menstruation and involves episodes of hypersomnolence that are linked to the menstrual cycle, with or without hyperphagia (Billiard, Guilleminault, & Dement, 1975). This is a rare disorder, and some consider it a variant of the Kleine-Levin syndrome. Billiard et al. (1975) found 15 cases in their literature search, and Guilleminault (1987c) reported 11 cases from his clinical experience (versus four cases of Kleine-Levin syndrome). Menstruation-linked periodic hypersomnia is not helped by amphetamine, but can be controlled with hormone therapy (Billiard et al., 1975).

4.2.3. Insufficient Sleep

American adolescents are chronically sleep deprived (Carskadon & Dement, 1987). In one survey of ninth through twelfth graders, two-thirds reported at least a moderate problem with "sleepiness during the day"; the average amount of sleep on school nights ranged from 7 hours in ninth graders to 6.5 hours in twelfth graders, with compensatory weekend sleep times averaging 9 to 9.5 hours (Carskadon & Mancuso, 1987). Although only 5% of the students in this survey reported "very great" difficulty with daytime sleepiness, nearly half (48%) reported falling asleep while reading or studying, and 31% reported struggling to stay awake during an exam. (Nine of the 240 students reported having falling asleep during an exam!) The reasons teenagers curtail sleep include social, academic, and economic pressures. The latter factor seems to have gained in importance in the last decade, as more and more teens have part-time jobs during the school year.

Although sleepiness arising from insufficient sleep may not be perceived as a clinical problem until the child's academic performance begins to suffer, it can have serious "subclinical" consequences. Even identifying an academic problem may be difficult in adolescents, since so many of the students may be sleepy. A major risk is that teens begin to self-medicate to achieve greater alertness. Many teens ingest high levels of caffeine in colas, coffee, and over-the-counter stimulants. We are tempted to speculate that some teenage drug abuse may be in part related to an attempt to overcome chronic sleepiness. A related problem concerns teenage experimentation with alcohol and its relationship to automobile accidents. How often does one hear of a tragic accident involving teenagers who just had one or two beers? A recent report suggests that sleepiness associated with insufficient or restricted nocturnal sleep interacts with alcohol, so that even a very low dose of alcohol may produce marked vulnerability (Lumley, Roehrs, Asker, Zorick, & Roth, 1987).

Management of insufficient sleep in adolescents is difficult for many reasons. Teenagers, as we have noted previously, enjoy staying up late and often do not realize fully the consequences of their behaviors. In today's world, the pressure for teens to be consumers is extremely great, and it is therefore difficult to persuade adolescents that they need sleep more than they need their part-time jobs. On the other hand, some motivated adolescents will respond positively when they are given enough information to make educated choices. Unfortunately, issues of sleep and wakefulness are not part of most educational programs, and teachers and parents are as ignorant of the facts as are teenagers.

5. REFERENCES

Anders, T. F., Carskadon, M. A., & Dement, W. C. (1980). Sleep and sleepiness in children and adolescents. In I. F. Litt (Ed.), *Pediatric Clinics of North America, 27*(1), 29–43.

Anders, T. F., & Keener, M. (1985). Developmental course of nighttime sleep–wake patterns in full-term and premature infants during the first year of life. I. *Sleep, 8,* 173–192.

Anders, T. F., Keener, M. A., & Kraemer, H. (1985). Sleep–wake state organization, neonatal assessment and development in premature infants during the first year of life. II. *Sleep, 8,* 193–206.

Association of Sleep Disorders Centers (ASDC). (1979). *Diagnostic classification of sleep and arousal disorders* (1st ed.). Prepared by the Sleep Disorders Classification Committee, H. P. Roffwarg (Chair). *Sleep, 2,* 1–137.

Baker, T., Foutz, A., McNerney, V., Mitler, M., & Dement, W. (1982). Canine model of narcolepsy: Genetic and developmental determinants. *Experimental Neurology, 75,* 729–752.

Baraitser, M., & Parkes, J. D. (1978). Genetic study of narcoleptic syndrome. *Journal of Medical Genetics, 15,* 254–259.

Billiard, M., Guilleminault, C., & Dement, W. (1975). A menstruation-linked periodic hypersomnia. Kleine-Levin syndrome or new clinical entity? *Neurology, 25,* 436–443.

Billiard, M., & Seignalet, J. (1985). Extraordinary association between HLA-DR2 and narcolepsy. *Lancet, 1,* 226–227.

Broughton, R. J. (1968). Sleep disorders: Disorders of arousal? *Science, 159,* 1070–1078.

Brouillette, R. T., Fernbach, S. K., & Hunt, C. E. (1982). Obstructive sleep apnea in infants and children. *Journal of Pediatrics, 100,* 31–40.

Brouillette, R., Hanson, D., David, R., Klemka, L., Szatkowski, A., Fernbach, S., & Hunt, C. (1984). A diagnostic approach to suspected obstructive sleep apnea in children. *Journal of Pediatrics, 105,* 10–14.

Brumback, R. A., & Weinberg, W. A. (1977). Childhood depression: An explanation of a behavior disorder of children. *Perceptual and Motor Skills, 44,* 911–916.

Busby, K., & Pivik, R. T. (1983). Failure of high intensity auditory stimuli to affect behavioral arousal in children during the first sleep cycle. *Pediatric Research, 17(10),* 802–805.

Carskadon, M. A. (1979). *Determinants of daytime sleepiness: Adolescent development, extended and restricted nocturnal sleep.* Unpublished doctoral dissertation, Stanford University.

Carskadon, M. A. (1982). The second decade. In C. Guilleminault (Ed.), *Sleeping and waking disorders: Indications and techniques* (pp. 99–125). Menlo Park, CA: Addison-Wesley.

Carskadon, M. A., & Dement, W. C. (1981). Cumulative effects of sleep restriction on daytime sleepiness. *Psychophysiology, 18,* 107–113.

Carskadon, M. A., & Dement, W. C. (1982a). The multiple sleep latency test: What does it measure? *Sleep, 5,* S67–S72.

Carskadon, M. A., & Dement, W. C. (1982b). Nocturnal determinants of daytime sleepiness. *Sleep, 5,* S73–S81.

Carskadon, M. A., & Dement, W. C. (1987). Sleepiness in the normal adolescent. In C. Guilleminault (Ed.), *Sleep and its disorders in children* (pp. 53–66). New York: Raven Press.

Carskadon, M. A., & Dement, W. C. (1987). Daytime sleepiness: Quantification of a behavioral state. *Neuroscience and Biobehavioral Reviews, 11,* 307–317.

Carskadon, M. A., Dement, W. C., Mitler, M. M., Roth, T., Westbrook, P., & Keenan, S. (1986). Guidelines for the multiple sleep latency test (MSLT): A standard measure of sleepiness. *Sleep, 9,* 519–524.

Carskadon, M. A., Harvey, K., & Dement, W. C. (1981). Multiple sleep latency tests in the development of narcolepsy. *Western Journal of Medicine, 135,* 414–418.

Carskadon, M. A., Harvey, K., Duke, P., Anders, T. F., Litt, I. F., & Dement, W. C. (1980). Pubertal changes in daytime sleepiness. *Sleep, 2,* 453–460.

Carskadon, M. A., Keenan, S., & Dement, W. C. (1987). Nighttime sleep and daytime sleep tendency in preadolescents. In C. Guilleminault (Ed.), *Sleep and its disorders in children* (pp. 43–52). New York: Raven Press.

Carskadon, M. A., & Mancuso, J. (1987). Reported sleep habits in boarding school students: Preliminary data. *Sleep Research, 16,* 173.

Carskadon, M. A., Orav, E. J., & Dement, W. C. (1983). Evolution of sleep and daytime sleepiness in adolescents. In C. Guilleminault & E. Lugaresi (Eds.), *Sleep/wake disorders: Natural history, epidemiology, and long-term evolution* (pp. 201–216). New York: Raven Press.

Ceroni, C. B. (1968). An episode of hypersomnia and megaphagia and its evolution to a narcoleptic syndrome. In Gastaut, H. (Ed.), *The abnormalities of sleep in man* (pp. 239–245). Proceedings of the 15th European meeting on Electroencephalography, Bologna: Gaggi.

Chase, M. H. (1983). Synaptic mechanisms and circuitry involved in motoneuron control during sleep. *International Review of Neurobiology, 24,* 213–258.

Clark, R. W., Schmidt, H. S., & Schuller, D. E. (1980). Sleep-induced ventilatory dysfunction in Down's syndrome. *Archives of Internal Medicine, 140,* 45–50.

Coons, S. (1987). Development of sleep and wakefulness during the first 6 months of life. In C. Guilleminault (Ed.), *Sleep and its disorders in children* (pp. 17–27). New York: Raven Press.

Critchley, M., & Hoffman, H. L. (1942). The syndrome of periodic somnolence and morbid hunger (Kleine-Levin syndrome). *British Medical Journal, 1,* 137–139.

Czeisler, C. A., Richardson, G. S., Coleman, R. M., Zimmerman, J. C., Moore-Ede, M. C., Dement, W. C., & Weitzman, E. D. (1981). Chronotherapy: Resetting the circadian clocks of patients with the delayed sleep phase syndrome. *Sleep, 4,* 1–21.

Czeisler, C. A., Zimmerman, J. C., Ronda, J. M., Moore-Ede, M. C., & Weitzman, E. D. (1980). Timing of REM sleep is coupled to the circadian rhythm of body temperature in man. *Sleep, 2,* 329–346.

Daly, D., & Yoss, R. (1959). A family with narcolepsy. *Proceedings of the Staff Meetings of the Mayo Clinic, 34,* 313–320.

Daniels, L. (1934). Narcolepsy. *Medicine, 34,* 1–122.

Dement, W. C., Carskadon, M. A., & Richardson, G. (1978). Excessive daytime sleepiness in the sleep apnea syndrome. In C. Guilleminault and W. C. Dement (Eds.), *Sleep apnea syndromes* (pp. 23–46). New York: Alan R. Liss.

Dement, W. C., & Kleitman, N. (1957). The relation of eye movements during sleep to dream activity: An objective method for the study of dreaming. *Journal of Experimental Psychology, 53,* 339–346.

Dement, W. C., Rechtschaffen, A., & Gulevich, G. (1961). The nature of the narcoleptic sleep attack. *Neurology, 16,* 18–33.

Duffy, J. P., & Davison, K. (1968). A female case of the Kleine-Levin syndrome. *British Medical Journal, 114,* 77–84.

Ferber, R. (1985). *Solve your child's sleep problem.* New York: Simon & Schuster.

Ferber, R. (1987a). The sleepless child. In C. Guilleminault (Ed.), *Sleep and its disorders in children* (pp. 141–163). New York: Raven Press.

Ferber, R. (1987b). Circadian and schedule disturbances. In C. Guilleminault (Ed.), *Sleep and its disorders in children* (165–179). New York: Raven Press.

Fisher, C., Kahn, E., Edwards, A., & Davis, D. M. (1973). A psychophysiological study of nightmares and night terrors: The suppression of stage 4 night terrors with diazepam. *Archives of General Psychiatry, 28,* 252–259.

Frank, Y., Braham, J., & Cohen, B. E. (1974). The Kleine-Levin syndrome. Case report and review of the literature. *American Journal of Diseases of Children, 127,* 412–413.

Frank, Y., Kravath, R. E., Pollack, C. P., & Weitzman, E. D. (1983). Obstructive sleep apnea and its therapy: Clinical and polysomnographic manifestations. *Pediatrics, 71,* 737–742.

Gilligan, B. S. (1973). Periodic megaphagia and hypersomnia—An example of the Kleine-Levin syndrome in an adolescent girl. *Proceedings of the Australian Association of Neurology, 9,* 67–72.

Guilleminault, C. (1987a). Disorders of arousal in children: Somnambulism and night terrors. In C. Guilleminault (Ed.), *Sleep and its disorders in children* (pp. 242–252). New York: Raven Press.

Guilleminault, C. (1987b). Obstructive sleep apnea syndrome in children. In C. Guilleminault (Ed.), *Sleep and its disorders in children* (pp. 213–224). New York: Raven Press.

Guilleminault, C. (1987c). Narcolepsy and its differential diagnosis. In C. Guilleminault (Ed.), *Sleep and its disorders in children* (pp. 181–194). New York: Raven Press.

Guilleminault, C., Connolly, S. J., & Winkle, R. A. (1983). Cardiac arrhythmia and conduction disturbances during sleep in 400 patients with sleep apnea syndrome. *American Journal of Cardiology, 52,* 490–494.

Guilleminault, C., Eldridge, F. L., Simmons, F. B., & Dement, W. C. (1975). Sleep apnea syndrome: Can it induce hemodynamic change? *Western Journal of Medicine, 123,* 7–16.

Guilleminault, C., Eldridge, F. L., Simmons, F. B., & Dement, W. C. (1976). Sleep apnea in eight children. *Pediatrics, 58,* 23–31.

Guilleminault, C., Korobkin, R., & Winkle, R. (1981). A review of 50 children with obstructive sleep apnea syndrome. *Lung, 159,* 275–287.

Guilleminault, C., Nino-Murcia, G., Heldt, G., Baldwin, R., & Hutchinson, D. (1986). Alternative treatment to tracheostomy in obstructive sleep apnea syndrome: Nasal continuous positive airway pressure in young children. *Pediatrics, 78,* 797–802.

Hawkins, D., Taub, J., & Van de Castle, R. (1985). Extended sleep (hypersomnia) in young depressed patients. *American Journal of Psychiatry, 142,* 905–910.

Hole, W., Lamoureaux, D., & Anders, T. F. (1987, April). *24 hour sleep–wake and crying behavior during the first month: Term and premature infants.* Paper presented at the biennial meeting of the Society for Research in Child Development, Baltimore, MD.

Hoppenbrouwers, T. (1987). Sleep in infants. In C. Guilleminault (Ed.), *Sleep and its disorders in children* (pp. 1–16). New York: Raven Press.

Jenkins, S., Owen, C., Bax, M., & Hart, H. (1984). Continuities of common behavior problems in pre-school children. *Journal of Child Psychology and Psychiatry and Allied Disciplines, 25,* 75–89.

Juji, T., Satake, M., Honda, Y., & Doi, Y. (1984). HLA antigens in Japanese patients with narcolepsy. *Tissue Antigens, 5,* 316–319.

Kahn, A., Rebuffat, E., Blum, D., Sottiaux, M., Van de Merckt, C., Dramaix, M., & Montauk, L. (1987). Difficulty in initiating and maintaining sleep associated with cow's milk allergy in infants. *Sleep, 10,* 116–121.

Kessler, S. (1976). Genetic factors in narcolepsy. In C. Guilleminault, W. C. Dement, & P. Passouant (Eds.), *Narcolepsy* (pp. 285–302). New York: Spectrum.

Kessler, S., Guilleminault, C., & Dement, W. C. (1974). A family study of 50 REM narcoleptics. *Acta Neurologica Scandinavica, 50,* 503–512.

Kleitman, N., & Englemann, T. (1953). Sleep characteristics of infants. *Journal of Applied Physiology, 6,* 269–282.

Kravath, R. E., Pollak, C. P., & Borowiecki, B. (1977). Hypoventilation during sleep in children who have lymphoid airway obstruction treated by nasopharyngeal tube and T and A. *Pediatrics, 59,* 865–871.

Kripke, D. (1983). Phase-advance theories for affective illness. In T. A. Wehr & F. K. Goodwin (Eds.), *Circadian rhythms in psychiatry*. Pacific Grove, CA: Boxwood Press.

Kupfer, D. J. (1976). A psychobiologic marker for primary depression disease. *Biological Psychiatry, 11*, 159–174.

Lahmeyer, H., Poznanski, E., & Bellur, S. (1983). EEG sleep in depressed adolescents. *American Journal of Psychiatry, 140*, 1150–1153.

Langdon. N., Welsh, K. I., vanDam, M., Vaughan, R. W., & Parkes, D. (1984). Genetic markers in narcolepsy. *Lancet, 2*, 1178–1180.

Lavie, P., Gadoth, N., Gordon, C. R., Goldhammer, G., & Bechar, M. (1979). Sleep patterns in Kleine-Levin syndrome. *Electroencephalography and Clinical Neurophysiology, 47*, 369–371.

Lavie, P., Gertner, R., Zomer, J., & Podoshin, L. (1981). Breathing disorders in sleep associated with "microarousals" in patients with allergic rhinitis. *Acta Otolaryngologia, 92*, 529–533.

Levine, O. R., & Simpser, M. (1982). Alveolar hypoventilation and cor pulmonale associated with chronic airway obstruction in infants with Down syndrome. *Clinical Pediatrics, 21*, 25–29.

Lind, M. G., & Lundell, B. P. W. (1982). Tonsillar hyperplasia in children. *Archives of Otolaryngology, 108*, 650–654.

Loughlin, G. M., Wynne, J. W., & Victorica, B. E. (1981). Sleep apnea as a possible cause of pulmonary hypertension in Down syndrome. *Journal of Pediatrics, 98*, 435–437.

Lumley, M., Roehrs, T., Asker, D., Zorick, F., & Roth, T. (1987). Ethanol and caffeine effects on daytime sleepiness/alertness. *Sleep, 10*, 306–312.

Mangat, D., Orr, W. C., & Smith, R. O. (1977). Sleep apnea, hypersomnolence, and upper airway obstruction secondary to adenotonsillar enlargement. *Archives of Otolaryngology, 103*, 383–386.

McNicholas, W. T., Tarlo, S., Cole, P., Zamel, N., Rutherford, R., Griffin, D., & Phillipson, E. A. (1982). Obstructive apneas during sleep in patients with seasonal allergic rhinitis. *American Review of Respiratory Disease, 126*, 625–628.

Menashe, V. D., Farrehi, C., & Miller, M. (1965). Hypoventilation and cor pulmonale due to chronic upper airway obstruction. *Journal of Pediatrics, 67*, 198.

Mikkelsen, E. J., & Rapoport, J. L. (1980). Enuresis and sleep. *Urologic Clinics of North America, 7*, 361–377.

Mitler, M. M., van den Hoed, J., Carskadon, M. A., Richardson, G. S., Park, R., Guilleminault, C., & Dement, W. C. (1979). REM sleep episodes during the multiple sleep latency test in narcoleptic patients. *Electroencephalography and Clinical Neurophysiology, 46*, 479–481.

Moore, T., & Ucko, L. E. (1957). Night waking in early infancy. *Archives of Disease in Childhood, 32*, 333–342.

Nino-Murcia, G., & Keenan, S. A. (1987). Enuresis and sleep. In C. Guilleminault (Ed.), *Sleep and its disorders in children* (pp. 253–267). New York: Raven Press.

Noonan, J. A. (1965). Reversible cor pulmonale due to hypertrophied tonsils and adenoids: Studies in two cases. *Circulation, 31/32*, 164.

Okawa, M., Nanami, T., Wada, S., Shimizu, T., Hishikawa, Y., Sasaki, H., Nagamine, H., & Takahashi, K. (1987). Four congenitally blind children with circadian sleep–wake rhythm disorder. *Sleep, 10*, 101–110.

Okawa, M., & Sasaki, H. (1987). Sleep disorders in mentally retarded and brain-imapried children. In C. Guilleminault (Ed.), *Sleep and its disorders in children* (pp. 269–290). New York: Raven Press.

Parkes, J. D. (1981). Day-time drowsiness. *Lancet, 2*, 1213–1218.

Price, V. A., Coates, T. J., Thoresen, C. E., & Grinstead, O. A. (1978). Prevalence and correlates of poor sleep among adolescents. *American Journal of Diseases of Children, 132*, 583–586.

Puig-Antich, J., Goetz, R., Hanlon, C., Davies, M., Thompson, J., Chambers, W., Tabrizi, M., & Weitzman, E. (1982). Sleep architecture and REM sleep measures in prepubertal children with major depression. A controlled study. *Archives of General Psychiatry, 39*, 932–939.

Puig-Antich, J., Goetz, R., Hanlon, C., Tabrizi, M., Davies, M., & Weitzman, E. (1983). Sleep architecture and REM sleep measures in prepubertal major depressives. Studies during recovery from the depressive episode in a drug-free state. *Archives of General Psychiatry, 40*, 187–192.

Ragins, N., & Schachter, J. (1971). A study of sleep behavior in 2 year old children. *Journal of the American Academy of Child Psychiatry, 10*, 464–480.

Reynolds, C. F., Kupfer, D. J., Christiansen, C. L., Auchenbach, R. C., Brenner, R. P., Sewitch, D. E., Taska, L. S., & Coble, P. A. (1984). Multiple sleep latency test findings in Klein-Levin syndrome. *Journal of Nervous and Mental Disease, 172*, 41–44.

Reynolds, C. F., Stool, S., Holzer, B., et al. (1980, Fall). Polysomnographic findings in children with adenotonsillar hypertrophy. *Transactions of the Pennsylvania Academy of Ophthalmology and Otolaryngology*, 182–187.

Richardson, M. A., Seed, A. B., Cotton, R. T., Bento, C., & Kramer, M. (1980) Evaluation of tonsils and adenoids in sleep apnea syndrome. *Laryngoscope, 90*, 1106–1110.

Richman, N. (1987). Surveys of sleep disorders in children in a general population. In C. Guilleminault (Ed.), *Sleep and its disorders in children* (pp. 115–127). New York: Raven Press.

Sours, J. (1963). Narcolepsy and other disturbances of the sleep-waking rhythm: A study of 115 cases with a review of the literature. *Journal of Nervous and Mental Disease, 137*, 525–542.

Spire, J. P., Kuo, P. C., & Campbell, N. (1983). Maxillo-facial surgical approach: An introduction and review of mandibular advancement. *Bulletin Europeen de Physiopathologie Respiratoire, 19*, 604–606.

Tanner, J. M. (1962). *Growth at adolescence* (2nd ed.). Oxford: Blackwell.

Taub, J., Hawkins, D., & Van de Castle, R. (1978). Electrographic analysis of the sleep cycle in young depressives. *Biological Psychiatry, 7*, 203–214.

Tilkian, A. G., Guilleminault, C., Schroeder, J. S., Lehrman, R. L., Simmons, F. B., & Dement, W. C. (1976). Hemodynamics in sleep induced apnea: Studies during wakefulness and sleep. *Annals of Internal Medicine, 85*, 714–719.

Webb, W. B., & Agnew, H. W., Jr. (1974). Regularity in the control of the free-running sleep–wake rhythm. *Aerospace Medicine, 45*, 617–622.

Wehr, T., & Wirz-Justice, A. (1982). Circadian rhythm mechanisms in affective illness and in antidepressant drug action. *Pharmacopsychiatry, 15*, 31–40.

Weissbluth, M. (1987). Sleep and the colicky infant. In C. Guilleminault (Ed.), *Sleep and its disorders in children* (pp. 129–140). New York: Raven Press.

Weissbluth, M., Davis, A. T., Poncher, J., & Reiff, J. (1983). Signs of airway obstruction during sleep and behavioral, developmental and academic problems. *Journal of Developmental and Behavioral Pediatrics, 4*, 119–121.

Weitzman, E. D., Czeisler, C. A., Coleman, R. M., Dement, W. C., Richardson, G. S., & Pollak, C. (1979). Delayed sleep phase syndrome: A biological rhythm disorder. *Sleep Research, 8*, 221.

Weitzman, E. D., Czeisler, C. A., Coleman, R. M., Spielman, A. J., Zimmerman, J. C., &

Dement, W. C. (1981). Delayed sleep phase syndrome: A chronobiological disorder with sleep-onset insomnia. *Archives of General Psychiatry, 38,* 737–746.

Wilkus, R. J., & Chiles, J. A. (1975). Electrophysiological changes during episodes of the Kleine-Levin syndrome. *Journal of Neurology, Neurosurgery, and Psychiatry, 38,* 1225–1231.

Yoss, R. E., & Daly, D. D. (1960). Narcolepsy in children. *Pediatrics, 25,* 1025–1033.

Zarcone, V. (1973). Narcolepsy. A review of the syndrome. *New England Journal of Medicine, 288,* 1156–1165.

Author Index

Subject Index

Printed in the United States
19550LVS00003B/3-4